AIDS and Neurology

Clinical Neurology and Neurosurgery Monographs

Titles in Print

Fenichel *Neonatal Neurology*
Halliday *Evoked Potentials in Clinical Testing* 2E

Forthcoming Titles

Neary *Lobar Cerebral Atrophy*

To Julie and Heather McArthur and to Heather,
John, Caroline and Iain Harrison

For Churchill Livingstone
Commissioning Editor Mike Parkinson
Project Editor Dilys Jones
Project Controller Nancy Arnott
Sales Promotion Executive Marion Pollock

AIDS and Neurology

Michael J. G. Harrison

DM FRCP

Professor of Neurology, Reta Lila Weston Institute of
Neurological Studies, UCL School of Medicine; Consultant
Neurologist, The Middlesex Hospital and The National
Hospital, Queen Square, London, UK

Justin C. McArthur MBBS MPH

Associate Professor of Neurology, Associate Professor of
Epidemiology, Neurology, The Johns Hopkins University,
Baltimore, USA

Foreword by
Richard T. Johnson MD
The Johns Hopkins University School of Medicine,
Baltimore, USA

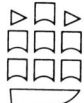

CHURCHILL LIVINGSTONE
EDINBURGH LONDON MADRID MELBOURNE NEW YORK AND TOKYO 1995

CHURCHILL LIVINGSTONE
Medical Division of Longman Group Limited

Distributed in the United States of America by
Churchill Livingstone Inc., 650 Avenue of the Americas, New York,
N.Y. 10011, and by associated companies, branches and
representatives throughout the world.

First published 1995

ISBN 0-443-048967

British Library Cataloguing in Publication Data
A catalogue record for this book is available from the British
Library.

Library of Congress Cataloging in Publication Data
A catalog record for this book is available from the Library
of Congress.

The
publisher's
policy is to use
**paper manufactured
from sustainable forests**

Produced by Longman Singapore Publishers (Pte) Ltd.
Printed in Singapore.

Contents

Foreword   vii
Acknowledgements   ix

1. Introduction   1
2. Seroconversion and the asymptomatic years   19
3. HIV-associated dementia complex   31
4. HIV infection in children   65
5. Spinal cord disease   77
6. Peripheral nerve disease   87
7 Muscle disease   109
8. Opportunistic infections – fungi   119

9. Opportunistic infections – viruses   133
10. Opportunistic infections – bacteria   151
11. Opportunistic infections – parasites   171
12. Neoplasms   183
13. Cerebrovascular disease   197
14. Common neurological symptoms in HIV infection   207
15. Investigations   219
16. Appendices   241

Index   255

Foreword

Human immunodeficiency virus (HIV) is unique among neurotropic viruses both in the unprecedented worldwide prevalence of nervous system infections and in the wide variety of different clinical syndromes associated with this infection. Experience with this newly discovered agent is in startling contrast to prior inquiries defining the causes of acute central nervous system infections in the 1950s and the exciting discovery of human slow infections associated with chronic neurological diseases in the 1960s.

The causes of acute viral meningitis and encephalitis were defined during the 1950s when practical cell culture systems were introduced into diagnostic laboratories and a variety of new viruses were recovered. Prior to this time only a handful of viruses had been associated with these acute neurological syndromes – rabies virus with hydrophobia, polioviruses with paralytic poliomyelitis, lymphocytic choriomeningitis virus and mumps virus with viral meningitis and herpes simplex virus and several arthropod-borne viruses with acute encephalitis. The recovery of enteroviruses and other agents in cultures led to the association of over 100 distinct different viruses with acute viral infection of the nervous system. The clinical syndrome of acute paralytic poliomyelitis proved, except on rare occasions, to be caused by the three serotypes of polioviruses. The clinical syndromes of acute viral meningitis and encephalitis were associated with a panoply of agents. Thus, these acute febrile illnesses with nuchal rigidity and a mononuclear cell pleocytosis with or without disturbance of consciousness and focal neurological signs proved to have remarkably diverse causes.

The concept of slow infections of the nervous system evolved in the 1960s. Chronic neurological diseases without signs of inflammation were associated with infections with both conventional viruses and with unconventional spongiform encephalopathy agents now referred to as prions. Between 1964 and 1969 four neurological diseases of unknown etiology proved to be slow infections – progressive multifocal leukoencephalopathy, subacute sclerosing panencephalitis, kuru and Creutzfeldt-Jakob disease. The concept was revolutionary, but despite the hope that viruses soon would be associated with a variety of common chronic neurological diseases including multiple sclerosis, amyotrophic lateral sclerosis, Parkinson's disease, Alzheimer's disease, and even schizophrenia, these hopes have not materialized although studies continue. Thus, a small number of agents was discovered which explained several rare diseases.

The association of human immunodeficiency virus with neurological disease represents a unique departure from these prior periods of searching for viral agents in acute and chronic neurological diseases. In the first years after the original descriptions of the acquired immunodeficiency syndrome (AIDS) neurological interest was limited to the unusual opportunistic infections of the nervous system, such as the unusual manifestations of toxoplasmosis and cryptococcosis and the singular frequency of progressive multifocal leukoencephalopathy, and the high rate of cerebral lymphomas. In 1985 this perspective changed with the recovery of HIV from brain, cerebrospinal fluid and peripheral nerve of patients with neurological diseases, the demonstration of HIV RNA and DNA in brain, and the documentation of intrathecal synthesis of anti-HIV antibodies in many patients; the same year HIV was shown to be a member of the lentivirus subfamily of retroviruses, and animal lentiviruses had consistently been associated with chronic encephalitis. Recognition that HIV invaded the nervous system early, in some cases at the time of seroconversion, established HIV as the most prevalent viral infection of the nervous system. Even more extraordinary is the variety of different clinical syndromes related to HIV infection involving both the central and peripheral nervous systems, occurring at time of seroconversion as well as after the onset of AIDS, and showing a variety of different pathological changes.

Over the coming decades neurological complications of HIV infections will be among the common diseases confronted by neurologists and internists. Michael Harrison and Justin McArthur were two of the first neurologists to become involved in the diagnosis and treatment of these complications, and their experience and knowledge can serve us all.

Baltimore 1995   R.T.J.

Acknowledgements

We would like to take this opportunity to express our gratitude to the patients and HIV-positive volunteers who have enthusiastically collaborated in the research described in this book. We are also indebted to our colleagues in the research teams, and in the clinics and wards, who share our attempts to care for patients with the neurological manifestations of HIV infection.

At the Middlesex Hospital, M.J.G.H. would particularly like to thank Professors Ian Weller and Stanton Newman and Dr Rob Miller for their constant help and support. Dr Brian Kendall, Dr Margaret Hall–Craggs and Mr John Brazier kindly provided illustrative material, and Teresa Fullam bore the heavy secretarial load with unfailing good humour.

At Johns Hopkins, J.C.M. wishes to thank his colleagues for innumerable discussions and their invaluable contributions, particularly Dr Richard Johnson for his guidance at many levels, Dr Jonathan Glass for providing many of the pathological sections, and Dr Jack Griffin for his advice in the peripheral nerve section. Dr Ola Selnes provided much of the neuropsychological material, and Dr Roland Lee, the neuroradiological images. Ms Nancy Rosenberg provided expert editorial assistance and prepared many of the diagrams and graphs. He would also like to acknowledge the dedication and continuing work of Dr John Bartlett and the many other members of the Johns Hopkins AIDS service, and recognize the role of Dr B. Frank Polk whose encouragement nurtured his initial involvement in HIV research.

The book would not have been possible without the help of Dilys Jones of Churchill Livingstone. The Middlesex Hospital studies are supported by the Medical Research Council of Great Britain, and those at Johns Hopkins by the National Institutes of Health (NS 26643 and AI 35042).

Finally, we would like to express our love and appreciation to our wives and families for their enthusiastic support and endurance during the completion of this project.

London and Baltimore 1995   M.J.G.H.
J.C.M.

1. Introduction

Early in 1981, five young men in the Los Angeles area developed pneumonia due to *Pneumocystis carinii* (PCP) (Fig. 1.1), an infection that had previously been confined to severely immuno-compromised patients. All were homosexuals, but none had any previously recognized disorder of the immune system (Masur et al 1981). They were found to have depressed levels of circulating T helper cells and impaired cellular immunity. Others were seen with chronic perianal ulcerative herpes simplex infection (Siegel et al 1981). At about the same time, clusters of cases of a hitherto rare cutaneous malignancy, Kaposi's sarcoma, were being reported from the male homosexual

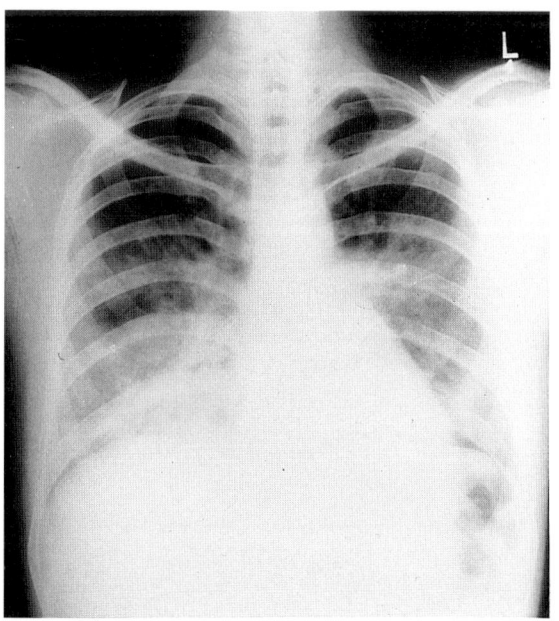

Fig. 1.1 Chest radiograph showing appearances of *Pneumocystis carinii* pneumonia (courtesy of Dr R. Miller).

communities of New York and San Francisco (Friedman-Klein et al 1982). Some of the patients with Kaposi's sarcoma also had severe infections with herpes simplex, PCP or cytomegalovirus (CMV). Within a few months, similar observations of PCP among injecting drug users were made. This evidence of an acquired disturbance in cellular immunity initially in male homosexuals and intravenous drug users strongly suggested a transmissible agent or a toxic effect of illicit drugs. Support for the concept of a transmissible agent came with the appearance of acquired immuno-deficiency syndrome (AIDS) with opportunistic infections and unusual tumours in haemophiliacs and other recipients of blood transfusions, and then children. In 1983 the causative agent, a retrovirus now called the human immunodefi-ciency virus or HIV-1, was discovered. Evidence from stored material suggested that HIV was first a cause of disease in the USA in the 1960s (Garry et al 1988). AIDS has since become a major public health menace, and the leading cause of death in some sections of the community (Barré-Sinoussi et al 1983). Within 3 years it is predicted that 20 million people will be infected and in some parts of Africa and the USA, AIDS has become the leading cause of death in the age range 25–44.

The worldwide distribution of AIDS has shown different patterns. Pattern 1 countries (North America, West Europe and Latin America) have a low level of seroprevalence in their communities, most of their cases are in homosexuals, and males predominate. Pattern 2 countries (Sub-Saharan Africa and the Caribbean) have a seroprevalence of >1%, males and females are equally affected, and most contacts are heterosexual. Pattern 3 countries (East Europe, Asia, Pacific and North

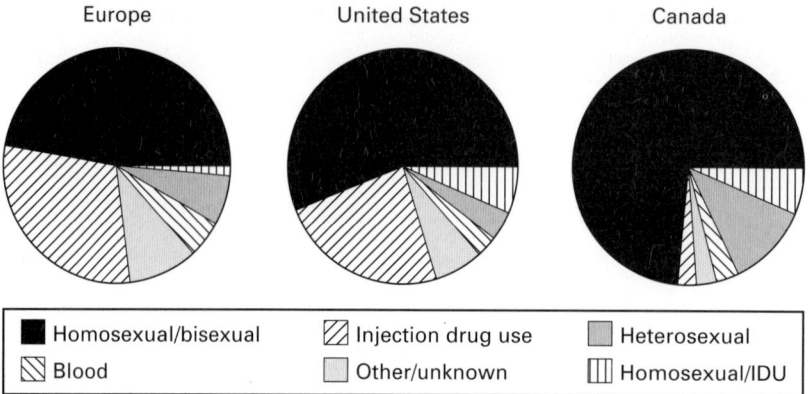

Fig. 1.2   Comparison of risk background for HIV infection in Western countries.

Africa) have the lowest seroprevalence, though the situation is changing in Thailand and India, for example.

The US data from 1990 (Janssen 1992) revealed that 87% of affected individuals were male; 55% were homosexual or bisexual and 25% intravenous drug users. Some small differences are seen when Europe, Canada and the USA are compared (Fig. 1.2). Most heterosexual acquired AIDS involves females, and a third of their children are infected by vertical transmission. Fifty per cent of such perinatally infected children develop AIDS within 3 years; 50% of infected adults develop AIDS in 8–10 years. Documented HIV seroconversion after occupational exposure has occurred in 36 healthcare workers up to March 1993 (Centers for Disease Control and Prevention 1993). Thirty-one workers had percutaneous exposure and eight have developed AIDS.

The national US prevalence of AIDS varies with location between rural low levels to high urban levels of up to 130/100 000 (in San Francisco). In the 25–44 year age group, AIDS is the second most common cause of death after trauma for males, and the fifth in females.

The development of reliable serological tests in 1985 facilitated the description of a clinically asymptomatic stage of infection before the onset of severe immunodeficiency. HIV stimulates an antibody response that develops usually within 2–6 months of primary infection. In some individuals, however, seroconversion may be delayed for up to 48 months (Wolinsky et al 1989). The virus

binds to T helper lymphocytes through their CD4 receptor (Klatzman et al 1984), and depletes their number through various mechanisms (Phillips et al 1991) (Fig. 1.3). These cells normally orchestrate the body's immune responses, so their loss leaves the patient susceptible to opportunistic infections by viruses, fungi, bacteria and parasites, and to an increased incidence of lymphomas. From an early stage it was clear that the nervous system was frequently involved in AIDS (Snider et al 1983). In 10–20% of HIV-infected patients, neurological illness is the presenting feature. At autopsy some 80% of brains and 100% of peripheral nerves are abnormal; in life some 30% have neurological symptoms or signs indicative of involvement of the neuraxis. Amongst the severe and life-threatening infections experienced by patients with cellular immunodeficiency were

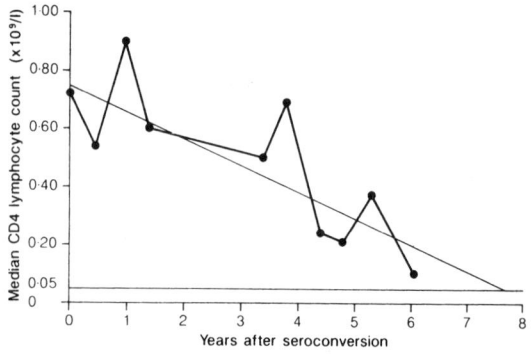

Fig. 1.3   Declining CD4 count during HIV infection. Serial CD4 lymphocyte counts since seroconversion are shown for one HIV-infected patient (root mean-square-error about fitted slope = 0.16×10^9l). (After Phillips et al 1991.)

brain abscesses due to *Toxoplasma gondii* and meningitis due to *Cryptococcus neoformans*. Other neurological manifestations emerged without signs of opportunistic infection suggesting that HIV was probably directly neurovirulent as well as lymphotropic and could lead to a number of 'primary' HIV-associated neurological disorders including dementia, myelopathy and sensory neuropathy. Most neurological disease occurs late in HIV infection, after systemic opportunistic infections have already developed. Therefore, as survival after AIDS lengthens, more neurological disease can be anticipated.

THE VIRUS

There are important parallels between these human conditions and the animal lentivirus infections, because all lentiviruses cause a degree of neurological damage from leucoencephalitis (Johnson et al 1988) (Table 1.1). The lentiviruses or 'slow viruses', of which HIV-1 is a member, share certain pathogenic similarities, including mechanisms by which they evade host defences and immune clearance and cause persistent infection. They typically have long incubation periods and are associated with chronic diseases occurring

Table 1.1 Properties of lentiviruses

Contain RNA genome and reverse transcriptase
Host specific
Prolonged incubation period
Persistent infections in natural hosts
Restricted viral replication
Cytopathic effects in vitro
Infect cells of the immune system

(After Kennedy 1992)

in nature. They comprise: visna virus, with which HIV-1 shares morphological and genomic characteristics; caprine arthritis encephalitis virus; equine infectious anaemia virus; bovine immunodeficiency virus; and feline immunodeficiency virus. Human infection with HIV-2 and simian disease with SIV-1, which produces an AIDS-like syndrome after experimental inoculation in macaques, complete the currently recognized list. HIV-2 is a retrovirus distinct from HIV-1, which is prevalent in parts of Western Africa (De-The et al 1989). Although there have been some reports of neurological disease associated with HIV-2, it does not appear to be frequent in the West.

HIV is a non-transforming retrovirus that produces a cytopathic or lytic effect on T cells, although the precise mechanisms for T cell deple-

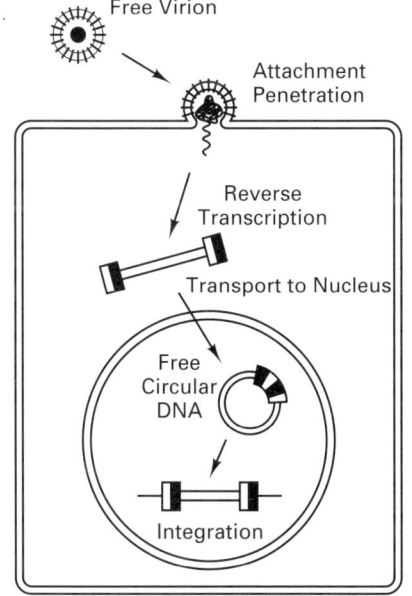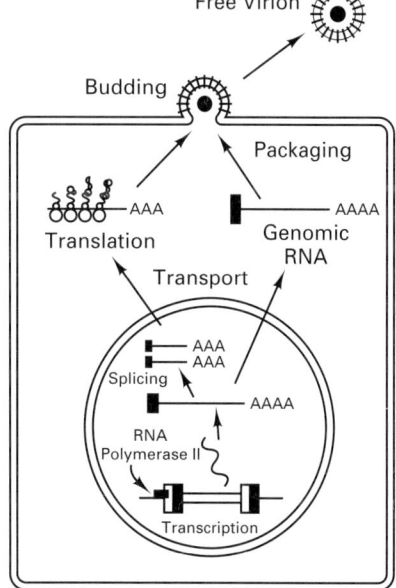

Fig. 1.4 Retrovirus replication. (After Haseltine 1989.)

tion are uncertain. The CD4 receptor is the principal target site for HIV; however, there may be other cellular receptors. Galactosyl ceramide and sulphatide serve as alternate receptors in neural cell lines (Harouse et al 1991), but the in vivo relevance of these findings is uncertain and there is no proof of latent or productive infection of human neurones in vivo. The replicative cycle of HIV produces an opportunity for rapid mutation, and differences among HIV strains may account for biological differences in tropism or cytopathic effect.

HIV structure and life cycle

The retrovirus family, retroviridae, is composed of three major sub-families: lentivirus, to which HIV belongs (lenti:slow); oncovirus, to which HTLV-I belongs (onco:tumour); and spumavirus (spuma:foam). Of these three sub-families, members of the lentivirus and oncoviruses have been linked to neurological disease in humans, but to date, spumaviruses do not appear to cause human disease. The retroviruses share genomic and morphological similarities and may have originally derived from an ancestral virus. The retroviruses

include a number of RNA viruses which replicate in a unique manner; their other distinguishing characteristics are listed in Table 1.1. The viruses are distinguished from other viruses because they carry a unique pair of enzymes: first, an RNA-dependent DNA polymerase (reverse transcriptase), which uses RNA as a template to make a complementary DNA strand, and a second enzyme (a ribonuclease) which breaks down the original RNA strand, thus allowing a complementary DNA strand to be synthesized on the remaining DNA strand (Fig. 1.4). After the double-stranded DNA has been synthesized, it is incorporated by the enzyme integrase into the host cell DNA and replicates with it. Once integrated into the host cell genome, it is termed a provirus, and may remain latent for months or years, without affecting cellular function. Alternatively, the provirus may separate from the host cell DNA to produce retrovirus mRNA, which directs viral protein synthesis.

The HIV virion is a relatively large, icosahedral structure with numerous external spikes (Fig. 1.5). The envelope spikes are composed of gp120 with a transmembrane component, gp41. The lipid bilayer is derived from host proteins during viral

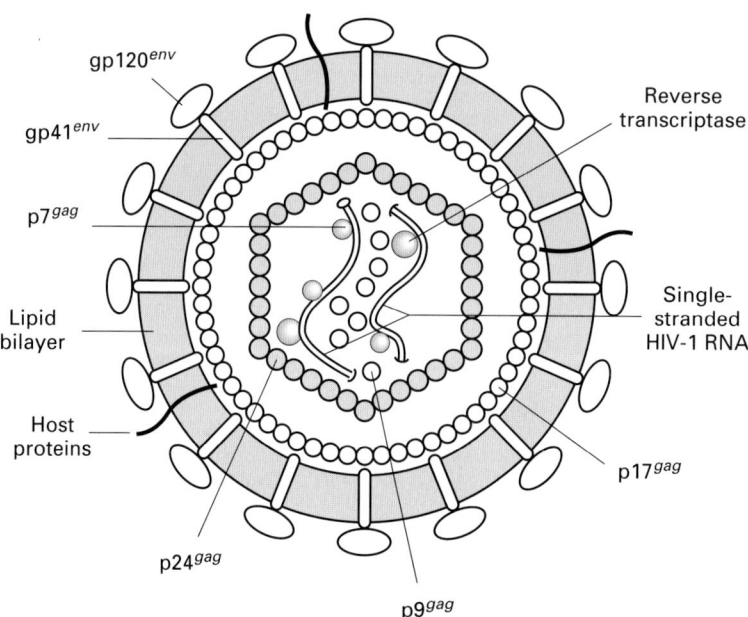

Fig. 1.5   Structure of the HIV-1 virion. (After Greene 1991.)

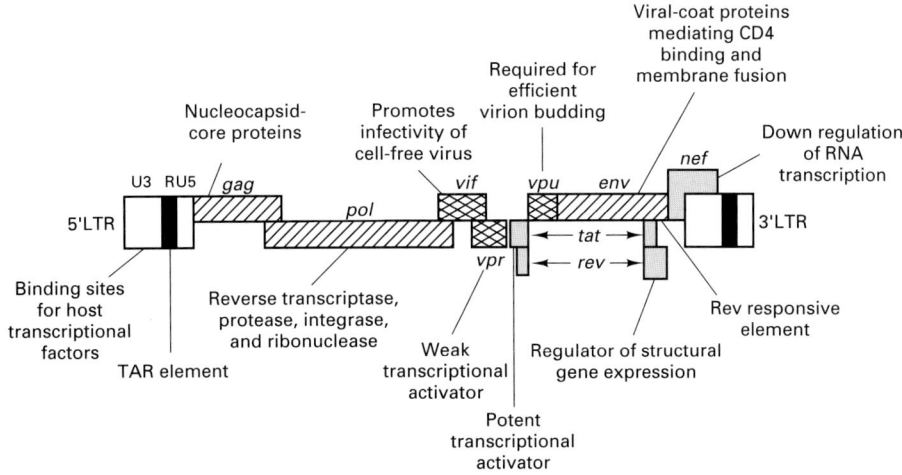

Fig. 1.6 Genome of HIV-1. (After Greene 1991.)

budding. The core is formed from four nucleic capsid proteins: p24 (the major component), p17, p9 and p7. Genomic structure of HIV includes genes that code for structural proteins and several genes that code for regulatory proteins (Fig. 1.6). The three groups of structural proteins are coded for by the gag, pol and env regions of the HIV gene. The env gene codes for the two major envelope proteins, gp120 and gp41; gp120 is a large glycoprotein that forms the surface spikes of the virion, while gp41 is a transmembrane glyco-protein. The two envelope proteins are critical for viral binding and cell fusion. The pol region codes for reverse transcriptase, a protease and an endonuclease. Endonuclease is critical for the integration of DNA into the host genome and the protease cleaves the polyproteins encoded for by gag and pol into their active forms. The gag region encodes for the core proteins, including p24, the nucleoid shell and several smaller proteins. Additional information is available in two reviews (Levy 1989, Greene 1991). At least five genes (tat, rev, nef, vif and vpr) are involved in the regulation of HIV's replication. The tat gene, a transactivating regulator of RNA translation, is thought to be expressed early in the replication phase to boost viral production after host cell activation. The rev gene may control the conversion from proviral state to active viral replication by modulating the expression of structural proteins. The nef gene appears to inhibit viral replication by down-regulating RNA transcription (hence 'nef' for 'negative factor'). However, the role of nef remains uncertain because both in vitro and in vivo studies have shown that the nef gene is not required for viral replication and the inhibitory effects of nef are relatively weak compared with the activating effects of tat. The vif

Table 1.2 Genomic structure of HIV: recognized genes and putative functions

Gene	Function
gag	Nucleocapsid proteins including nucleoid shell (p24), matrix protein and nucleic acid binding protein
pol	Reverse transcriptase, endonuclease (integrase) and protease
env	Envelope glycoproteins – surface protein recognizing cell surface receptors (gp120) and transmembrane protein (gp41); gp120 responsible for attachment to all surfaces via CD4 receptor; gp41 responsible for cell entry through fusion with cell membrane.
tat	Potent transcriptional activating function
rev	Regulates viral protein transcription, essential for activation of the cytoplasmic expression of mRNA
nef	Relatively negative factor for virus replication. Not essential for viral replication
vif	Maturation of cell proteins during budding. Promotes infectivity of cell-free virus
vpr	Weak transcriptional activator, which may induce cell differentiation
vpx	Possibly weak transcriptional activator
vpu	Possibly required for efficient virion budding

(After Greene 1991)

gene is responsible for the maturation of viral proteins during budding, and vpr may function as a weak transcriptional activator, which may induce cell differentiation and cellular factors needed for efficient viral replication (Levy et al 1993). Table 1.2 summarizes the functions of proteins encoded by the structural and regulatory genes of HIV-1. The function of the other viral genes that have been identified (Fig. 1.6) is unknown.

Knowledge of the life cycle of HIV shows that there are several potential targets (Fig. 1.7) for antiretroviral drugs to work at from viral attachment to budding (Table 1.3). Furthest on in development have been inhibitors of reverse transcriptase, protease and the regulatory tat gene (Hirsch & D'Aquila 1993). Of the transcriptase inhibitors, zidovudine was the first to show antiretroviral activity in vitro and in clinical trials, followed by dideoxyinosine (ddI), dideoxycytidine (ddC) and dideoxyglyceropentenofuranosyl thymine (d4T). Zidovudine is converted into a triphosphate in the cell, and incorporated into an elongating nucleic acid by the viral reverse transcriptase. There it prevents normal linkage of residues at the 3' and 5' positions on the five carbon sugar moieties. This terminates proviral DNA chain growth. Viral expression in the cell can be inhibited by disturbing the role of the tat protein made by the tat gene. Tat protein binds to a specific HIV-1 RNA sequence increasing the rate of transcription. Some benzodiazepines, e.g. Ro24-7429, antagonize this function. Inhibiting the role of HIV-1 protease (in cleaving gag and pol polyproteins) leads to the production of non-infectious particles of low reverse transcriptase activity. Protease inhibitors like Ro31-8959 are under trial. The use of soluble CD4 to inhibit cell binding by virus and of viral envelope proteins to enhance host responses has also been tested unsuccessfully. Viral mutation and drug resistance are major problems, and sequential or combination regimens are increasingly likely to be necessary.

HIV-1 is tropic for CD4+ lymphocytes and macrophages. However cells that do not express CD4 receptor can be infected in vitro. The CD4 receptor on T lymphocytes (Dalgleish et al 1984) is also present on monocytes and macrophages and is assumed to be critical for the entry of the virus into these cells (Ho et al 1986). There may be other receptors in neural cells; for example, gal-C may act as an alternative receptor in the nervous system (Harouse et al 1991). The viral

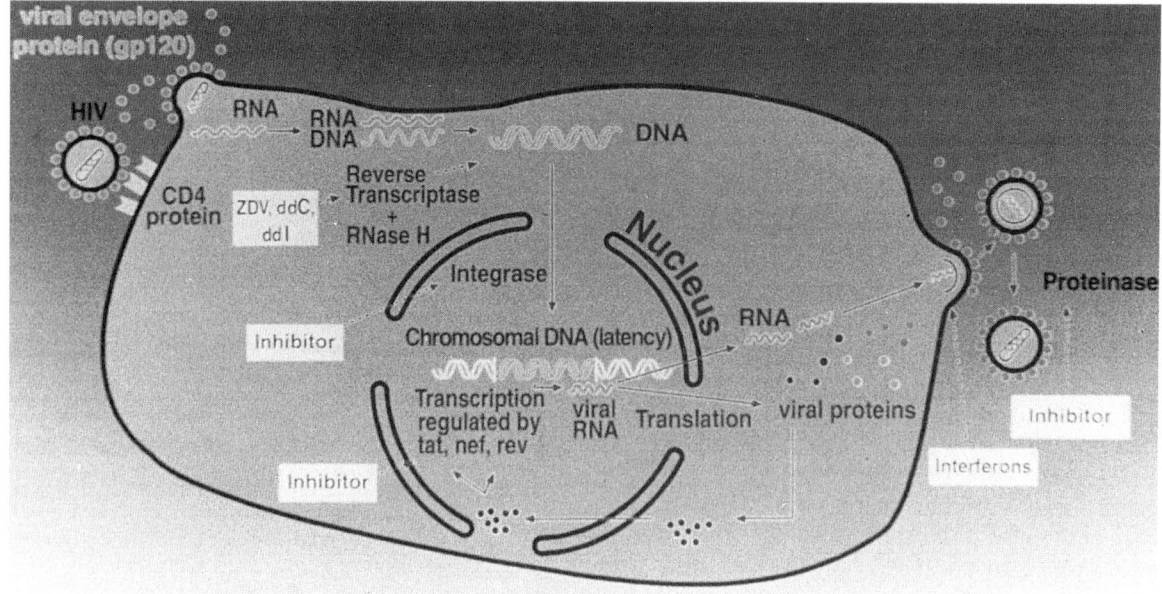

Fig. 1.7   Life cycle of HIV-1 and site of action of antiviral drugs. (Reproduced by kind permission of Hoffman-La Roche.)

Table 1.3 Life cycle of HIV and targets for therapeutic intervention

Stage	Possible intervention	Agents
Binding to host cell	Block HIV binding or cell receptor	CD4 analogues, HIV or cell receptor analogues, peptide T(?) vaccines
Entry into host cell	Drugs that block fusion or uncoating	
Transcription of RNA to DNA by reverse transcriptase	Reverse transcriptase inhibitors	Nucleoside and non-nucleoside agents (AZT, ddI, ddC, foscarnet, zalcitabine, nevaripine, TIBO)
Integration of viral DNA into host DNA	Inhibitors of HIV topoisomerase	
Transcription of DNA into RNA	Inhibition of transcription	Ribavirin
Viral gene expression	Inhibitors of tat or rev expression; amplifiers of nef expression	Tat-inhibitor (Roche Ro24-7429) Antisense oligonucleotides
Virion packaging	Protease, glycosylating and myristylating inhibitors	Castanospermine Protease inhibitors (Roche Ro31-8959)
Virus budding	Inhibitors	Interferons, particularly alpha HIV antibodies

(After Hirsch & D'Aquila 1993)

envelope glycoprotein gp120 binds to the CD4 receptor leading to conformational changes in other viral membrane proteins (e.g. gp41), which causes fusion of the virus and cell (Fig. 1.4). This in turn triggers disruption of the viral core with release of RNA (Grewe et al 1990). This RNA is converted by the viral enzyme reverse transcriptase into DNA, which then integrates into the host cell DNA forming proviral DNA.

Initially, it was thought that after infection and integration of HIV DNA into the host cell genome, there followed a long period of latency. Recent work suggests that this is not a true latent infection and that even during the long incubation period of HIV infection, there may be viral transcription with production of new active virions (Michael et al 1992). Most patients show a slow decline in CD4 counts during this period, with annual decrements in CD4 of 50–100/mm^3. Some HIV-infected individuals, however, show remarkable stability in CD4 for many years,

suggesting that their HIV infection is held under closer control. Studies of lymph nodes from HIV-infected persons confirm that there is no true latency but rather a progressive increase in viral burden, which may be confined to the follicular centres of lymph nodes during the asymptomatic phase. Eventually the virus 'escapes', overwhelming the lymphoreticular system and the rapid increase in HIV burden is associated with the onset of symptomatic disease (Pantaleo et al 1993b). Although depletion of CD4 cells is at the core of immunodeficiency seen in AIDS, HIV RNA synthesis as proof of cell invasion is only detected in a minority of CD4 lymphocytes. Even sensitive methods such as polymerase chain reaction (PCR) to detect HIV DNA only detect proviral infection in 1/1000 of CD4+ cells in asymptomatic patients and 1/100 in those with AIDS (Schnittman et al 1989). The concentrations of HIV DNA do not reflect the amount of transcription and virion production and measurements of HIV RNA using reverse transcriptase PCR show a steadily increasing amount of HIV RNA during AIDS, implying that the viral burden increases in parallel with disease progression (Michael et al 1992). During the years after infection, CD4 cell numbers fall, the rate presumably being a major factor in the variable natural history. Some patients appear to have had no more than a few months between infection and AIDS, whilst others remain asymptomatic for at least 13 years. By 10 years, some 60% show clinical evidence of immunological impairment (Bacchetti & Moss, 1989). The fall in CD4 cell numbers is the best predictor of the time to appearance of immunosuppression clinically (Lange et al 1989). Other useful surrogate markers in the blood are the levels of β_2-microglobulin and neopterin, markers of monocyte–macrophage activation (Fahey et al 1990).

EFFECTS ON CELLULAR IMMUNITY

HIV has been isolated from peripheral blood T cells, macrophages, plasma, bone marrow, semen and also from brain, spinal cord, peripheral nerve and cerebrospinal fluid (CSF) (Ho et al 1985). HIV produces a cytopathic or lytic effect on T cells in vitro, but it remains uncertain exactly how it leads to such profound depletion of CD4+ cells in vivo. Proposed mechanisms include CD4 cell killing with viral budding, leading to the death of single cells, cell fusion with syncytia formation, virus-specific immune responses, including re-actions of natural killer cells, antibody-dependent cellular cytotoxicity and cytotoxic T lymphocytes. Other proposed mechanisms include autoimmune mechanisms based on the homology between HLA-DR and HLA-DQ molecules and the envelope glycoprotein or the development of super-antigens. Super-antigens are antigens capable of binding to the majority of T cells, binding only to the variable β region of the T cell antigen receptor and inducing a broad expansion of T cells, followed by dilution or anergy. Finally, programmed cell death or apoptosis induced by cell activation without direct infection may play a role in CD4 cell depletion. These mechanisms are comprehensively reviewed in a recent summary (Pantaleo et al 1993a).

The process of cell death in infected cell lines is not entirely clear. In many cases the creation of multinucleated cells or syncytia presages cell lysis, but high rates of viral replication can prove fatal to a cell without this (Stevenson et al 1988). Furthermore, the fusion of envelope gp120 alone with CD4 can lead to cell death, so accumulation of foreign RNA and DNA in the cell is not a necessary condition for cell failure (Lifson et al 1986). The role of gp120 in activating immune cells such as macrophages leading to the production of cytokines may be especially relevant to the effect of HIV on neuronal function (see later).

Infection of CD4 lymphocytes has a series of important effects on cellular immunity because these cells serve a critical role in orchestrating the immune system. Some of the immunological functions of CD4 lymphocytes are listed in Table 1.4. The formation of syncytia makes the cells ineffective ('combat ineffective') (Dalgleish 1992) and infected cells show down-regulation of their CD4 receptors. Because these are critical in the normal interaction of T cells with antigen-presenting cells and B cells, the effect is widespread. T cell responses to mitogens and proliferative responses become blunted in a similar manner to the immunological abnormalities observed during measles (Griffin 1991). During

Table 1.4   Immunological functions of CD4 lymphocytes

Activation of macrophages
Induction of cytotoxic T lymphocyte function
Induction of natural killer cell function
Induction of suppressor cell function
Induction of B cell function
Secretion of factors inducing non-lymphoid cell function
Secretion of haematopoietic colony stimulating factors
Secretion of growth and differentiation factors for lymphoid cells

the period of clinical latency, there is evidence of chronic T cell activation with persistent elevation in the blood of a variety of markers of immune activation, including soluble CD4, CD8 and IL-2 receptor, IL-6, neopterin and β_2-microglobulin. Early in infection, activated CD4 T cells are of Th1 type, which produce interferon γ, IL-2, tumour necrosis factor (TNF-α) and lymphotoxin, which activates macrophages. Later in infection, Th2 cells predominate, which produce IL-4, IL-6 and IL-10 lymphokines, which deactivate macrophages and regulate the production of other cytokines including TNF-α and IL-1 (Shearer & Clerici 1992). This dysregulation may lead to the overproduction of TNF-α and IL-1 and other cytokines that may stimulate HIV replication. Other cytokines are affected in AIDS, for example, IL-2 and interferon production is impaired (Murray et al 1985). The concept is emerging that in AIDS there is an activation of macrophages with the overproduction of monokines, which may be pathogenic or contribute to some of the systemic and neurological manifestations (Poli & Fauci 1992). For example, there is evidence that TNF-α, as well as recruiting macrophages in response to infection, also increases virus production (Rosenberg & Fauci 1990) and may underlie the frequent fevers, wasting, cachexia and anaemia. The advent of opportunistic infections presumably magnifies this process and TNF-α may contribute to the accelerating phase of terminal disease and be a factor in the cachexia and the neurological disease. The role of lymphokines and monokines in regulating HIV infection and producing pathophysiological effects is extremely complex and is incompletely understood at this point. Several cytokines, including TNF-α and IL-6, appear to up-regulate HIV expression, while other cytokines, particularly the interferons and TGF-β, may down-regulate HIV production in infected cells. The balance of these cytokines may therefore be relevant to the control or stimulation of HIV infection, and the development of symptomatic disease.

THE HOST RESPONSE TO HIV INFECTION

After infection, core antigens such as p24 become detectable in the blood (Fig. 1.8). The level falls rapidly as the production of neutralizing antibodies (both IgM and IgG) is stimulated. Antibodies to envelope constituents such as gp120, gp41 and gp160 are initially at low titre but increase (Dalgleish 1992). However, the antibodies are not able to clear the virus completely, probably because of its intracellular sequestration. The time between infection and seroconversion varies and is usually 2 –6 months. The 'window' of seroconversion can be as long as 48 months, which creates difficulties in diagnosis and has led to transfusion of infectious but seronegative blood products. As the immunodeficiency develops, antibodies to p24 decline and p24 antigen may reappear. Quantitation of virus with cultures (Coombs et al 1989) or PCR (Michael et al 1992) shows that viral burden rises dramatically in the later phases of infection (Fig. 1.9). It is unclear how important the neutralizing properties of anti-HIV antibodies are in controlling infection early. An additional potential protective role of antibodies is in the

production of antibody-dependent cellular cytotoxicity (ADCC) after binding to natural killer cells, leading to the killing of HIV-infected cells. HIV-specific cytotoxic T lymphocytes may also contribute to the control of HIV infection. Levy (1993) has suggested that CD8 cells are important in controlling HIV expression, and a decline in CD8 cell numbers precedes the development of increases in HIV load. Some of the humoral response may be harmful, rather than protective, with the development of cross-reactivity to host constituents and the stimulation of immune-mediated disorders. Such factors may underlie the thrombocytopenia or inflammatory demyelinating neuropathies occasionally seen. The same mechanisms may underlie the elimination of HIV-infected cells, including lymphocytes, macrophages and follicular dendritic cells in the lymph nodes, and may contribute to progressive immune deterioration (Pantaleo et al 1993b).

The reason for the long period of asymptomatic infection in so many affected individuals is difficult to explain. It has been suggested that the virus is capable of hiding from the immune responses, by down-regulating its replication rate or by its ability to evolve genomically. Alternatively, the rate of loss of CD4 cells simply determines the progressive loss of immune containment of the virus. Host factors may be important too, with particular HLA haplotypes predisposing to more rapid disease progression. Two ancestral haplotypes, 8.1 and 35.2, carry susceptibility genes

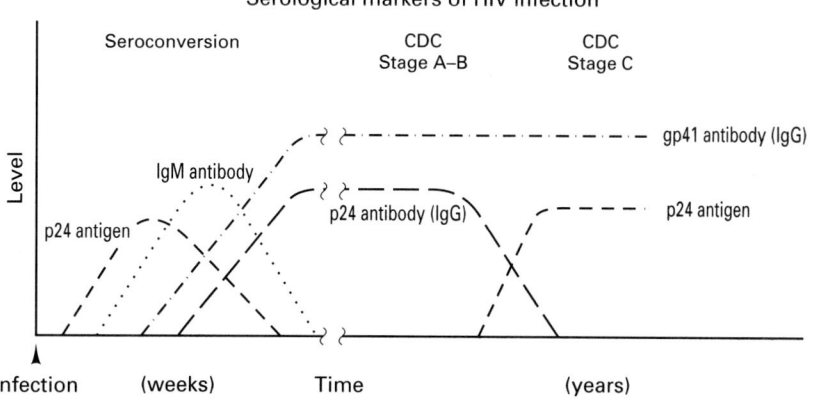

Fig. 1.8 Serological markers of HIV infection at different clinical stages. (From a poster by Wellcome Foundation.)

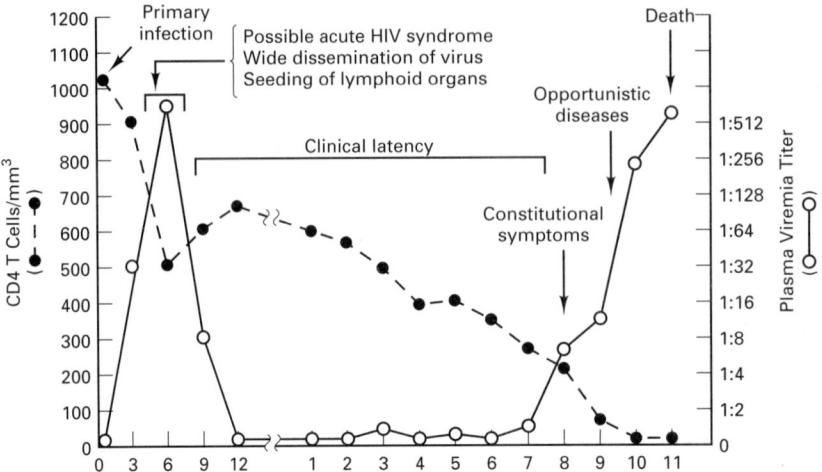

Fig. 1.9 Relationship of CD4 count and plasma viraemia to stage of HIV infection and clinical consequences. (After Pantaleo et al 1993.)

for rapid development of immunodeficiency after HIV infection (French et al 1992). Clerici and Shearer (1993) have found that progression to AIDS is characterized by loss of IL-2 and gamma interferon production concomitant with increases in IL-4 and IL-10 (Th2 response dominant). On the other hand, many seronegative but HIV-exposed individuals generate strong Th1-type responses to HIV antigens. In addition, co-infections with other viruses, such as CMV or HTLV-1, may accelerate the course of HIV infection. HIV-infected macrophages increase their production of TNF-α, and in an autocrine-paracrine fashion, TNF-α can up-regulate transcription of integrated HIV and therefore a cycle of increasing replication can occur once macrophage activation occurs.

A striking feature of HIV infection is the development of polyclonal hyperglobulinaemia (Amadori & Chieco-Bianchi 1990). Most of this is due to IgG, but not all is due to antibodies to HIV. Some, for example, are non-specific anti-phospholipid antibodies. Though total IgG is increased, IgG_2 may be decreased and play a role in susceptibility to pneumococcal infections. These are a particular problem in African AIDS, and in children where there can, however, be a pan hypogammaglobulinaemia. The frequent occurrence of lymphadenopathy in the early years of the disease is also a pointer to immune stimulation before immunosuppression. Indeed, some features of HIV infection with lymphadenopathy,

skin disease, diarrhoea, falling CD4 cell counts, appearance of B cell lymphomas and opportunistic infections are reminiscent of graft-versus-host disease (GVHD). Dalgleish (1992) has suggested that the immune system might 'see' the HIV envelope as an allo-epitope and create the circumstances of GVHD.

VIRAL MUTATION AND STRAIN DIFFERENCES

The virus displays great genomic variability because point mutations occur frequently during the replication cycle of HIV. The reverse transcriptase step is particularly prone to error and most of the point mutations occur here. There appear to be several 'dominant' strains worldwide, which differ from country to country. In the USA, for example, the most common strain is HIV-MN, while in Thailand there are two distinct strains (HIV-MN and HIV-E). Even isolates taken from the same patient at different times may show differences in their cytopathogenicity and their rate of in vitro replication (Cheng-Mayer et al 1988). It is tempting to propose that some of the clinical heterogeneity in severity and course of the human disease may relate to the emergence of more virulent strains in some individuals. It is suggested that the initial infection is 'monoclonal', but that the viral DNA becomes more heterogenous with time. It has also been suggested that patients whose viral isolates are highly cytopathic in vitro and show fast replication rates have a worse prognosis (Schnittman et al 1989). HIV isolates can be grouped into either macrophage tropic, non-syncytium producing (NSI) or T cell tropic, syncytium producing (SI) classes based on their ability to replicate in macrophages or established T cell lines (Koyanagi et al 1987). The macrophage tropic class of isolates dominate in the asymptomatic carriers. Syncytial inducing isolates are highly cytopathic, and have higher replication rates in vitro than non-syncytial inducing strains (Tersmette et al 1989). The syncytial inducing isolates tend to be found in patients with more rapid loss of CD4 cells and a shorter survival. Progression to AIDS may be related to a shift from macrophage to T cell tropic virus population with accelerated loss of T cells (Koot et al 1993). This relationship between course of disease and the ability of HIV to produce syncytia remains unproven, however, and the virological or immunological cause for the emergence of such variants during the course of the disease is largely unknown. Macrophage tropic virus is still likely to play a role in depletion of CD4 cells (Xiao Fang Yu, personal communication). The genomic variability poses great difficulties for the development of successful vaccines.

CLINICAL DISEASE: STAGING AND DEFINITIONS

Although the course of HIV infection varies considerably among infected individuals, a 'typical' course with recognizable stages has now been accepted by most investigators. This includes the following stages: first, primary infection, usually asymptomatic but sometimes accompanied by an HIV seroconversion illness (see below). This phase is followed by a prolonged period of clinical latency, which, as discussed above, is accompanied by steady immunological deterioration and an increase in viral load, predominantly within lymphoid tissue. Then, after a variable incubation period averaging 8–10 years, constitutional symptoms begin to appear, including fever, weight loss, diarrhoea, fatigue and infections indicative of cellular immunodeficiency – shingles and oral thrush. As the CD4 count declines further and cellular immunodeficiency deepens, more serious opportunistic infections develop characterizing the period of 'full blown' AIDS. The neurological illnesses attributed to a primary effect of HIV typically occur during this phase of infection (Figs 1.10, 1.11). Table 1.5 lists the CD4 range and typical duration of these various stages.

HIV infection has been defined, staged and classified in a number of different ways (see Appendix 1 for criteria). Since the beginning of the epidemic, the Centers for Disease Control (CDC) have developed surveillance definitions for AIDS, which have been used primarily for epidemiological purposes. The CDC classification system for HIV infection relies primarily on clinical findings rather than CD4 count, and has been widely used both in clinical and research settings. These definitions of AIDS indicator illnesses are widely used to establish disability benefits. The most recent version of the CDC AIDS definition includes four additional AIDS-defining criteria: severe HIV-related immunosuppression with a CD4 count of less than 200 cells/mm^3 or CD4 percentage less than 14%, pulmonary tuberculosis, recurrent pneumonia or invasive cervical cancer. This revision resulted in an additional approximately 12 000 cases in the USA for the period from April 1992 to March 1993. Of these, the majority (over 7000) were diagnosed on the basis of severe immunosuppression, 708 from pulmonary tuberculosis, 157 from recurrent pneumonia and 25 from invasive cervical cancer.

The policy of considering a CD4 count of less than 200 cells/mm^3 poses several important problems. First there is significant interlaboratory variability in performing T subset analyses, and often quite dramatic intraindividual variation (Hoover et al 1992). For this reason, it has been recommended that two determinations be made. Second, in many parts of the world T cell subset analyses are beyond the reach of health resources. The CDC estimates that, as of January 1992, between 115 000 and 170 000 US residents had severe immunosuppression with CD4+ T cell counts less than 200 without a diagnosis of AIDS. Only about 50 000 of these persons were receiving medical care for HIV-related conditions. The number of persons with severe immuno-

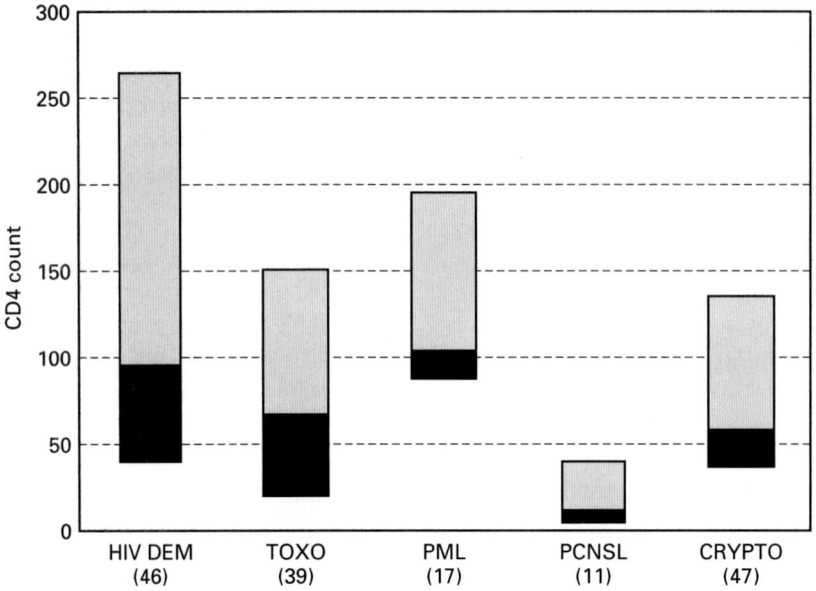

Fig. 1.10   Distribution of CD4 counts (interquartile range and median) within 9 months of HIV-related neurological diagnosis. (Data from Multicentre AIDS Cohort Study March 1993, courtesy of Lisa Jacobson.) HIV DEM, HIV dementia ($n = 46$); TOXO, toxoplasmosis; PML, progressive multifocal leucoencephalopathy; PCNSL, primary CNS lymphoma; CRYPTO, cryptococcosis.

suppression is expected to increase from 130 000 to 205 000 by January 1995 and the expanded AIDS surveillance definition is predicted to result in an increase of approximately 75% in the number of persons reported during 1993 (Centers for Disease Control 1992).

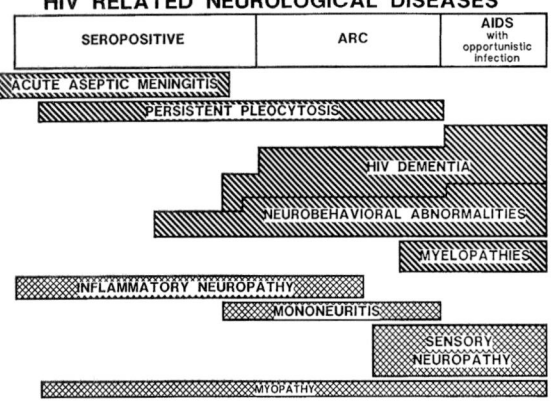

Fig. 1.11   Relative timing of HIV-related neurological disease with respect to systemic disease and relative frequency (width of bar). (Reproduced from Johnson et al 1988 with permission of The FASEB Journal.)

The World Health Organization (WHO 1990), recognizing that the manifestations of HIV infection may vary worldwide, and that the availability of medical services may affect diagnostic precision, has developed a second staging system. The joint CDC/WHO classification system for HIV disease in adolescents and adults is tabulated in Appendix 1 and incorporates both clinical conditions and CD4 count. It is similar in some respects to the Walter Reed staging system, which is less commonly used (Redfield et al 1986). It links the severity of clinical illness to the extent of

Table 1.5   Disease stage, CD4 range and typical duration

Stage	Typical range of CD4 counts (cells/mm^3)	Typical duration
Acute syndrome	1000–500	1–4 weeks
Asymptomatic	750–200	2–15+ years
Early symptomatic	500–100	1–4+ years
Late symptomatic	200–50	1–4+ years
Advanced disease	50–0	0–2+ years

(After Choi et al 1993)

immune system dysfunction, and was developed initially for military use. It has been used in research studies, but because of its complexity it is less widely used today.

NERVOUS SYSTEM INVOLVEMENT

From early in the epidemic, it has been obvious that HIV targets not only CD4 lymphocytes, but also the nervous system. This tropism for the nervous system, or 'neurotropism', is compounded by other biological characteristics of HIV: it can invade the nervous system, presumably through the ingress of infected monocytes or macrophages ('neuroinvasive') and it can cause damage to the nervous system ('neurovirulent'). These three elements of HIV's biology – neurotropism, neuroinvasiveness and neurovirulence – underlie its role in inducing the 'primary' neurological diseases. The strains of HIV that have been isolated from brain tend to be macrophage-tropic rather than lymphocyte-tropic (see Chapter 3). There are parallels between HIV and the other lentiviruses, which have similar characteristics. For example, HIV is morphologically and genetically related to visna, a neurotropic and lymphotropic lentivirus that causes nervous system damage in sheep (Kennedy et al 1989). Infectious HIV has been recovered from cultures of CSF, brain and spinal cord (Ho et al 1985), and in some patients initial infection with HIV-1 is accompanied by acute meningitis, representing central nervous system (CNS) infection as an early feature of HIV infection. These signs of CNS involvement at the time of seroconversion suggest that the CNS may be 'seeded' from the start. Some patients have unique oligoclonal IgG bands in the CSF and demonstrate intrathecal synthesis of specific IgG, implying active CNS infection. The frequency of intrathecal synthesis of HIV IgG rises with increasing duration of infection (Van Wielink et al 1990). CSF samples taken from asymptomatic individuals within 2 years of seroconversion (Appleman et al 1988) show a cellular reaction in one-third, positive virus culture in one-half and a related IgG rise in two-thirds, all confirming early low-grade infection of the CNS long before immunosuppression or CNS symptoms appear. SIV-infected macaques show a similar early CSF pleocytosis, again indicating CNS invasion in the first few weeks of infection. In man, brain invasion has been documented within 15 days of infection. This occurred after the accidental injection of HIV-positive blood as part of a nuclear medicine procedure. The recipient died from unrelated disease and had positive HIV immunostaining in the brain (Davis et al 1992). Finally there is the simple point that many patients with nervous system manifestations have no evidence of any other identifiable pathogen. However, this neglects the possibility that new pathogens may be discovered and that interactions with known pathogens can produce atypical clinical pictures.

The immune deficiency produced by HIV infection makes patients susceptible to infection by a variety of organisms, including viruses, bacteria, fungi and parasites, that are of low pathogenicity in the normal individual and of variable prevalence in different parts of the world. The usual CD4 count at the time of presentation with the various infections is shown in Fig. 1.10. Some of these opportunistic infections in fact reflect reactivation of a previous infection rather than a 'true' opportunistic process. Thus, the patient's prior exposure to these organisms determines the risk of symptomatic infection when immune deficiency supervenes. Thus in areas where exposure to *Toxoplasma gondii* is widespread, e.g. Haiti, Florida and France, the risk of developing *Toxoplasma* encephalitis in AIDS may be as high as 30%. In the UK and most of the USA, where only 10–20% of young adults have serological evidence of prior exposure, the incidence of *Toxoplasma* brain abscesses appears to be much lower.

The immune deficiency state not only influences the type of infectious agent that becomes a symptomatic pathogen, but also modifies the response (Table 1.6). Thus inflammation may be minimal and in intracranial infections there may be no fever or meningism. Furthermore, the CSF response may be muted with minimal pleocytosis. HIV infection impairs humoral as well as cellular immunity, so antibody production can be defective. This reduces the value of antibody titres in the diagnosis of opportunistic infections, and in the late stages of AIDS the HIV antibody tests

Table 1.6 Special features of opportunistic infections in AIDS

Blood	Reduced leucocytosis
	Reduced antibody response
CSF	Reduced pleocytosis
	Chronic abnormalities from HIV
Organisms	Parasites (toxoplasmosis)
	Fungi (cryptococci)
	Viruses (papova, CMV, herpes simplex, herpes zoster)
	Bacteria (spirochaetes, mycobacteria)
Pathology	Less tissue inflammatory response
	Multiple pathogens
Treatment	Long courses
Relapse	Common lifelong maintenance therapy

Table 1.7 Epidemiological features of CNS infections in AIDS

Infection	Epidemiological features
Opportunistic infections/lymphoma	IVDU > Homosexual
	Adults > Children
Cryptococcal meningitis	IVDU > Homosexual
	Black > Caucasian
	New Jersey > New York
Cerebral toxoplasmosis	Hispanic > Non-Hispanic
	Florida > Rest of USA
PML	Uniform distribution
Primary lymphoma	Uniform distribution

PML, progressive multifocal leucoencephalopathy; IVDU, intravenous drug user.

themselves are occasionally negative. Tissue responses also differ, so the normal abscess wall seen in immunocompetent individuals does not always develop and this affects neuroimaging characteristics. Multiple pathologies are common and the same patient may well have systemic and specific nervous system problems. At any one time a patient may have two or more intracranial infections, or have the combination of an infection and a lymphoma.

Little is yet known about the possibility that the risk factors for HIV infection may influence its manifestations (Table 1.7). There are some known differences. It already appears that Black patients and injecting drug users are more prone to develop cryptococcal meningitis. It is also possible that a prior experience of other sexually transmitted diseases or the septicaemic episodes associated with the use of unsterile needles may affect the response to an opportunistic infection or to HIV itself. Haemophiliacs have a background of repeated immunological challenge through frequent transfusion and injections of foreign proteins, in contrast to the situation when infection occurs with a single transfusion. Whether these differences are clinically important is not yet clear. The neuropathological findings in AIDS following haemophilia (Esiri et al 1989) differ, but it is possible that this is simply due to patients dying of their haemophilia rather than of their AIDS with the result that the CNS lesions represent those seen at an earlier stage of HIV-related disease.

The recent discovery that HTLV-1 can be responsible for a chronic myelopathy, particularly in the tropics and Japan, and that AIDS can be due to HIV-2 suggests that the full spectrum of human illnesses resulting from this family of retroviruses has not yet been seen. All human retroviruses studied to date have been lymphotropic. Whether they will all prove to cause disease of the nervous system is not yet known. This latest 'experiment of nature' also promises to illuminate the pathogenesis of some familiar neurological disorders such as the Guillain-Barré syndrome and polymyositis, which may complicate HIV infection. The effect of profound immunodeficiency on coincidental illnesses such as multiple sclerosis and myasthenia gravis may also emerge from the chance association of these diseases with AIDS.

NEUROLOGICAL MANIFESTATIONS

Particular clinical manifestations tend to occur at different stages in the evolution of HIV infection (Fig. 1.11). Thus early on, conditions in which there is a prominent inflammatory response, such as acute demyelinating neuropathy of Guillain-Barré type and polymyositis, are more likely, whereas opportunistic infections, HIV dementia and axonal neuropathies are only common when there is evidence of immune deficiency. In the CNS, infection with HIV is established very early in the infection; however, HIV either remains dormant or there is only a low level of HIV replication until immune deficiency develops.

Table 1.8 Common brain diseases complicating AIDS: clinical differentiation

Disorder	Presentation	Alert	Fever/HA	Focal exam
Toxoplasmosis	< 2 weeks	↓	+	+++
Lymphoma	2–8 weeks	↓ or NL	0	+
PML	weeks/months	NL	0	++
Cryptococcosis	< 2 weeks	↓	+++	0
HIV dementia	weeks/months	NL	0	0
CMV encephalitis	< 2 weeks	↓ or NL	+	0

PML, progressive multifocal leucoencephalopathy; NL, normal; HA, headache.
(After Price R, American Academy of Neurology 1990.)

After this, productive HIV infection within brain macrophages and microglia accelerates, leading to activation of non-infected macrophages that may indirectly cause the 'primary' neurological manifestations of HIV – dementia, myelopathy and sensory neuropathy. The local release of soluble factors, including cytokines, arachidonic acid metabolites and potentially other toxins, may stimulate further HIV transcription, amplifying the process, or cause damage to neural cells directly (Epstein & Gendelman 1993).

Physicians are ever increasingly being confronted with conditions they hitherto considered neurological curiosities, and are having to become expert in the care of infections that were previously the confine of the transplant teams. Bedside diagnosis is very difficult and often confounded by the co-occurrence of multiple neurological problems. Criteria are listed in Appendices 2–5. The clinical presentation of many problems, e.g. toxoplasmosis, lymphoma, progressive multifocal leucoencephalopathy and HIV dementia, overlaps (McArthur 1987), although there are some pointers to be found in the presence or absence of fever, changed conscious level, focal deficit and

length of history (Table 1.8). Neuroradiological and microbiological investigation is indicated on the merest suspicion of intracranial neurological disease with detailed study of the blood and CSF (Table 1.9). Furthermore, multiple pathology is common: for example, multiple focal brain lesion on a CT scan may prove to be due to the simultaneous development of lymphoma and *Toxoplasma* abscesses or tuberculosis (Fig. 1.12). The same patient may have a CNS infection, an axonal neuropathy, and a drug-related myopathy, complicating the interpretation of the neurological examination.

Table 1.9 Evaluation of intracranial lesions in HIV infection

• Blood	HIV serology/CD4
	CMV cultures
	Cryptococcus antigen (>95% PPV)
	Toxoplasma serology (<85% PPV)
• CSF	Cryptococcosis/tuberculosis/neurosyphilis
	Cytology – lymphoma, CMV
• Imaging	Number/location
	Oedema
	Enhancement

PPV, positive predictive value.

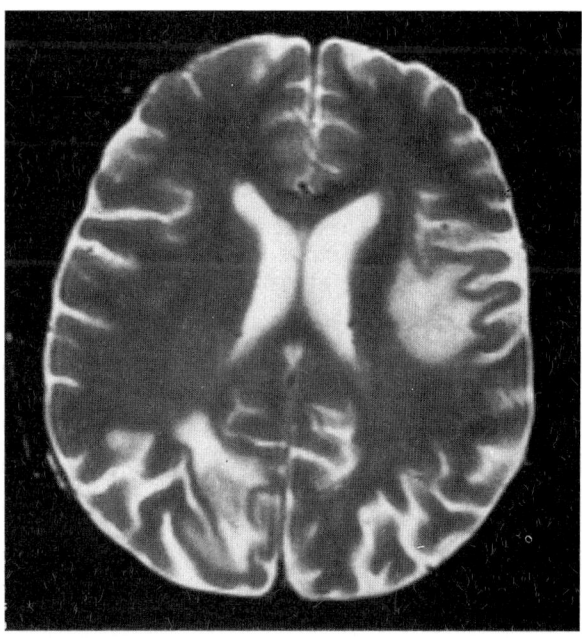

Fig. 1.12 MRI scan (T2-weighted) showing coincident PML in the right hemisphere and toxoplasmosis in the left occipital lobe.

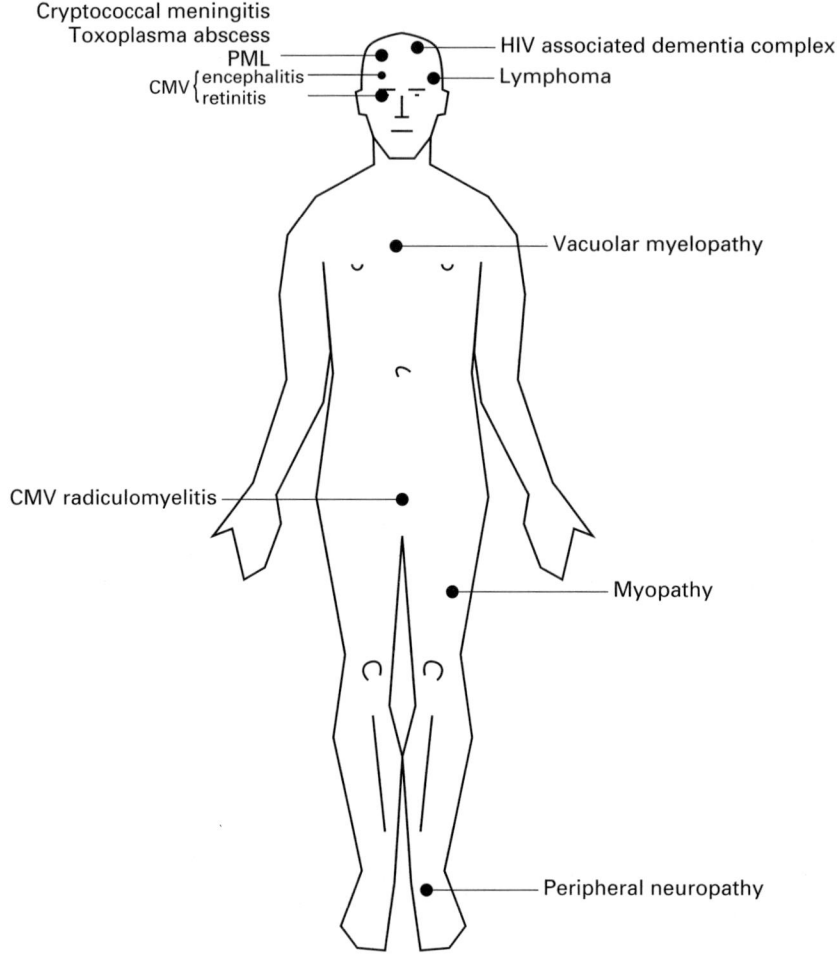

Cryptococcal meningitis
Toxoplasma abscess
PML
CMV {encephalitis / retinitis}

HIV associated dementia complex
Lymphoma

Vacuolar myelopathy

CMV radiculomyelitis

Myopathy

Peripheral neuropathy

Fig. 1.13   Schematic representation of main neurological complications.

Table 1.10   AIDS indicator neurological diseases diagnosed in the USA (1991/1992) (Percentages of all AIDS cases)

	1991	1992
HIV encephalopathy	2705 (6%)	2949 (6%)
Primary CNS lymphoma	303 (1%)	302 (1%)
Cerebral toxoplasmosis	2326 (5%)	2340 (5%)
Progressive multifocal leucoencephalopathy	386 (1%)	415 (1%)
Extrapulmonary cryptococcosis	2439 (5%)	2543 (5%)
Disseminated coccidiomycosis	74 (<1%)	119 (<1%)
CMV disease other than retinitis	1670 (4%)	2132 (5%)

(Reproduced from Centers for Disease Control and Prevention 1993)

As the full spectrum (Fig. 1.13) of neurological manifestations is still emerging, and diagnostic criteria are still undergoing modification, the present account can only reflect current understanding and clinical practice. The unique effects of HIV infection will be discussed first, whilst later chapters will consider the consequences of immunosuppression per se. The relative frequency of the different neurological manifestations is revealed by the 1991/1992 USA data shown in Table 1.10.

REFERENCES

Amadori A A, Chieco-Bianchi L. B cell activation and HIV-1 infection. Immunology Today 1990; 11: 374 (abstr.)

Appleman M E, Marshall D W, Brey R L. Cerebrospinal fluid abnormalities in patients without AIDS who are seropositive for the human immunodeficiency virus. J Infect Dis 1988; 158: 193–198

Bacchetti P, Moss A R. Incubation time of AIDS in San Francisco. Nature 1989; 338: 251–253

Barre-Sinoussi F, Nugeyre M, Dauguet C. Isolation of a T-lymphotropic retrovirus from a patient at risk for acquired immune deficiency syndrome. Science 1983; 220: 868–871

Centers for Disease Control. Projections of the number of persons diagnosed with AIDS and the number of immunosuppressed HIV-infected persons – United States 1992–1994. Morbidity and Mortality Weekly Report 1992; 41: RR1–RR29

Centers for Disease Control and Prevention. HIV/AIDS Surveillance Report 1993; 5: 3–19

Cheng-Mayer C, Seto D, Tateno M, Levy J A. Biologic features of HIV-1 that correlate with virulence in the host. Science 1988; 240: 80–82

Choi S S, Lagakos S W, Schooley R T, Volberding P A. CD4+ lymphocytes are an incomplete surrogate marker for clinical progression in persons with asymptomatic HIV infection taking zidovudine. Ann Intern Med 1993; 118: 674–680

Clerici M, Shearer G M. A Th1–Th2 switch is a critical step in the etiology of HIV infection. Immunol Today 1993; 14: 107–110

Coombs R W, Collier A C, Allain J P, et al. Plasma viremia in human immunodeficiency virus infection. New Engl J Med 1989; 321: 1626–1631

Dalgleish A G. The immunology of retrovirus disease. In: Rudge P (ed). Baillière's Clinical Neurology 1992; 1: 23–40

Dalgleish A G, Beverly P C L, Clapham P R. The CD4 antigen is an essential component of the receptor for the AIDS retrovirus. Nature 1984; 312: 763–767

Davis L E, Hjelle B L, Miller V E, et al. Early viral brain invasion in iatrogenic human immunodeficiency virus infection. Neurology 1992; 42: 1736–1739

De-The G, Giordano C, Gessain A, et al. Human retroviruses HTLV-I, HIV-1, and HIV-2 and neurological diseases in some equatorial areas of Africa. J Acquired Immunodeficiency Syndromes 1989; 2: 550–556

Epstein L G, Gendelman H E. Human immunodeficiency virus type 1 infection of the nervous system: pathogenetic mechanisms. Ann Neurol 1993; 33: 429–436

Esiri M M, Scaravilli F, Millard P R, Harcourt-Webster J N. Neuropathology of HIV infection in haemophiliacs: comparative necropsy study. Br Med J 1989; 299: 1312–1315

Fahey J L, Taylor J M G, Detels R, et al. The prognostic value of cellular and serologic markers in infection with human immunodeficiency virus type 1. New Engl J Med 1990; 322: 166–172

French M, Abraham L, Mallal S, et al. MHC genes and HIV. Today's Life Sci 1992; 32–36

Friedman-Klein A E, Laubenstein L J, Rubinstein P. Disseminated Kaposi's sarcoma in homosexual men. Ann Intern Med 1982; 96: 693–700

Garry R F, Witte M H, Gottlieb A A, et al. Documentation of an AIDS virus infection in the United States in 1968. JAMA 1988; 260: 2085–2086

Greene W C. The molecular biology of human immunodeficiency virus type 1 infection. New Engl J Med 1991; 324: 308–317

Grewe C, Beck A, Gelderblom H R. HIV: early virus–cell interactions. J Acquired Immunodeficiency Syndromes 1990; 33: 965–973

Griffin D E. Immunologic abnormalities accompanying acute and chronic viral infections (review). Rev Infect Dis 1991; 13(suppl): S129–S133

Harouse J M, Bhat S, Spitalnik S L, et al. Inhibition of entry of HIV-1 in neural cell lines by antibodies against galactosyl ceramide. Science 1991; 253: 320–323

Hirsch M S, D'Aquila R T. Therapy for human immunodeficiency virus infection. N Engl J Med 1993; 328: 1686–1695

Ho D D, Rota T R, Hirsch M S. Infection of monocyte/macrophages by HTLV-III. J Clin Invest 1986; 77: 1712–1715

Ho D D, Rota T R, Schooley R T, et al. Isolation of HTLV-III from cerebrospinal fluid and neural tissues of patients with neurologic syndromes related to the acquired immunodeficiency syndrome. New Engl J Med 1985; 313: 1493–1497

Hoover D R, Graham N M H, Chen B, et al. Effect of CD4+ cell count measurement variability on staging HIV-1 infection. J Acquired Immunodeficiency Syndromes 1992; 5: 794–802

Janssen R S. Epidemiology of human immunodeficiency virus infection and the neurological complications of the infection. Sem Neurol 1992; 12: 10–17

Johnson R T, McArthur J C, Narayan O. The neurobiology of human immunodeficiency virus infections. FASEB J 1988; 2: 2970–2981

Kennedy P G E. Neurological aspects of human retroviruses. In: Rudge P (ed). Baillière's Clinical Neurology vol. 1, issue 1. London: Baillière Tindall, 1992: 41–59

Kennedy P G E, Narayan O, Zink M C. The pathogenesis of Visna, a lentivirus-induced immunopathologic disease of the central nervous system. In: Gilden D H, Lipton H L, eds. Clinical and molecular aspects of neurotropic virus infection. Boston: Kluwer Academic, 1989: 393–421

Klatzman D, Barre-Sinoussi F, Nugeyre M. Selective tropism of lymphadenopathy-associated virus (LAV) for helper-inducer T-lymphocytes. Science 1984; 225: 59–62

Koot M, Keet I P M, Vos A H V, et al. Prognostic value of HIV-1 syncytium-inducing phenotype for rate of CD4+ cell depletion and progression to AIDS. Ann Intern Med 1993; 188: 681–688

Koyanagi Y, Milse S, Mitsuyasu R T, et al. Dual infection of the central nervous system by AIDS viruses with distinct cellular tropisms. Science 1987; 236: 819–822

Lange J M A, de Wolf F, Goudsmit J. Markers for progression in HIV infection. AIDS 1989; 3(suppl): S153–S160

Levy D N, Fernandes L S, Williams W V, Weiner D B. Induction of cell differentiation by human immunodeficiency virus 1 vpr. Cell 1993; 72: 541–550

Levy J A. Human immunodeficiency viruses and the pathogenesis of AIDS (review). JAMA 1989; 261: 2997–3006

Levy J A. Pathogenesis of human immunodeficiency virus infection. Microbiol Rev 1993; 57: 183–289

Lifson J D, Feinberg M B, Reyes G R. Induction of CD4 dependent cell fusion by the HTLV-III envelope glycoprotein. Nature 1986; 323: 725–728

Masur H, Michelis M A, Greene J B. An outbreak of community acquired *Pneumocystis carinii* pneumonia. Initial manifestations of immune dysfunction. New Engl J Med 1981; 305: 1431–1438

McArthur J C. Neurologic manifestations of AIDS. Medicine (Baltimore) 1987; 66: 407–437

Michael N L, Vahey M, Burke D S, Redfield R R. Viral DNA and mRNA expression correlate with the stage of human immunodeficiency virus (HIV) type 1 infection in humans: evidence for viral replication in all stages of HIV disease. J Virol 1992; 66: 310–316

Murray H, Welte K, Jacobs J H. Production of and in vitro response of IL-2 in AIDS. J Clin Invest 1985; 76: 1959–1964

Pantaleo G, Graziosi C, Fauci A S. The immunopathogenesis of human immunodeficiency virus infection. New Engl J Med 1993a; 328: 327–335

Pantaleo G, Graziosi C, Demarest J F, et al. HIV infection is active and progressive in lymphoid tissue during the clinically latent stage of disease. Nature 1993b; 362: 355–358

Phillips A N, Lee C A, Elford J, et al. Serial CD4 counts and the development of AIDS. Lancet 1991; 337: 389–392

Poli G, Fauci A S. The role of monocyte/macrophages and cytokines in the pathogenesis of HIV infection. Pathobiology 1992; 60: 246–251

Redfield R R, Wright D C, Tramont E C. The Walter Reed staging classification for HTLV-III/LAV infection. New Engl J Med 1986; 314: 131–132

Rosenberg Z F, Fauci A S. Immunopathogenic mechanisms of HIV infection: cytokine induction of HIV expression. Immunol Today 1990; 11: 176

Schnittman S M, Psallidopoulos M C, Lane H C. The reservoir of HIV-1 in human peripheral blood is a T cell that maintains expression of CD4. Science 1989; 245: 305–308

Shearer G M, Clerici M. T helper cell immune dysfunction in asymptomatic, HIV-1-seropositive individuals: the role of Th1-Th2 cross-regulation (review). Chem Immunol 1992; 54: 21–43

Siegel F P, Lopez C, Hammer G S, et al. Severe acquired immunodeficiency in male homosexuals manifested by chronic perianal ulcerative herpes simplex lesions. N Engl J Med 1981; 305: 1439–1444

Snider W D, Simpson D M, Nielsen S, et al. Neurological complications of acquired immune deficiency syndrome: analysis of 50 patients. Ann Neurol 1983; 14: 403–418

Stevenson M, Meier C, Mann A M. Envelope glycoprotein of HIV induces interference and cytolysis resistance in CD4+ cells: mechanism of persistence in AIDS. Cell 1988; 53: 483–486

Tersmette M, Gruters R A, de Wolf F, et al. Evidence for a role of virulent human immunodeficiency syndrome: studies of sequential HIV isolates. J Virol 1989; 63: 2118–2125

Van Wielink G, McArthur J C, Moench T, et al. Intrathecal synthesis of anti-HIV-IgG: correlation with increasing duration of HIV-1 infection. Neurology 1990; 40: 816–819

WHO. AIDS interim proposal for WHO staging system for HIV infection and disease. Weekly Epidemiol Rec 1990; 65: 221–224

Wolinsky S M, Rinaldo C R, Kwok S, et al. Human immunodeficiency virus type 1 (HIV-1) infection a median of 18 months before a diagnostic western blot. Evidence from a cohort of homosexual men. Ann Intern Med 1989; 111: 961–972

2. Seroconversion and the asymptomatic years

Primary HIV infection was first recognized in 1985 (Cooper et al 1985) and generally presents as a mononucleosis-like syndrome with or without aseptic meningitis, associated with seroconversion for HIV antibody. This illness has been reported in all major groups at risk for HIV infection, although it is less well defined in children.

Some patients are acutely ill at the time of their original infection with HIV, others have relatively mild symptoms, or the seroconversion is unrecognized. Retrospective studies of seroconverters have shown that most individuals who undergo seroconversion, in fact, have a recognized acute clinical syndrome. Perhaps the most useful heralding symptoms are lymphadenopathy, persistent fatigue and lethargy, and truncal rash (Fox et al 1987, Tindall et al 1988) (Table 2.1). The syndrome usually takes the form of a glandular fever-like illness with the familiar combination of myalgias, pyrexia, sore throat, arthropathy and gastrointestinal symptoms. A maculopapular rash over the trunk and extremities is not uncommon. Aphthous ulcers or oral candidiasis can occur and some patients develop cervical or axillary lymphadenopathy typically in the second week of the syndrome. The erythrocyte sedimentation rate (ESR) is often raised and there may be a prominent atypical lymphocytosis. HIV antibodies are initially negative but p24 antigen can be detected in blood and/or cerebrospinal fluid (CSF) (Fig. 1.8, Chapter 1). In one case studied over the time of seroconversion, a meningoencephalitis coincided with the appearance of a pleocytosis and markers of immune stimulation in the CSF before HIV antibodies were detectable (Fig. 2.1) (Griffin et al 1990). Several studies with repeated serology during and after a seroconversion illness have

Table 2.1 Clinical manifestations of primary HIV infection

Mononucleosis-like
Fever
Pharyngitis
Lymphadenopathy
Arthralgia, myalgia
Headache, retro-orbital pain
Lethargy, malaise
Anorexia, weight loss
Nausea, vomiting
Diarrhoea

Neuropathic
Meningitis
Encephalitis
Peripheral neuropathy
Radiculopathy
Guillain-Barré syndrome
Cognitive or affective impairment

Dermatological
Erythematous maculopapular rash
Roseola-like rash
Diffuse urticaria
Desquamation
Alopecia
Palatal or gingival ulceration

(Reproduced from Sande & Volberding 1988 with permission of W B Saunders Company)

shown that in most individuals, specific HIV antibodies are detectable within 2 weeks of the beginning of the acute seroconversion illness. IgM antibodies appear first, followed by IgG, and immunofluorescence assay (IFA) appears more sensitive than enzyme-linked immunosorbent assay (ELISA). The width of the 'window' between initial infection and reliable seropositivity varies. Data from the Multicenter AIDS Cohort Study (MACS) indicate that in some patients this window of seronegativity following infection may last up to 48 months (Wolinsky et al 1989). For

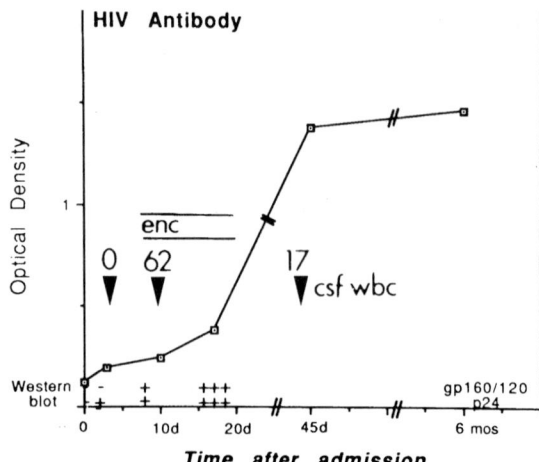

Fig. 2.1   Time course of seroconversion illness. Patient admitted with delirium tremens, which cleared in a few days. Initially HIV ELISA was negative, Western blot indeterminate, and on day 3 the CSF contained no pleocytosis. Developed fever, lymphadenopathy, a generalized rash, atypical lymphocytosis and meningoencephalitis on day 8 (enc) with CSF pleocytosis of 62 WBCs, rise in HIV antibody titre and development of bands on Western blot.

individuals in whom HIV seroconversion illness is suspected, the measurement of p24 antigen, HIV cultures or the use of polymerase chain reaction (PCR) may be useful for confirmation.

A variety of neurological manifestations may be seen during or immediately after these systemic effects of the initial infection. A meningoencephalitis is perhaps the most usual (McArthur 1987). The patient may have headache out of keeping with the degree of fever and have mild meningism and photophobia. Cranial nerve palsies (usually a peripheral facial weakness) may accompany this meningitic illness. The condition is self-limiting, recovery being usual within a couple of months or so. Others have an encephalitic illness (Carne et al 1989, Griffin et al 1990). After a prodrome of fever and malaise, complaints of poor memory and concentration, irritability, seizures and personality change come to dominate the clinical picture. Recovery is prompt even from coma and no other cause such as herpes simplex is found. Investigation reveals little but for diffusely abnormal electroencephalograms (EEGs). The CSF may show a pleocytosis and elevated protein and be p24 positive.

Less commonly, individual patients have experi-

enced a myelopathy with paraparesis (Denning et al 1987), or a radiculopathy with sciatica, reflex loss in the legs, weakness and sphincter disturbance such as that caused in AIDS by cytomegalovirus (CMV). The most common peripheral nervous system manifestation appears to be a Guillain-Barré peripheral neuropathy (Vendrall et al 1986). There are also reports of an asymmetrical bilateral painful brachial neuritis (Calabrese et al 1989) and of an individual with a progressive sensory ataxia due to ganglioneuritis immediately after seroconversion (Elder et al 1986). One patient developed rhabdomyolysis at the same time as their primary HIV infection (Mahe et al 1989), and another a cerebellar syndrome (Portegies & Brew 1991).

Some of these manifestations may reflect direct invasion of the nervous system by the HIV. This early invasion is tragically documented in a recent accidental infection. A report of a patient who died 15 days after accidentally receiving an intravenous injection of white blood cells (during a nuclear medicine test) from a patient with AIDS showed that HIV was present in the brain (Davis et al 1992). Mild perivascular cuffing and a mild lymphocytic meningitis were seen without glial nodules, giant cells or white matter abnormalities. HIV antigen was detected in rare infiltrating cells within perivascular and subpial spaces. In another study of HIV-infected individuals dying before AIDS, Gray et al (1993) examined 11 brains of patients who died from drug overdoses. The HIV-seropositive cases had lymphocytic meningitis, granular ependymitis, myelin pallor with reactive astrocytosis, and microglial proliferation, although immunocytochemistry for HIV antigens was negative. Other investigators have detected HIV DNA using PCR in brains from similar patients dying from accidental deaths before AIDS (Scaravilli et al 1993).

Other complications appear more likely to be immunologically triggered, for example in the case of Guillain-Barré neuropathy in the way that it follows *Campylobacter* infections.

In all these situations the management depends on exclusion of alternative causes such as herpes simplex meningoencephalitis by virological tests, and on supportive care. There is an argument for the short-term use of an antiviral drug, which theoretically might shorten the duration of the meningitic illness, for example. The main problem is often of recognizing the seroconversion status of the patient when routine diagnostic serology is as yet negative. If there is a high index of suspicion in an at-risk patient, the antigenic tests or culture and PCR should be carried out and the antibody tests repeated weekly.

THE 'ASYMPTOMATIC' PERIOD

This is a somewhat confusing term as patients may develop a variety of conditions. What is referred to is the lack of constitutional symptoms related to immunosuppression. Generally, asymptomatic patients with (previously termed CDC stage III) and without (previously termed CDC stage II) lymphadenopathy are considered together because the presence of lymphadenopathy is not indicative of a different course or prognosis (Appendix 1).

CDC stage A defines the interval between seroconversion and symptomatic immunosuppression (AIDS). It is highly variable in duration, but commonly lasts 8–10 years (Fig. 1.9, Chapter 1). Risk factors for progression were discussed in Chapter 1. Because of the length of this phase of the infection and the relatively imprecise criteria used for its definition, the term 'asymptomatic' individual is an artificial term that is sometimes more confusing than helpful. For example, before the recent expansion of the CDC AIDS definitions, two asymptomatic individuals, one with a normal CD4 count and the second with a CD4 count less than 100, would both be classified as asymptomatic. While not necessarily important from a clinical perspective, this has undoubtedly led to some confusion in comparison of research studies purporting to study similar 'asymptomatic' individuals who in fact have very different levels of immunodeficiency. This may account for some of the discrepancies in some of the neurological and neuropsychological testing during this phase of the infection (see below). The most common clinical manifestation during these years is the development in about one in three of a non-specific persistent generalized lymphadenopathy, which previously defined CDC stage III. Nodes over 1 cm in diameter are felt in more than two

non-contiguous extrainguinal sites. They are non-tender and mobile. If the nodes enlarge, become painful or are accompanied by fever or weight loss, a biopsy is needed to exclude a systemic lymphoma. Usually a benign follicular hyperplasia is all that is found, and the lymphadenopathy is not a risk factor for the rapidity of progression to AIDS. For this reason the old terms CDC stages II and III are considered equivalent, and are now together referred to as defining the 'asymptomatic' phase of the illness (CDC stage A).

During clinical latency, HIV accumulates in the lymphoid organs associated with follicular dendritic cells and replicates actively despite a low viral burden and low to absent replication in peripheral blood cells (Pantaleo et al 1993). The peripheral blood therefore does not accurately reflect the actual state of HIV infection. Embretson et al (1993) used in situ PCR of lymph nodes to show large numbers of latently infected CD4+ lymphocytes and macrophages. They argue that this is enough to explain immune depletion.

Neurological conditions developing during the asymptomatic phase

During this so-called asymptomatic stage, neurological conditions may occur in which there is a prominent inflammatory response. For example, an acute demyelinating neuropathy of Guillain-Barré type and an acute polymyositis may occur and may herald seroconversion. The acute inflammatory demyelinating neuropathy is clinically indistinguishable from that seen in non-HIV infected individuals, though one characteristic difference is the presence of a CSF pleocytosis (Cornblath et al 1987). Treatment considerations are discussed in Chapter 6. An acute meningitic illness with headache and cranial nerve palsies can also be seen at this time (Fig. 1.10, Chapter 1). These patients develop headache and malaise or may present with a Bell's palsy or other cranial nerve palsies. The CSF shows a persistent pleocytosis of about 20 cells, and no pathogens other than HIV are cultured. There is only anecdotal evidence of the value of antiviral therapy, which is usually instituted. Many asymptomatic HIV-seropositive patients have a chronic pleocytosis, which in some is accompanied by mild chronic neurological symptoms, including headache and minor cognitive symptoms (McArthur 1987, Hollander & Stringari 1987). This chronic meningitis is generally low grade and studies of repeated lumbar punctures have defined the temporal profile of these CSF changes (Chapter 15).

Multiple sclerosis

There was much interest in the possibility that the profound immunosuppression of AIDS might have revealing effects on the natural history of multiple sclerosis (MS) in the likely eventuality of the two conditions occurring in the same patient. Berger et al in 1989 described four patients in whom MS seemed to have been present for several years before seroconversion to HIV. The disease in these patients seemed unchanged by the HIV infection.

The same authors also reported three cases in which an acute MS-like illness including optic neuritis and myelitis occurred in close relationship to the development of seropositivity suggesting more than a chance association. A subsequent case had a relapsing and remitting illness affecting brain, cord and optic nerve (Berger et al 1992). Gray et al (1991) added two more pathologically examined cases. The association appeared more than chance because one patient came from a low-risk area for MS, and the other had an acute onset at the age of 66 years, which is highly unusual for routine MS. The brains showed scattered but well-demarcated areas of demyelination in the hemispheres and brainstem. There was some perivenous cuffing and reactive gliosis. The pathological account makes it clear, however, that Gray's patients also had typical perivenular demyelination, which is perhaps more typical of post-infectious demyelination than 'ordinary' MS. There were no multinucleated cells or microglial nodules, and there was no staining for HIV, so it seems unlikely that the lesions were a manifestation of acute HIV encephalitis.

It thus remains possible that these florid cases of rapidly progressive widespread demyelination soon after seroconversion are rather different from MS and not a useful model of that disease. HIV testing may be appropriate for patients with a rapid deteriorating illness, with magnetic resonance (MR) images suggestive of widespread MS-like plaques. Steroids and interferon β may be appropriate therapeutic options.

Cognitive impairment during the asymptomatic phase

The early recognition of the frequency of dementia and neuropathological changes in patients with AIDs raised the issue of whether a subclinical decline in cognitive performance occurs early in the course of HIV infection. There has been much subsequent debate over whether there is any subtle neuropsychological deterioration during the years before immunosuppression is obvious clinically or by laboratory markers. Fig. 2.2 illustrates some of the different hypotheses, depending on whether deterioration is precipitous or gradual, and on whether it precedes or only follows the onset of immunosuppression.

The first study by Grant et al (1987) suggested that there were detectable differences in performance on a neuropsychological test battery when asymptomatic HIV positive and negative subjects were compared. The finding of a high rate of neuropsychological impairment among asymptomatic seropositive individuals suggested that manifestations of CNS infection with HIV might develop frequently during the asymptomatic phase (Fig. 2.2, 'X'). There were immediate and long-lasting public health and employment practice concerns. One result of this study was the decision by the US military to remove asymptomatic seropositive personnel from flight duty and other technically 'complex' positions because of the perceived risk for cognitive impairment. In 1988, the World Health Organization reviewed this and other studies and came to the conclusion that 'at present there is no evidence for an increase of clinically significant neuropsychiatric abnormalities in CDC groups II or III HIV seropositive (i.e. otherwise asymptomatic) individuals compared to HIV seronegative controls' (World Health Organization 1988).

More than 40 studies have now addressed this issue. Some have claimed to have shown a significant difference, but others have seen no such evidence (Table 2.2). A review of the published

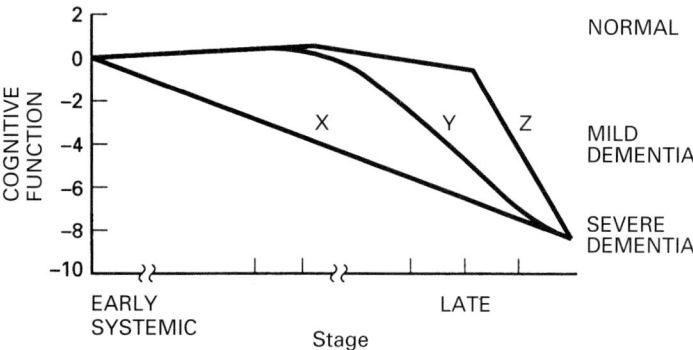

Fig. 2.2   Theoretical temporal profiles of cognitive decline towards
HIV-1 dementia. 'X' represents slow, steadily progressive cognitive
impairment beginning during the asymptomatic phase. This pattern is
rare. 'Y' represents a more typical pattern with a more rapid decline in
cognitive function beginning after AIDS or with advanced
immunosuppression.

data (Newman et al 1994) was prompted by this
continued confusion, which has important implications both in terms of patient care and in understanding the pathogenesis of the fully developed
dementia in later stages. A literature search
focused on studies in which neuropsychological
testing of asymptomatic HIV patients was
reported. In each case a note was made of the
tests administered, the definitions of abnormality
employed and the number of subjects studied.
Odds ratios with 95% confidence limits were
calculated wherever adequate data were detailed
in the published account. Forty-two studies were

found in the literature, employing such a diversity
of neuropsychological tests that 85 different tests
were detected in the reports (Table 2.3). There
were many different definitions of impairment.
Odds ratios were calculated in 16 studies that
gave appropriate data and calculated an overall
index of impairment (Table 2.4). Their relationship to the size of the study and control groups is
shown in Figure 2.3.

The most striking finding of this review of test
results in seropositive and seronegative groups is
seen in the relationship of the odds ratio for each
study and the size of the experimental group.
Studies with less than about 80 subjects had
diverse odds ratios ranging up to 12. Over 80
subjects were examined in eight studies in which
an overall definition of impairment was provided.
These show odds ratios so close to unity that the

Table 2.2   Cross-sectional neuropsychological studies in
asymptomatic HIV infection

Author (year)	Cases/controls
Grant et al (1987) ⋆	44/11
Poutiainen al (1988) ⋆	13/10
Fitzgibbon et al (1989) ⋆	25/25
Perry et al (1989) ⋆	20/20
Krikorian et al (1990) ⋆	38/16
Wilkie et al (1990) ⋆	46/13
Helmstaedter et al (1988)	181/28
Tross et al (1988)	100/20
Goethe et al (1989)	83/18
Miller et al (1990)	727/769
Arday et al (1991)	1283/6415

⋆ These studies have suggested an increased frequency of
cognitive impairment in asymptomatic HIV seropositive
individuals; the other studies have not.

Table 2.3   Types of neuropsychological test in published
studies of HIV infection

Verbal and language skills	20
Memory and learning	24
Attention and concentration	14
Visual and spatial skills	11
Visuomotor and manual skills	9
Executive function	4
Numerical skills	1
Composite measures	2

(Reproduced from Newman et al 1994)

Table 2.4 Summary of comparison of neuropsychological testing in asymptomatic seropositive and seronegative subjects

Study	n	OR	CI
Grant et al (1987)	27	4.96	0.95 – 25.80
Tross et al (1988)	36	10.10	0.60 –172.00
Carne et al (1989)	33	12.80	0.74 – 22.00
Lunn et al (1991)	40	2.08	0.53 – 8.20
Perry et al (1989)	40	4.74	1.28 – 17.50
Saykin et al (1988)	44	9.07	2.30 – 35.80
Wilkie et al (1990)	59	4.64	1.31 – 16.60
Brown & Sesel (1992)	62	6.79	1.98 – 23.30
Clifford et al (1990)	83	0.90	0.37 – 2.19
McArthur et al (1990)	107	0.94	0.37 – 2.40
McAllister et al (1992)	112	1.42	0.56 – 3.56
Naber et al (1989)	200	1.41	0.68 – 2.92
Janssen et al (1989)	231	1.27	0.70 – 2.30
McArthur et al (1990)	463	0.90	0.53 – 1.52
Miller et al (1990)	946	1.18	0.92 – 1.52
Miller et al (1990)	1496	1.14	0.92 – 1.40

OR, odds ratio; CI, 95% confidence interval.
(Reproduced from Newman et al 1994.)

conclusion must be that no increased prevalence of neuropsychological deficit has been proven. The controversy, it is suggested, lies in undue attention being paid to small data sets. Of course, there may well be an element of selection bias. The difficulties in arriving at a consensus view about this important issue thus prove to be mostly methodological. A wide spectrum of tests has been used and the definition of abnormality has varied widely. Many studies give no overall definition of impairment, and others fail to use an appropriate control group. Seronegative individuals from the same at-risk background with comparable educational level are preferable to non-risk controls or laboratory or literature norms. When large numbers of asymptomatic seropositive subjects are studied and compared with appropriate controls, there is no widespread evidence of significant cognitive impairment or 'subclinical dementia'. Clearly, HIV dementia can occasionally develop during the asymptomatic phase; however, its frequency is very low. In cross-sectional data from the MACS, studying 279 asymptomatic seropositive patients, only one had evidence of mild dementia – a prevalence rate of 3.7 per 1000 (McArthur et al 1989). A recent

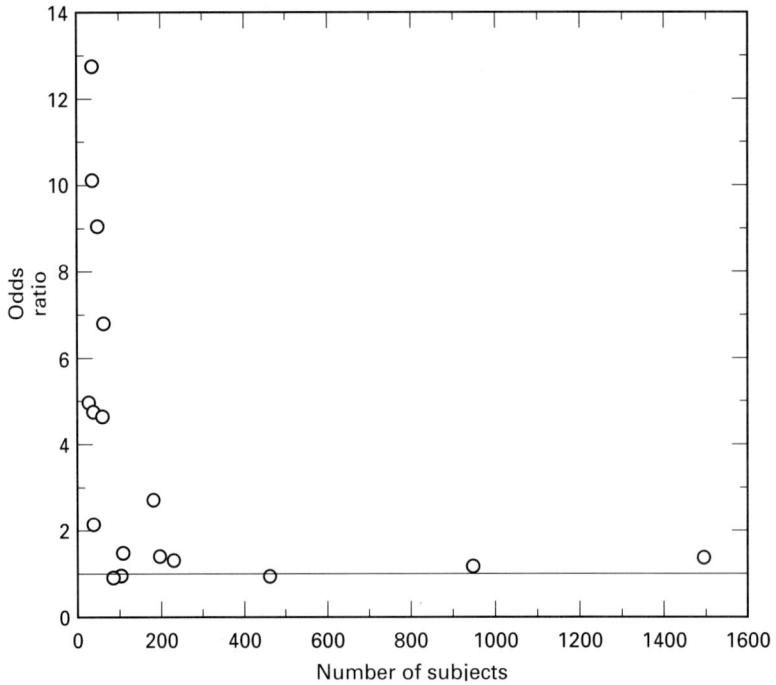

Fig. 2.3 Relationship of 'evidence' of cognitive impairment in asymptomatic HIV seropositive subjects to numbers of subjects in study.

study by Bornstein et al (1993) compared 77 HIV-negative controls with 233 HIV-positive homosexual or bisexual men. Asymptomatic positives (mean CD4 count 549) were different from the controls in some of the tests. Most cross-sectional studies reported to date that have demonstrated apparent neurocognitive abnormalities have not followed the abnormalities over time. It is unclear, therefore, whether these abnormalities would remain stable, worsen or possibly even improve given repeated testing. A number of longitudinal studies have in fact been completed in several different risk behaviour groups (Table 2.5). Perhaps the most compelling evidence that the frequency of significant (and progressive) cognitive impairment is low during the asymptomatic phase of infection comes from these longitudinal studies. Universally, they have reached the same conclusion: that cognitive *decline* is not a feature of this phase of infection. Longitudinal studies such as the MACS, and those including studies in drug users and haemophiliacs, reach the same conclusion, because they fail to demonstrate any decline in cognitive performance throughout the asymptomatic period (Selnes et al 1990, 1992a). Indeed, preliminary analysis suggests that decline is unlikely until CD4 counts have fallen to around 50 (Selnes et al 1992b). The practical conclusions are important and apply to decisions

about driving, legal competence, business acumen and whether to HIV test well subjects in responsible or technically complex jobs, etc. In addition the findings imply that though the virus is detectable in the CNS at an early stage, there is little evidence of major damage until the patient is immunosuppressed.

Other methods of testing neurological functioning of HIV-positive individuals have sought indirect evidence of CNS impairment at an early stage. Careful examination with recording of findings to a protocol has been carried out in a number of cohort studies that have included appropriate seronegative controls (Royal et al 1991, McAllister et al 1992). The study by Royal et al is representative, and examined 109 seropositive and 51 seronegative intravenous drug users. Symptoms referrable to the nervous system were common, but of equal prevalence in the two groups (Fig. 2.4); 21% of seropositive and 17% of seronegative individuals had three or more such symptoms. Neurological signs were also common, with depressed leg reflexes and sensory findings more frequent than findings more suggestive of central problems. Again there was no evidence that these features were related to serostatus (Fig. 2.4). The high prevalence rate is not due to the choice of an intravenous drug user cohort. McAllister et al (1992) examined 110 asymptomatic homosexual men. Clinical neurological abnormalities were found in 32% of seropositive and 25% of seronegative subjects (not significant). Again sensory signs and symptoms suggesting a possible neuropathy predominated, though brisk reflexes were seen in eight individuals. 'Hard' neurological signs were rare in both of these studies. Jansen et al (1989) also found that neurological abnormality was associated with symptomatic, not asymptomatic, HIV infection.

Cognitive evoked potentials (Chapter 15), which correlate with progression of dementia in Alzheimer's disease, have been found abnormal in some studies (Goodin et al 1990), but not others (Goodwin et al 1990). With seronegative controls from at-risk backgrounds, and adjustment for level of intelligence quotient (IQ), there seem to be no changes except in patients with AIDS (Table 2.6). Visual, auditory and somatosensory

Table 2.5 Longitudinal neuropsychological studies in asymptomatic HIV infection

Author (year)	Cohort	Follow-up (months)	Cases/ controls
Selnes et al (1990)	Homosexuals	18	238/170
Saykin et al (1991)	Homosexuals	18	21/21
Gastaut et al (1990)	Homosexuals	6–18	50/8
Selnes et al (1992a)	Injecting drug users	12	37/69
Helmstaedter et al (1992)	Haemophiliacs	20	62/–
Whitt et al (1992)	Haemophiliacs	24	25/25
Robertson et al (1992)	Homosexuals	24	118/0
Karlsen et al (1993)	Homosexuals	24	36/–
Selnes et al (1992b)	Injecting drug users	36	19/40

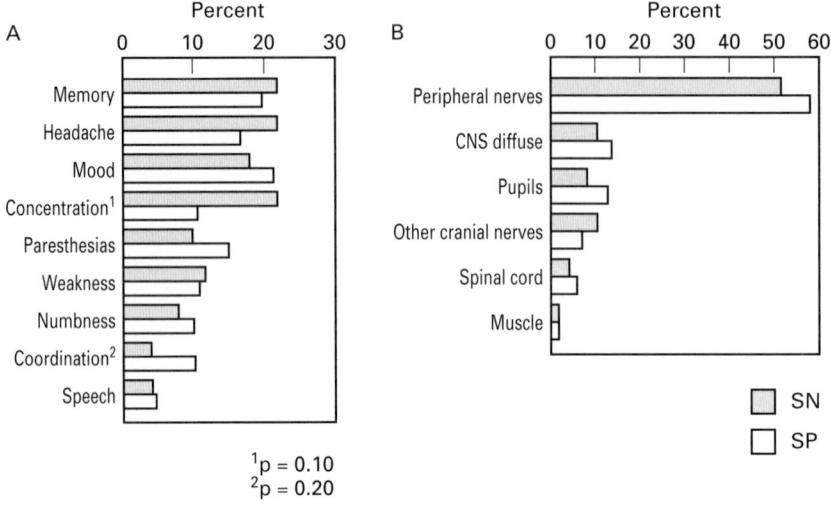

Fig. 2.4   Prevalence of neurological symptoms (A) and signs (B) in seropositive and seronegative injecting drug users. (Reproduced from Royal et al 1991.)

Table 2.6   Cognitive evoked potentials

	Latency auditory P300 (ms) ± SD		
	Seronegative (n = 23)	Asymptomatic seropositive (n = 45)	
Frontal	319 ± 29.5	330 ± 34.1	NS
Central	321 ± 29.8	333 ± 37.8	NS
Parietal	335 ± 38.1	348 ± 38.1	NS

NS, not significant.
(Middlesex Hospital data, reproduced from Connolly et al 1994 with permission of Annals of Neurology)

evoked potentials from the limbs (which might be expected to reflect cerebral or cord pathology) have proved normal in asymptomatic individuals (Smith et al 1988, McAllister et al 1992, Jabbai et al 1993) (Table 2.7). EEG (including quantitative) studies have also addressed the issue of subclinical change. Parisi et al (1989) found that an abnormal record in an asymptomatic patient was predictive of progression to symptomatic disease, but the MACS data (Nuwer et al 1992) on a much larger cohort that compared EEG findings in seropositive and seronegative individuals found no difference in mean dominant frequency or abundance of slow activity.

Magnetic resonance imaging (MRI), both qualitative and quantitative, has also been applied to the search for subclinical changes. Cerebral

imaging reveals abnormalities in seropositive individuals that are no more prevalent than in normal populations. For example, seronegative people from the same background also show a

Table 2.7   Visual, auditory and lumbar somatosensory evoked potentials

	Latency (ms) ± SD		
	Control	Asymptomatic seropositive	
VER P100*	110.7 ± 4.7	113.4 ± 7.5	NS
AER I–V interval*	4.14 ± 0.09	4.06 ± 0.19	NS
LLSEP P40**	41.8 ± 2.4	42.1 ± 2.6	NS
	(26)	(56)	

VER, visual evoked response; AER, auditory evoked response; LLSEP, lower limb somatosensory evoked potential.
Figures in parentheses are the number of subjects.
* Data from Farnarier & Somma-Mauvais (1990).
** Middlesex Hospital data.

Table 2.8   Incidence of MRI findings (visual rating)

	Seronegatives	Asymptomatic seropositives	
Atrophy, sulci	6/23	4/34	NS
Atrophy, ventricles	4/23	1/34	NS
White matter lesions	7/23	4/34	NS
Development of atrophy over 12 months	1/22	1/35	NS

(Middlesex Hospital data)

Table 2.9 Calculated CSF/intracranial volume (ICV) ratios from quantitative MRI

	Seronegatives ($n = 28$)	Asymptomatic seropositives ($n = 32$)	
CSF/ICV ratio	0.128 ± 0.02	0.126 ± 0.02	NS

(Middlesex Hospital data)

Table 2.10 Magnetic resonance spectroscopy: N-acetyl aspartate (NAA)/choline ratios in occipital white matter

	Seronegatives ($n = 56$)	Asymptomatic seropositives ($n = 22$)	
NAA/total	0.54 ± 0.03	0.52 ± 0.04	NS

(Middlesex Hospital data)

comparable prevalence of small white-matter intensities, or 'atrophy' (McArthur et al 1990, Jernigan et al 1993) (Table 2.8). When patients develop AIDS there is more evidence of atrophy than in the other groups, and more specific white matter changes become apparent (see Chapter 15). Relaxation measurements and volume calculations also show no significant differences between positive and negative cases in the UK study (Table 2.9). Proton spectroscopy has revealed decreased N-acetyl-aspartate (NAA) peaks in the posterior white matter of AIDS patients. Although normal controls show the highest ratios (e.g. NAA/choline), the differences between seronegative and seropositive individuals are not significant (Table 2.10). The body of data currently available is compatible with the simple hypothesis that the overt manifestations of brain infection with HIV develop only late in infection after immunodeficiency is advanced.

Peripheral nervous system abnormalities in the asymptomatic phase

Nerve conduction studies (Table 2.11) and various quantitative sensory testing devices measuring temperature and vibration thresholds (QST) (Table 2.12) have sought evidence of subclinical neuropathy in asymptomatic seropositive subjects analogous to the subclinical neuro-

Table 2.11 Nerve conduction studies

	Seronegative ($n = 29$)	Asymptomatic seropositive ($n = 55$)	
Sural SAP (μV)	12.0 ± 5.1	9.9 ± 5.2	NS
Post. tib. MCV (m/s)	46.0 ± 4.6	44.0 ± 5.0	NS
Post. tib. F wave (m/s)	52.7 ± 4.5	53.0 ± 5.2	NS

SAP, sensory action potential; post. tib., posterior tibial nerve; MCV, motor conduction velocity.
(Middlesex Hospital data)

pathy in diabetic subjects. Here many studies report a small frequency of abnormal results both for temperature thresholds and sural nerve sensory action potentials (Fuller et al 1991). Winer et al (1992) found neurophysiological signs in seven AIDS and eight asymptomatic patients with clinical signs of neuropathy. In addition, using the Middlesex Hospital thermal testing device (Chapter 15), he found abnormal thresholds in 14 out of 15 of the neuropathic patients and in 10 subjects with no clinical abnormality. Gastaut et al (1989) also reported neurophysiological signs of a predominantly subclinical sensory neuropathy in 13 out of 18 asymptomatic seropositive subjects, though no controls were studied and the results depend on the use of 'norms'. The data from the Middlesex Hospital cohort (unpublished) reveal subtle signs of a sensory neuropathy in some as yet neurologically asymptomatic patients with AIDS. The most frequently abnormal measurements are the amplitude of the sural sensory action potential, and thermal thresholds. It is unclear whether these abnormal results are in fact related to HIV infec-

Table 2.12 Quantitative sensory testing

	Seronegative (n)	Asymptomatic seropositive (n)	
Thermal threshold			
Warm	1.3 ± 1.8 (18)	2.2 ± 2.6 (23)	NS
Cold	0.44 ± 0.38 (19)	0.39 ± 0.31 (23)	NS
Vibration threshold			
Foot	7.0 ± 2.9 (27)	8 ± 4 (55)	

(Middlesex Hospital data)

tion, or might stem from other peripheral nerve insults common to people at risk for HIV infection particularly alcohol and other toxins.

MANAGEMENT PLAN

Acute neurological illness in a patient at risk for HIV infection may prove to be associated with seroconversion. The suspicion would be increased by a pleocytosis in the CSF. If antibodies to HIV are negative, antigen should be sought, and p24 serology repeated serially. These illnesses are self-limiting, but antiviral treatment should be given in the short term. During asymptomatic HIV infection, polymyositis, demyelinating neuropathy, an MS-like illness and a meningitic illness with cranial nerve palsies may be seen. Steroids are appropriate for a florid myositis or MS, plasmapheresis for demyelinating neuropathy, and antiviral treatment for meningitis. The existence of subclinical involvement of the nervous system is controversial and unlikely to cause practical problems. The opportunity should be taken to identify the patient's antibody status against *Toxoplasma*, and to consider prophylaxis when the CD4 count falls. It may in the future prove valuable to screen for JC virus infection in circulating lymphocytes.

REFERENCES

Arday D R, Brundage J F, Gardner L I, et al. The effect of human immunodeficiency virus type 1 antibody status on military applicant aptitude test scores. Am J Epidemiol 1991; 133; 1210–1219

Berger J R, Sheramata W A, Resnick L, et al. Multiple sclerosis like illness occurring with human immunodeficiency virus infection. Neurology 1989; 39: 324–329

Berger J R, Tornatore C, Major E O, et al. Relapsing and remitting human immunodeficiency virus associated leukoencephalomyelopathy. Ann Neurol 1992; 31: 34–38

Bornstein R A, Nasrallah H A, Para M F, et al. Neuropsychological performance in symptomatic and asymptomatic HIV infection. AIDS 1993; 7: 519–524

Brown F O, Sesel J. Neuropsychological impairment in South African HIV patients: preliminary prevalence data. VIIIth Int Conf AIDS, Amsterdam 1992; POB 3553 (abstr)

Calabrese L H, Estes M, Yen-Lieberman B, et al. Systemic vasculitis in association with human immunodeficiency virus infection. Arthritis Rheum 1989; 32: 569–576

Carne C A, Stibe C, Bronkhurst A, et al. Subclinical neurological and neuropsychological effect of infection with HIV. Genitourin Med 1989; 65: 151–156

Clifford D B, Jacoby R G, Miller J P, et al. Neuropsychometric performance of asymptomatic HIV-infected subjects. AIDS 1990; 4: 767–774

Connolly S, Manji H, McAllister R H, et al. Long-latency event-related potentials in asymptomatic HIV-1 infection. Ann Neurol 1994; 35: 189–196

Cooper D A, Gold J, Maclean P, et al. Acute AIDS retrovirus infection: definition of a clinical illness associated with seroconversion. Lancet 1985; i: 537–540

Cornblath D R, McArthur J C, Kennedy P G, et al. Inflammatory demyelinating peripheral neuropathies associated with human T-cell lymphotropic virus type III infection. Ann Neurol 1987; 21: 32–40

Davis L E, Hjelle B L, Miller V E, et al. Early viral brain invasion in iatrogenic immunodeficiency virus infection. Neurology 1992; 42: 1736–1739

Denning D W, Anderson J, Rudge P, Smith H. Acute myelopathy associated with primary infection with human immunodeficiency virus. Br Med J 1987; 294: 143–144

Elder G, Dalakas M, Pezeshkpour G, Sever J. Ataxic neuropathy due to ganglioneuritis after probable acute human immunodeficiency virus infection. Lancet 1986; ii: 1275–1276

Embretson J, Zupancic M, Ribas J L, et al. Massive covert infection of helper T-lymphocytes and macrophages by HIV during the incubation period of AIDS. Nature 1993; 362: 359–362

Farnarier G, Somma-Mauvais H. Multimodal evoked potentials in HIV infected patients. EEG Clin Neurophysiol 1990; suppl 41: 355–369

Fitzgibbon M L, Cella D F, Munfleet G, et al. Motor slowing in asymptomatic HIV infection. Percept Mot Skills 1989; 68: 1331–1338

Fox R, Eldred L J, Fuchs E J, et al. Clinical manifestations of acute infection with human immunodeficiency virus in a cohort of gay men. AIDS 1989; 1: 35–38

Fuller G N, Jacobs J M, Guiloff R J. Subclinical peripheral nerve involvement in AIDS: an electrophysiological and pathological study. J Neurol Neurosurg Psychiatr 1991; 54: 318–324

Gastaut J L, Bolgert F, Brunet D, et al. Early intellectual impairment in HIV seropositive patients. A longitudinal study (abstract). Neurol Neuropsychol Complications HIV Infect 1990; 1: 95

Gastaut J L, Gastaut J A, Pellissier J F, et al. Neuropathies peripheriques au cours de l'infection par le virus de l'immunodefience humaine. Une etude prospective de 56 sujets. Rev Neurol 1989; 145: 451–459

Goethe K E, Mitchell J E, Marshall D W, et al. Neuropsychological and neurological function of human immunodeficiency virus seropositive asymptomatic individuals. Arch Neurol 1989; 46: 129–133

Goodin D S, Aminoff M J, Chernoff D N, et al. Long latency event related potentials in patients infected with human immunodeficiency virus. Ann Neurol 1990; 27: 414–419

Goodwin G M, Chiswick A, Egan V, et al. The Edinburgh cohort of HIV-positive drug users: auditory event-related potentials show progressive slowing in patients with Centre for Disease Control stage IV disease. AIDS 1990; 4: 1243–1250

Grant I, Hampton Atkinson J, Kesselink J R, et al. Evidence of early central nervous system involvement in the acquired immunodeficiency syndrome (AIDS) and other human immunodeficiency. Ann Intern Med 1987; 107: 828–836

Gray F, Chimelli L, Mohr M, et al. Fulminating multiple sclerosis-like leukoencephalopathy revealing human immunodeficiency virus infection. Neurology 1991; 41: 105–109

Gray F, Gherardi R, Lescs M C, et al. Early brain changes in HIV infection: neuropathologic study of 11 HIV-seropositive, non-AIDS asymptomatic cases (abstr). Neuroscience of HIV infection: Basic and Clinical Frontiers. Clin Neuropathol 1993; 12 (Suppl 1): S11

Griffin D E, McArthur J C, Cornblath D R. Soluble interleukin-2 receptor and soluble CD8 in serum and cerebrospinal fluid during human immunodeficiency virus-associated neurologic disease. J Neuroimmunol 1990; 28: 97–109

Helmstaedter C, Riedel R, Marzhauser S T, et al. Reduced vigilance and verbal memory deficits in psychometric evaluation of HIV-positive hemophiliacs (abstract). Neurology 1988; 38 (suppl 1): 298

Helmstaedter C, Hartmann A, Niese C, et al. Stage-independence and individual outcome of neuro-cognitive deficits in HIV. A follow-up study of 62 HIV-positive hemophilic patients. Nervenarzt 1992; 63: 88–94

Hollander H, Stringari S. Human immunodeficiency virus-associated meningitis. Clinical course and correlations. Am J Med 1987; 83: 813–816

Jabbai B, Coats M, Salazar A, et al. Longitudinal study of EEG and evoked potentials in neurologically asymptomatic HIV infected subjects. EEG Clin Neurophysiol 1993; 86: 145–151

Janssen R S, Saykin A J, Cannon L, et al. Neurological and neuropsychological manifestations of HIV-1 infection: association with AIDS-related complex but not asymptomatic HIV-1 infection. Ann Neurol 1989; 26: 592–600

Jernigan T L, Archibald S, Hesselink J R, et al. Magnetic resonance imaging morphometric analysis of cerebral volume loss in human immunodeficiency virus infection. Arch Neurol 1993; 50: 250–255

Karlsen N R, Reinvang I, Froland S S. A follow-up study of neurophysiological function in asymptomatic HIV-infected patients. Acta Neurol Scand 1993; 87: 83–87

Krikorian R, Wrobel A J, Meinecke C, et al. Cognitive deficits associated with human immunodeficiency virus encephalopathy. J Neuropsychiatry Clin Neurosci 1990; 2: 246–260

Lunn S, Skydsbjerg M, Schulsinger H, et al. A preliminary report on the neuropsychologic sequelae of human immunodeficiency virus. Arch Gen Psychiatr 1991; 48: 139–142

Mahe A, Bruet A, Chabin E, Fendler J-P. Acute rhabdomyolysis coincident with primary HIV-1 infection. Lancet 1989; ii: 1454–1455

McAllister R H, Herns M V, Harrison M J G, et al. Neurological and neuropsychological performance in HIV seropositive men without symptoms. J Neurol Neurosurg Psychiatr 1992; 55: 143–148

McArthur J C, Neurologic manifestations of AIDS. Medicine (Baltimore) 1987; 66: 407–437

McArthur J C, Cohen B A, Selnes O A, et al. Low prevalence of neurological and neuropsychological abnormalities in otherwise healthy HIV-1 infected individuals: results from the Multicenter AIDS Cohort Study. Ann Neurol 1989; 26: 601–611

McArthur J C, Kumar A J, Johnson D W, et al. Incidental white matter hyperintensities on magnetic resonance imaging in HIV-1 infection. Multicenter AIDS Cohort Study. J Acquired Immunodeficiency Syndromes 1990; 3: 252–259

Miller E N, Satz P, Visscher B. Computerized and conventional neuropsychological assessment of HIV-1-infected homosexual men. Neurol 1991; 41: 1608–1616

Miller E N, Selnes O A, McArthur M B, et al. Neuropsychological performance in HIV-1 infected homosexual men: the Multicenter AIDS Cohort Study (MACS). Neurology 1990; 40: 197–203

Naber D, Perro C, Schick U, et al. Psychiatrische symptome und neuropsychologische Auffalligkeiten bei HIV-infizierten. Nervenarzt 1989; 60: 80–85

Newman S P, Lunn S, Harrison M J G. Neuropsychological testing of HIV infected subjects in the literature 1994. AIDS, in press

Nuwer M R, Miller E N, Visscher B R, et al. Asymptomatic HIV infection does not cause EEG abnormalities. Neurology 1992; 42: 1214–1219

Pantaleo G, Graziosi C, Demarest J F, et al. HIV infection is active and progressive in lymphoid tissue during the clinically latent stage of disease. Nature 1993; 362: 355–358

Parisi A, Di Perri G, Strosselli M, et al. Usefulness of computerized electroencephalography in diagnosing, staging and monitoring AIDS-dementia complex. AIDS 1989; 3: 209–213

Perry S, Belsky-Barr D, Barr W B, Jacobsberg L. Neuropsychological function in physically asymptomatic, HIV seropositive men. J Neuropsychiatr 1989; 1: 296–303

Portegies P, Brew B J. Update on HIV-related neurological illness. AIDS 1991; S5 (suppl): S211–S217

Poutiainen E, Iivanainen M, Elovaara I, et al. Cognitive changes as early signs of HIV infection. Acta Neurol Scand 1988; 78: 49–52

Robertson K R, Wilkins J, Robertson W, Hall C D. Neuropsychological changes in HIV seropositive subjects over time; one and two year follow-up (abstract). Neurosci HIV Infect: Basic Clin Frontiers 1992; 1: 129

Royal W, Updike M, Selnes O A, et al. HIV-1 infection and nervous system abnormalities among a cohort of intravenous drug users. Neurology 1991; 41: 1905–1910

Sande M A, Volberding P A. The medical management of AIDS. Philadelphia: W B Saunders, 1988

Saykin A J, Janssen R S, Sprehn G C, et al. Neuropsychological dysfunction in HIV-infection: characterization in a lymphadenopathy cohort. J Clin Neuropsychol 1988; 10: 82–95

Saykin A J, Janssen R S, Sprehn G C, et al. Longitudinal evaluation of neuropsychological function in homosexual men with HIV infection: 18-month follow-up. J Neuropsychiatr 1991; 3: 286–298

Scaravilli F, Sinclair E, Gray F, Ciardi A. PCR detection of HIV proviral DNA in the brain of asymptomatic HIV-positive patients; correlation with morphological changes. Clin Neuropathol 1993; 12: S13 (abstr)

Selnes O A, Miller E, McArthur J C, et al. HIV-1 infection: no evidence of cognitive decline during the asymptomatic stages. Neurology 1990; 40: 204–208

Selnes O A, McArthur J C, Royal W, et al. HIV-1 infection and intravenous drug use: longitudinal neuropsychological evaluation of asymptomatic subjects. Neurology 1992a; 42: 1924–1930

Selnes O A, Updike M, Nance-Sproson T, et al. Long-term neurophysiological follow-up of HIV-infected intravenous drug users (abstract). Neurosci HIV Infect: Basic Clin Frontiers 1992b; 1: 61 (abstr)

Selnes O A, McArthur J C, Concha M, et al. Neurocognitive abnormalities with progression to AIDS: association with low CD4+ levels. VIII Int Conf AIDS/STD 1992c (abstr)

Smith T, Jacobsen J, Gaub J, et al. Clinical and electrophysiological studies of human immunodeficiency virus-seropositive men without AIDS. Ann Neurol 1988; 23: 295–297

Tindall B, Barker S, Donovan B, et al. Characterization of the acute clinical illness associated with human immunodeficiency virus infection. Arch Intern Med 1988; 148: 945–949

Tross S, Price R W, Navia B, et al. Neuropsychological characterisation of the AIDS dementia complex. AIDS 1988; 2: 81–88

Vendrall J, Heredia C, Pujol M, et al. Guillain-Barré syndrome associated with seroconversion for anti-HTLV-III. Neurology 1986; 37: 544

Whitt J K, Hooper S R, Tennison M B, et al. Neuropsychologic functioning of human immunodeficiency virus-infected children with hemophilia. J Pediatr 1993; 122: 52–59

Wilkie F L, Eisdorfer C, Morgan R, Loewenstein D A, Szapoecznik J. Cognition in early immunodeficiency virus infection. Arch Neurol 1990; 47: 433–440

Winer J B, Bang B, Clarke J R, et al. A study of neuropathy in HIV infection. Q J Med 1992; 83: 473–488

Wolkinsky S M, Rinaldo C R, Kwok S, et al. Human immunodeficiency virus type 1 (HIV-1) infection a median of 18 months before a diagnostic western blot. Evidence from a cohort of homosexual men. Ann Intern Med 1989; 111: 961–972

World Health Organization. Report on the consultation on the neuropsychiatric aspects of HIV infection. Geneva: WHO, 1988

3. HIV-associated dementia complex

INTRODUCTION

In the early days of the AIDS epidemic in the USA, isolated reports appeared of neurological complications of what was then called the 'gay-related immunosuppressed disease' or 'GRID'. Horowitz et al (1982) and Britton et al (1982) described cases of encephalopathy, including some with an organic psychosis, which they attributed to cytomegalovirus (CMV) encephalitis. In the first authoritative review, Snider et al (1983) described 18 patients with an encephalitic illness characterized by the development of cognitive changes accompanied by malaise, lethargy, loss of libido and social withdrawal. Most progressed to severe dementia with confusion, incontinence, paraparesis and coma. These patients too were thought to have a form of CMV encephalitis. It soon became recognized that this was a common form of neurological morbidity in AIDS, adding to the impact of the central nervous system (CNS) opportunistic processes such as cryptococcal meningitis, toxoplasmosis, progressive multifocal leucoencephalopathy (PML) or cerebral lymphoma.

TERMINOLOGY AND DEFINITIONS

HIV dementia was originally termed 'subacute encephalitis' (Snider et al 1983). Later, Navia and Price first used the term 'AIDS dementia complex' (Navia et al 1986a, b). This phrase indicates the association with *AIDS*, the predominance of cognitive impairment and *dementia* in the syndrome, but the additional term *'complex'* indicates the frequency of motor deficits and myelopathy. The Centers for Disease Control (CDC) added the term 'HIV encephalopathy' to

the list of AIDS-defining illnesses in 1987 (Centers for Disease Control 1987), and in 1991 the American Academy of Neurology AIDS Task Force (Janssen et al 1991) developed terminology and definitional criteria for AIDS dementia, myelopathy, neuropathy and minor forms of cognitive impairment (Table 3.1) to aid research into clinicopathological correlations and in order to monitor natural history and response to antiretroviral therapy. The terms AIDS dementia complex, HIV dementia, HIV encephalopathy and the most recent term, HIV-associated dementia complex, are synonymous. Minor degrees of cognitive and motor impairment that are not sufficient to diagnose dementia are termed 'HIV-associated minor cognitive/motor disorder'. It is still uncertain whether this minor impairment always progresses to frank dementia, whether patients can remain cognitively stable with these minor deficits for years, or whether improvement can occur. The term 'HIV encephalitis' should be reserved for the pathological features of multinucleated giant cell encephalitis with HIV identified in the brain and not used to describe the clinical syndrome. Similarly, while HIV-associated dementia complex can develop concurrently with other HIV-associated neurological disorders such as myelopathy and neuropathy, it appears that these are all discrete disorders with different manifestations, courses and pathogenetic mechanisms. Thus, the concept of classifying all of these disorders together as 'neuroAIDS' is simplistic and erroneous.

These new diagnostic criteria enable the relative contributions of dementia, motor and behavioural abnormalities to be documented. They also highlight the importance of excluding the confounding

Table 3.1 Simplified version of 1991 American Academy of Neurology definitional criteria for HIV neurological CNS disorders

HIV-1-associated dementia complex
Probable (must have *each* of the following):
1. Acquired abnormality in two or more cognitive domains, present for at least 1 month *and* cognitive dysfunction impairing work or activities of daily living, not solely attributable to systemic illness
2. Acquired abnormality in motor function or performance, verified by clinical examination and/or neuropsychological tests *and/or*
   Decline in motivation, emotional control or change in social behaviour
3. Absence of clouding of consciousness, for a period of time sufficient to establish criterion 1
4. No other aetiology present (e.g. medical, psychiatric, substance abuse, CNS infection or neoplasm)

Possible (must have one of the following):
1. Criteria 1, 2 and 3 above are present, but an alternative aetiology is present and the cause of criterion 1 is not certain
2. Criteria 1, 2 and 3 above are present, but the aetiology is not certain due to an incomplete evaluation

HIV-1-associated minor cognitive/motor disorder
Probable (must have *each* of the following):
1. Acquired cognitive/motor/behavioural abnormalities, verified by both a reliable history and neurological/neuropsychological tests
2. Mild impairment of work or activities of daily living
3. Does not meet criteria for HIV dementia or HIV myelopathy
4. No other aetiology present

Possible (must have one of the following):
1. Criteria 1, 2 and 3 above are present, but an alternative aetiology is present and the cause of criterion 1 is not certain
2. Criteria 1, 2 and 3 above are present, but the aetiology of criterion 1 cannot be determined due to incomplete evaluation

Levels of cognitive dysfunction
Mild: Decline in work and home activities noticeable to others, but person not totally dependent on others. Incapable of more complicated daily tasks. Self-care intact
Moderate: Unable to work, including in the home. Requires assistance in activities of daily living
Severe: Unable to perform any activities of daily living without assistance. Requires continual supervision

Levels of myelopathic dysfunction
Mild: Ambulatory, but requires constant unilateral support
Moderate: Requires constant bilateral support for walking
Severe: Unable to walk even with assistance

(After Janssen et al 1991)

effects of depression, psychological stress, drug side-effects, systemic illness and CNS opportunistic processes. Symptoms must be persistent over at least a month to exclude transient metabolic effects. Subtle difficulties with cognitive tasks not interfering with normal independence in daily life are defined separately as HIV-associated minor cognitive/motor disorder. It is not yet known whether such findings predict subsequent development of functionally important deficits and frank dementia. Only prospective studies will define the course of minor cognitive impairment and how frequently it develops into more limiting cognitive dysfunction.

Because of the apparent frequency of mild cognitive impairment occurring in association with other systemic illnesses, as well as AIDS (Gutierrez et al 1993), the 10th revision of the International Classification of Diseases has proposed adding a new category F06.7 – 'mild cognitive disorder' and DSM-4 may add 'mild neurocognitive disorder' defined as a decline in cognitive performance with memory impairment or difficulties in learning or concentration.

EPIDEMIOLOGY

Reports of the prevalence of dementia in HIV infection have varied from 7 to 66% depending on the referral population studied and the selection criteria used. Navia and Price, looking at a retrospective autopsied group, found 66% to have been demented. McArthur (1987) described dementia in 16% from a neurological referral population consisting predominantly of individuals with advanced HIV infection, and community-based estimates are of the order of 7–15% (Levy et al 1985). In a multicultural study of neurocognitive disorders in HIV infection organized by the World Health Organization, the prevalence of dementia was 7% overall in six centres in Thailand, Africa, Germany and the USA (Maj et al 1991). The prevalence of HIV dementia was the same (7%) among individuals with AIDS in California (1989–1991) (Reardon et al 1992). Table 3.2 summarizes the current prevalence figures for HIV dementia. It is important to bear in mind that the prevalence of HIV dementia reflects not only the incidence rate but the survival, thus the prevalence of a condition like HIV dementia with a short survival will be lower than for a condition such as Kaposi's sarcoma (KS) with a longer survival.

Table 3.2 Approximate prevalence of HIV dementia

	%
Asymptomatic carriers (CDC A)	<1
First AIDS condition	3
Symptomatic HIV (CDC B)	5–10
Advanced HIV disease (CDC C)	20–30

Although it is uncommon for HIV dementia to develop during the asymptomatic period, HIV dementia can occasionally develop as the initial AIDS-defining event, even in individuals with relatively intact immune systems. Surveillance figures from the CDC have shown a stable incidence rate of about 3% over the last 5 years for HIV dementia as a first AIDS illness (Fig. 3.1). Navia et al (1989) were among the first to recognize this and described 29 patients who developed HIV dementia before other AIDS-defining illnesses, six of whom were asymptomatic at the time of onset of dementia. It is our impression that when HIV dementia develops during the asymptomatic phase it is frequently milder than dementia occurring in patients with advanced immunosuppression, and the course is less rapidly progressive. In patients with HIV dementia followed in the Multicenter AIDS Cohort Study (MACS), those who developed HIV dementia as the first AIDS-defining illness tended to have a lengthy period of cognitive stability followed by a gradual and relatively modest decline in cognitive

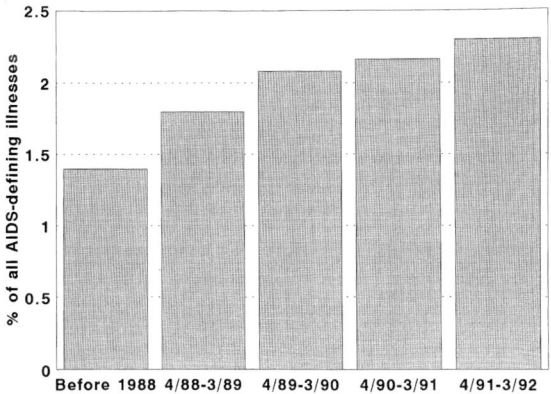

Fig. 3.1 HIV dementia (encephalopathy) as first AIDS-defining illness. (Data from Centers for Disease Control and Prevention 1993.)

performance (McArthur et al unpublished data). By contrast, those who developed dementia as a secondary illness all had a long period of relative cognitive stability, but this was followed by an abrupt, steep decline in cognitive performance occurring an average of 15 months after the initial AIDS-defining illness (Fig. 3.2). These observations suggest that while HIV dementia can occur before immune suppression, its progression is more rapid in more advanced HIV infection.

While the prevalence of dementia has been reasonably defined, up to now estimates of the incidence of dementia have been lacking, although tremendous efforts have been made in large-scale natural history studies of HIV-infected cohorts. The surveillance figures from the CDC are useful, but provide estimates that only apply to dementia as the *initial* manifestation of AIDS because the CDC reporting system does not usually identify secondary diagnoses occurring after AIDS. These surveillance figures have shown that, in the USA, HIV dementia is reported in about 7% of patients with AIDS, but is only the initial AIDS-defining illness in 2.8% (Fig. 3.1) In 1990, in persons 20–59 years old, the incidence of HIV dementia was 1.9 per 100 000 population (Janssen et al 1992). Reardon et al (1992), in a survey in California, found that dementia was more common among older individuals, gay and bisexual men rather than injection drug users, and was less likely to be diagnosed among Latinos, Haitians and women.

Day et al (1992) estimated an annual incidence of 14% in a small prospective study of 32 subjects with AIDS, and recent incidence data from the MACS have provided more accurate projections for the incidence of HIV dementia after AIDS (McArthur et al 1993). The onset of HIV dementia was uncommon before other AIDS-defining illnesses and developed concurrently in only 3% of AIDS cases. The annual incidence was approximately 7% during the 2 years after AIDS. Anaemia, low body mass index, older age and the description of more constitutional symptoms before onset of AIDS were all predictive of an increased risk for the subsequent development of HIV dementia. The strongest predictor of HIV dementia was anaemia *before* AIDS, an association that did not simply reflect stage of immune

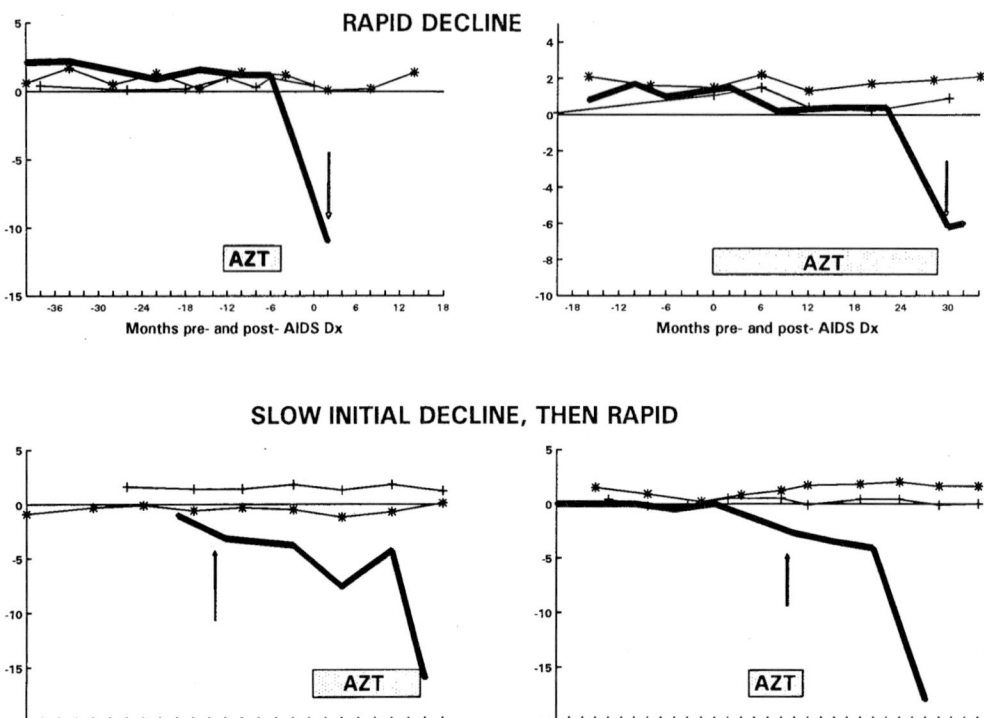

Fig. 3.2   Examples of patterns of longitudinal decline in psychomotor speed in four cases of incident HIV dementia (heavy line). In all cases, dementia was a secondary AIDS diagnosis. Time in months before and after AIDS is shown on the x-axis. Performance on a test of psychomotor speed in z-score units is shown on the y-axis. Performance of seronegative (*) and seropositive controls (+) is also shown (light lines).

deficiency or zidovudine usage (Fig. 3.3). The association may indicate a link between the inhibition of haematopoiesis and the development of neurological disease. The overproduction of cytokines by chronic activation of macrophages may play an important role both in myelosuppression (Fuchs et al 1991b) and in the pathogenesis of HIV dementia (Price and Brew 1988, Fuchs et al 1991a, Lipton 1991, Matsuyama et al 1991, Merrill and Chen 1991). The fact that cytokines can induce weight loss and other constitutional effects is also interesting because of the association noted in this study between dementia, low weight and increased constitutional symptoms before AIDS.

As survival times after AIDS have increased with improvements in antiretroviral treatments (Friedman et al 1991, Moore et al 1991, Piette et al 1991, Graham et al 1992) and prophylaxis of opportunistic infections has improved, some have

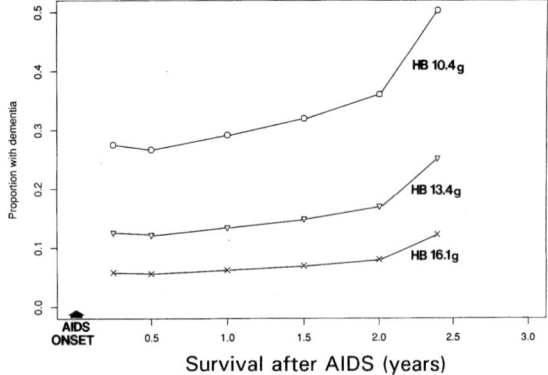

Fig. 3.3   Probability of developing HIV dementia stratified by haemoglobin level 1–6 months prior to AIDS onset, and post-AIDS survival time. Haemoglobin levels shown represent 10.4 g/dl (5th percentile, O), 13.4 g/dl (50th percentile, V) and 16.1 g/dl (95th percentile, X). (Reproduced from McArthur et al 1993.)

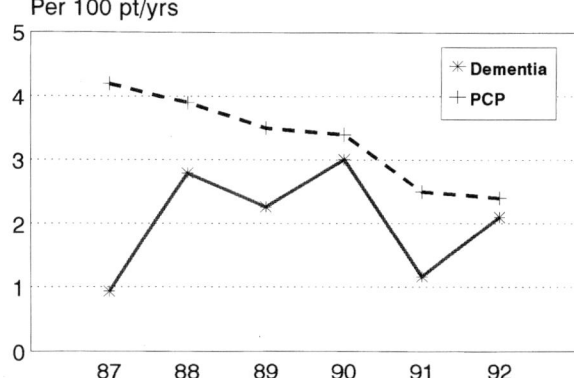

Fig. 3.4 Crude incidence rates for HIV dementia in the Multicentre AIDS Cohort Study compared with *Pneumocystis carinii* pneumonia (PCP).

suggested that the incidence of neurological disorders will increase. For dementia, the widespread and earlier use of zidovudine was initially thought to have reduced the incidence of HIV dementia with an encouraging and dramatic fall in the incidence of HIV dementia after AIDS from about 53% before zidovudine was available to 10% after its initiation (Portegies et al 1989a). This trend does not appear to have held up with subsequent studies because data from both the CDC and the MACS suggest that the incidence of HIV dementia has stabilized in the last few years (Bacellar et al 1994) (Fig. 3.4). In the MACS prospective study, McArthur et al (1993) found no protective effect from zidovudine therapy started before AIDS. Other reports have suggested that early zidovudine therapy may prevent dementia (Hamilton et al 1992, Nordic Medical Research Councils HIV Therapy Group 1992). The differences are unexplained, but the studies suggesting a 'neuroprotective' effect of antiretroviral therapy all used daily doses of zidovudine of 1000 mg or more while the average daily dose in the MACS was only around 600 mg. Thus the dose of zidovudine may be critical with respect to the prophylactic efficacy for dementia.

CLINICAL FEATURES

The influential pair of papers by Navia et al (1986a, b) led to the concept of an 'AIDS dementia complex', a phrase that stresses the association with *AIDS*, the prominence of *dementia* in the

syndrome, and the co-occurrence or predominance of other neurological signs such as myelopathy – *complex*. They reviewed 70 autopsied patients of whom 46 had been seen by a neurologist and diagnosed as demented in life. However, not all showed marked cognitive impairment. They hypothesized that variable combinations of cognitive impairment, motor disability and behavioural disturbance were all manifestations of the direct effects of the virus in the brain, and were commonly related to encephalitis. In general, the clinical severity of dementia correlated with the density of multinucleated giant cells; however, some demented patients showed few pathological abnormalities. By contrast, not all patients with pathological features of encephalitis had been noted to be cognitively impaired in life, suggesting some discordance between clinical and pathological findings.

In a recent clinical pathological study of prospectively characterized AIDS patients with and without HIV dementia, multinucleated giant cells or diffuse myelin pallor were specific for HIV dementia, being found at autopsy only in those patients with clinically recognized dementia (Glass et al 1993). However, one or both of these pathological changes occurred in only 50% of patients with dementia, suggesting that other pathological or pathophysiological phenomena underlie the clinical features of HIV dementia.

Early symptoms (Table 3.3) of HIV dementia consist of increasing forgetfulness and difficulty with concentration, loss of libido, apathy, inertia and waning interest in work and hobbies, resulting in social withdrawal. These symptoms are non-specific, but when developing after AIDS or in severely immunosuppressed patients should prompt consideration of HIV dementia. In adults, the clinical manifestations of HIV dementia suggest a predominantly subcortical involvement initially (Navia et al 1986a), although considerable variability in presentation has been reported. Symptoms particularly fall into the areas of cognition, behavioural change and motor dysfunction. Patients complain of losing track of conversations and the plots of books and films, and of taking longer to complete more complex daily tasks. Impaired short-term memory causes difficulties with remembering appointments, medications and telephone numbers. Motor complaints include

Table 3.3   Early symptoms of AIDS dementia complex in 44 patients

	No.of patients
Cognitive	29
Motor	20
Forgetfulness	17
Behavioural	17
Apathy, withdrawal	16
Loss of balance	15
Loss of concentration	11
Confusion	10
Leg weakness	9
Slowness of thought	8
Poor handwriting	6
Headache	6
Mood change	5
Seizures	3
Psychosis, etc.	2
Miscellaneous	9

(Reproduced from Navia et al 1986b with permission of Annals of Neurology)

poor handwriting, insecure balance, and a tendency to drop things easily. Driving is affected frequently with a tendency to have accidents even with simple activities like parking. Friends and partners report shifts in personality with apathy and social withdrawal, and blunting of emotional responsiveness. Significant depression, however, is not common, although the blunting of affect often mistakenly suggests it. A small proportion of patients develop agitation or mania as an early feature and the new onset of mania with no previous history should raise the suspicion of an evolving HIV dementia (Lyketsos et al 1993, unpublished study). The psychological response to the diagnosis of HIV infection or the development of AIDS can include anger, agitation, panic or hopelessness and fearful uncertainty as described by patients with cancer (Faulstich 1987). Cognitive symptoms can be features of this state, but do not necessarily reflect an incipient dementia. Reassurance is particularly important in this situation because the fear of dementia can be almost as limiting for some patients as dementia itself. The neuropsychological features of HIV dementia reflect the prominence of subcortical involvement early, characterized by (a) memory loss selective for impaired retrieval, (b) impaired manipulation of acquired knowledge, and (c) a general slowing of psychomotor speed and thought processes (Table 3.4). Five to

Table 3.4   Cognitive domains most affected in HIV dementia

- Psychomotor slowing
- Verbal and visual memory impairment
- Complex sequencing
- Mental flexibility
- Visuo-constructional difficulties

ten per cent of patients develop seizures; however, these are not usually difficult to control or persistent. Myoclonus is not a typical feature, although a non-specific sustension tremor develops in some patients. Drowsiness is not usual and, when prominent or accompanied by headache, usually indicates an opportunistic process.

The differential diagnosis of complaints of poor concentration and of lapses in memory in the early stages of HIV dementia (Table 3.5) includes the effects of bereavement, anxiety, sensitivity to medication, recreational drugs and toxic confusional states, for example, related to the hypoxia of *Pneumocystis carinii* pneumonia (PCP). Certain medications are particularly common causes of cognitive symptoms: tricyclic antidepressants, anxiolytics and hypnotics, narcotic analgesics and muscle relaxants.

Later (Table 3.6) the presence of overt dementia is clear with cognitive difficulties clearly out of

Table 3.5   Differential diagnosis of early HIV-associated dementia complex

- Bereavement
- Depression
- Anxiety
- Alcohol
- Recreational drugs
- Medication
- Metabolic encephalopathy

Table 3.6   Late features of HIV-associated dementia complex

- Global cognitive impairment
- Mutism
- Abulia
- Severe psychomotor retardation
- Reduced insight/denial
- Hallucinations
- Spastic weakness (myelopathy)
- Decorticate posture
- Ataxia
- Myoclonus
- Seizures

proportion to the degree of systemic disease or affective change. Progressive slowing of thought processes with psychomotor retardation becomes prominent. Insight and judgment are affected, short-term memory deteriorates, and in late HIV dementia, denial of cognitive symptoms is typical.

Although the mental state changes are often accompanied by complaints of difficulty walking, tremor and clumsiness, the neurological examina-tion may reveal nothing in early or mild HIV dementia, or merely raise suspicions of non-specific incoordination and slowing, and hyper-reflexia. It has been suggested that subtle signs such as the errors made in a task involving antisaccadic eye movements (Merrill et al 1991), along with slowness in repetitive hand movements and slight unsteadiness of gait, may be the first motor signs accompanying the dementing process,

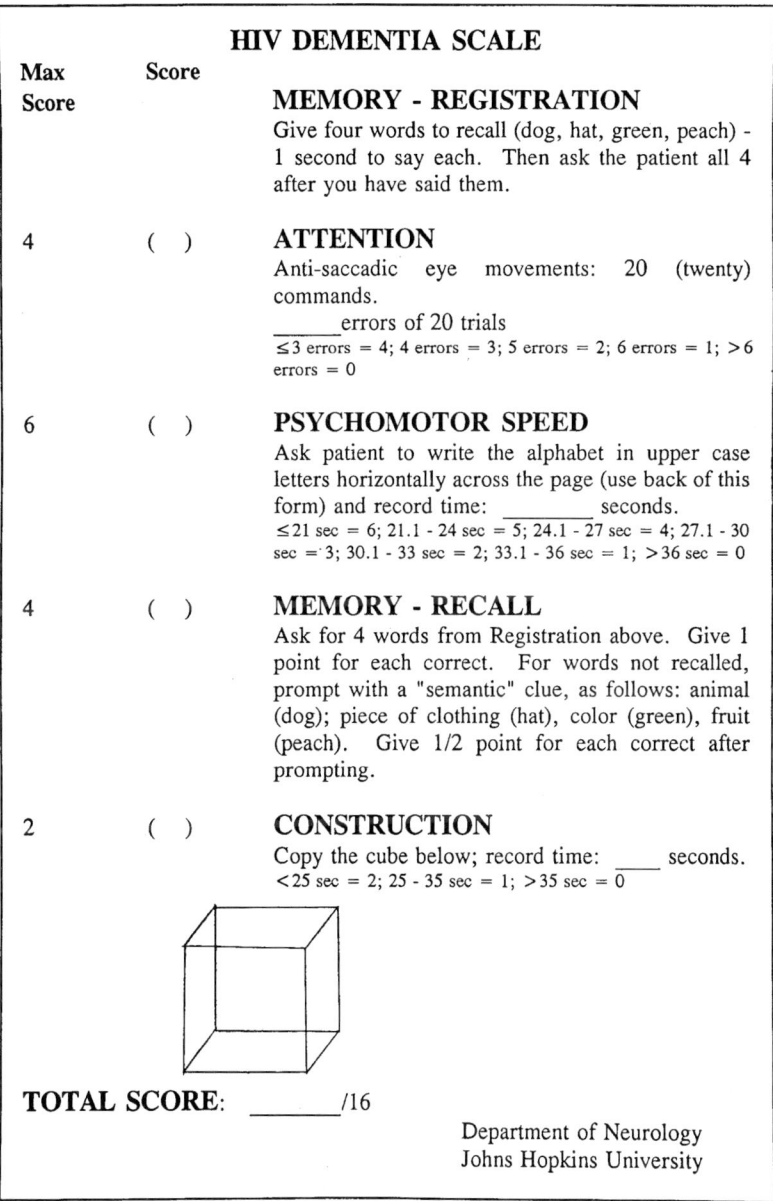

HIV DEMENTIA SCALE

Max Score	Score	
		MEMORY - REGISTRATION Give four words to recall (dog, hat, green, peach) - 1 second to say each. Then ask the patient all 4 after you have said them.
4	( )	**ATTENTION** Anti-saccadic eye movements: 20 (twenty) commands. _____errors of 20 trials ≤3 errors = 4; 4 errors = 3; 5 errors = 2; 6 errors = 1; >6 errors = 0
6	( )	**PSYCHOMOTOR SPEED** Ask patient to write the alphabet in upper case letters horizontally across the page (use back of this form) and record time: _____ seconds. ≤21 sec = 6; 21.1 - 24 sec = 5; 24.1 - 27 sec = 4; 27.1 - 30 sec = 3; 30.1 - 33 sec = 2; 33.1 - 36 sec = 1; >36 sec = 0
4	( )	**MEMORY - RECALL** Ask for 4 words from Registration above. Give 1 point for each correct. For words not recalled, prompt with a "semantic" clue, as follows: animal (dog); piece of clothing (hat), color (green), fruit (peach). Give 1/2 point for each correct after prompting.
2	( )	**CONSTRUCTION** Copy the cube below; record time: ____ seconds. <25 sec = 2; 25 - 35 sec = 1; >35 sec = 0

TOTAL SCORE: _____ /16

Department of Neurology
Johns Hopkins University

Fig. 3.5 HIV Dementia Scale. (From Power et al 1994.)

and are therefore helpful in detecting early dementia. These soft signs are difficult to interpret in patients who are febrile or cachectic. The presence of 'primitive' reflexes such as the pout or snout reflex are not diagnostic of HIV dementia, because these signs can be elicited in normal individuals. Later, tremor, grasp reflexes, hyperreflexia and clonus may be obvious. Terminally, the patient is bedbound, incontinent, abulic and mute, with decorticate posturing. The role of myelopathy in these signs is difficult to disentangle, however. The patients often also have concurrent sensory neuropathy. However, it is unclear whether dementia and neuropathy are truly associated or simply occur together in the later stages of HIV infection. Focal motor or sensory signs implying structural hemisphere disease should suggest a diagnosis other than HIV-associated dementia complex. We have developed a simple scale (the HIV Dementia Scale) (Fig. 3.5), which provides a rapid screening for the memory deficits and psychomotor slowing typical of HIV dementia (Power et al 1994). Table 3.7 lists some of the common CNS opportunistic infections and other medical conditions and appropriate exclusionary tests. Table 3.8 lists clinical features useful in diagnosis of HIV dementia.

Price and Brew have devised a severity scale or staging system for HIV dementia (Table 3.9), which is widely used in both clinical and research arenas. The scale combines the functional impact

Table 3.7 Differential diagnosis in HIV dementia and exclusionary tests

Disorder	Exclusionary test
Toxoplasmosis	MRI/CT
Lymphoma	
CMV encephalitis	
Progressive multifocal leucoencephalopathy	
Cryptococcal/TB meningitis	CSF analysis
	Serum cryptococcal antigen
Neurosyphilis	Serum FTA
Medication side-effects	History
Substance abuse	Toxicology screen
Depression/other psychiatric conditions	Psychiatric evaluation
Thyroid/B_{12} deficiency	Appropriate laboratory tests

CMV, cytomegalovirus; TB, tuberculosis; MRI, magnetic resonance imaging; CT, computed tomography; FTA, fluorescent treponemal antibody.

Table 3.8 Clinical features useful for diagnosis of HIV-1 related dementia

- HIV-1 seropositivity (Western blot confirmation)
- History of *progressive* cognitive/behavioural decline with apathy, memory loss, slowed mental processing
- Neurological examination: diffuse CNS signs including slowed rapid eye/limb movements, hyperreflexia, hypertonia and release signs
- Neuropsychological assessment: progressive deterioration on serial testing in at least two areas including frontal lobe, motor speed and non-verbal memory
- CSF analysis: elevated β_2-microglobulin, non-specific abnormalities of IgG and protein, exclusion of neurosyphilis and cryptococcal meningitis
- Imaging studies: diffuse cerebral atrophy with ill-defined white matter hyperintensities on MRI in the absence of opportunistic processes
- *Absence* of major psychiatric disorder or intoxication
- *Absence* of metabolic derangement, e.g. hypoxia, sepsis
- *Absence* of active CNS opportunistic processes

Table 3.9 HIV-associated Dementia Scale

Dementia severity

Stage 0 (normal):   Normal mental and motor function. Neurological signs are within the normal age-appropriate spectrum
Stage 0.5 (equivocal or subclinical):   Absent, minimal or equivocal symptoms without impairment of work or capacity to perform activities of daily living (ADL). Examination may be normal or mildly abnormal signs may include reflex changes (e.g. generalized increase in deep tendon reflexes with active jaw jerk, snout or glabellar sign) or mildly slowed ocular movements, but without clear slowing of extremity movements or loss of their dexterity or strength
Stage 1 (mild):   Able to perform all but the more demanding aspects of work or ADL but with unequivocal evidence (symptoms or signs including performance on neuropsychological testing) of intellectual or motor impairment. The abnormal motor signs usually include slow or clumsy movements of extremities
Stage 2 (moderate):   Able to perform basic activities of self-care at home but cannot work or maintain more demanding aspects of daily life (e.g. maintain finances, read text more complex than a tabloid newspaper)
Stage 3 (severe):   Major intellectual incapacity (cannot follow news or personal events, cannot sustain complex conversation, considerable slowing of all output) or motor disability
Stage 4 (end stage):   Nearly vegetative. Intellectual and social comprehension and output are at a rudimentary level. Nearly or absolutely mute

Myelopathy severity

Stage 0:   Normal
Stage 1:   Tandem gait may be impaired, but the patient can walk without assistance
Stage 2:   Ambulatory, but may require single prop (e.g. cane)
Stage 3:   Cannot walk unassisted, requiring walker or personal support, usually with slowing and clumsiness of arms as well
Stage 4:   Paraparetic or paraplegic with double incontinence

(After Price & Brew 1988)

of both cerebral and spinal cord dysfunction; however, we have found it more useful to separate out the two areas and grade each separately because myelopathy can present with minimal or no dementia, and vice versa. Thus, in practice, a severely demented patient with only mild myelopathy would be categorized as MSK 3 (dementia), MSK 1 (myelopathy). The sub-clinical stage 0.5 is a stage where neurocognitive deficits may be present but frank dementia is not apparent. 'HIV-associated minor cognitive motor impairment' could be graded in this fashion. This clinical staging system correlates well with performance on psychomotor speed measures and is useful to track progression and response to therapy.

The prognosis of HIV dementia is very poor (Fig. 3.6), averaging 6 months from onset of symptoms to death, usually from secondary complications of the neurological disease. The course has some variability, however, which may depend on the immune state at onset or the effect of antiretroviral therapy. Thus, some patients have a 'typical' progression with worsening neurological deficits over 3–6 months, while others remain only mildy demented and cognitively stable right up until death.

NEUROPSYCHOLOGICAL TESTING IN HIV DEMENTIA

Neuropsychological testing is tremendously useful in the diagnosis and management of HIV dementia and serves as an important adjunct to the neurological evaluation. The principal cognitive domains affected in HIV dementia have been defined by several groups and the most useful tests for diagnosis and following the course of HIV dementia are those that examine psychomotor speed and memory (Tables 3.4 and 3.10) (Tross et al 1988, Van Gorp et al 1989) (also see Chapter 15). The principal neuropsychological abnormalities in HIV dementia include psychomotor slowing, verbal and non-verbal memory,

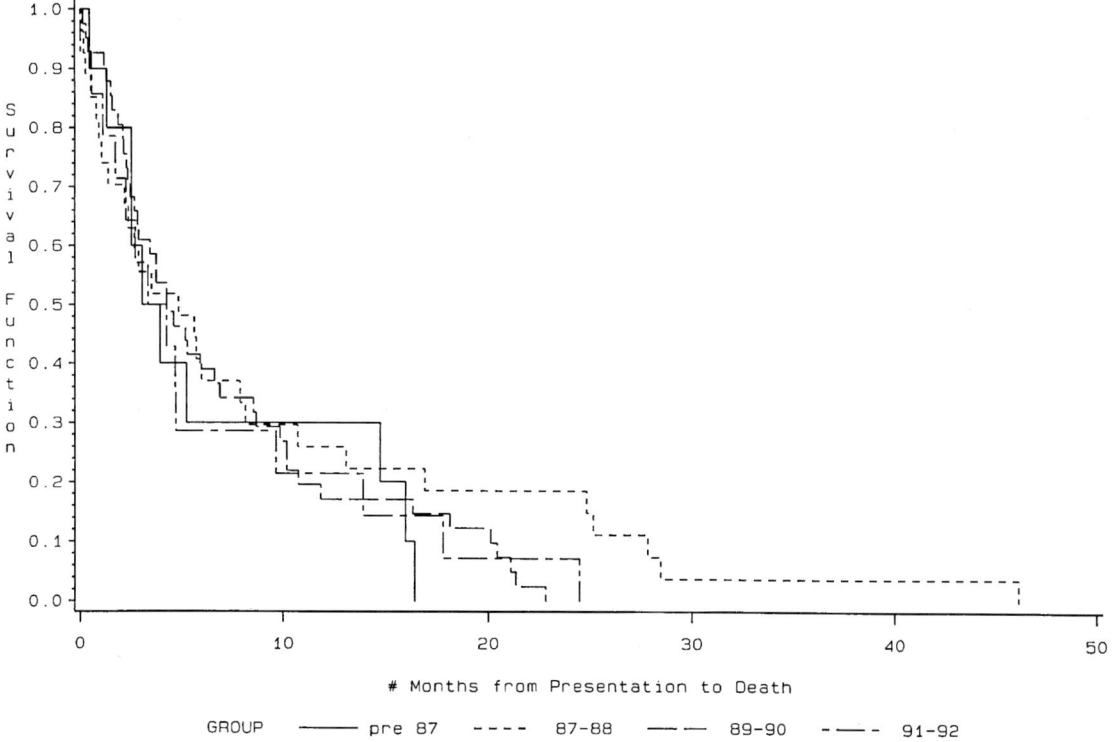

Fig. 3.6 Survival curves for 142 patients with HIV dementia followed at the Johns Hopkins University, stratified by date of diagnosis: 1991/92, 1989/90, 1987/88, pre-1987. Median survival is 4.3 months overall with no significant lengthening of survival over this time period. (Courtesy of Dr L. Nance-Sproson.)

Table 3.10 Neuropsychological battery used in the Multicentre AIDS Cohort Study

Test	Domain
Symbol digit test (paired recall)	Psychomotor speed, attention
Trailmaking Test A and B	Psychomotor speed
Grooved Pegboard	Motor speed
Rey Auditory Verbal Learning Test (immediate/delayed recall)	Verbal memory
Rey Complex Figure (immediate/delayed recall)	Visuo-constructional
Reaction time	Reaction time
Stroop Test	Frontal lobe/executive

Table 3.11 NIMH recommendations: neuropsychological battery

A	Vocabulary; National Adult Reading Test
B	Digit Span; Visual Span
C	Sternberg Search Task; Simple/Choice Reaction Times; Paced Auditory Serial Addition Test
D	California Verbal Learning Test; Working Memory Test; Modified Visual Reproduction Test (WMS)
E	Category Test; Trails Making Test A and B
F	Boston Naming Test; Letter/Category Fluency Test
G	Embedded Figures Test; Roadmap Test; Digit Symbol Substitution
H	Block Design; Tactual Performance
I	Grooved Pegboard; Finger Tapping Test; Grip Strength
J	Diagnostic Interview Schedule (DIS); Hamilton Depression Scale; Stait-Trait Anxiety Scale; Mini-Mental State Examination

(After Butters et al 1990)

difficulties with complex sequencing and mental flexibility, and visuo-constructional impairment. Attention, language, praxis and calculation are usually preserved. These features fit with the pattern of subcortical dementia as encountered in disease such as Huntington's chorea, Parkinson's disease and normal pressure hydrocephalus. Some imaging data support this subcortical involvement with evidence of a correlation between measured atrophy of the caudate nuclei and HIV dementia (Dal Pan et al 1992). Hestad et al (1993) found significant correlation between caudate atrophy as measured by enlargement of the bicaudate ratio (BCR) and impaired performance on several measures of neurocognitive performance, including Grooved Pegboard, Verbal Fluency and Trailmaking Test, suggesting that subcortical damage and particularly caudate region atrophy underlies the subcortical pattern of neuropsychological impairment.

Neuropsychological testing aids the neurological evaluation of suspected HIV dementia by quantifying the severity of cognitive impairment and defining the patterns of involvement. For example, attention, concentration and language are usually not affected in HIV dementia, at least in the early stages, so abnormalities in these areas should suggest other conditions, e.g. anxiety, depression or delirium (Fig. 3.7). Memory impairments, both verbal and non-verbal, and in particular deficits in psychomotor speed are characteristic and are typically more severe than deficits in other cognitive domains. As with other subcortical dementias, there is frequently a discrepancy between recall and recognition memory,

with relative preservation of the latter. These different patterns can be appreciated in Fig. 3.7 showing examples of neuropsychological profiles from patients with HIV dementia, HIV dementia and previous alcohol impairment, and a patient before and after treatment of depression.

It has to be remembered that abnormalities of neuropsychological testing are not necessarily specific, and premorbid conditions, including previous head trauma, learning disability and the effects of systemic illness or substance abuse, need to be considered carefully when interpreting results of neuropsychological testing. Age and education are both critical variables that influence neuropsychological performance independently. It is therefore critical to use appropriate age- and education-specific normative data (Selnes et al 1991a, b, Concha et al 1992, unpublished data).

The National Institute of Mental Health has developed recommendations for a lengthy battery for use in HIV-infected patients (Table 3.11), but in practice this is far too long for most patients to tolerate. Table 3.10 includes the battery used in the MACS, which is a short, sensitive battery that can be completed in 30 minutes, and which tests the major domains affected in HIV dementia. If a shorter battery is necessary, Trailmaking, Grooved Pegboard and Symbol-Digit can be completed in less than 10 minutes.

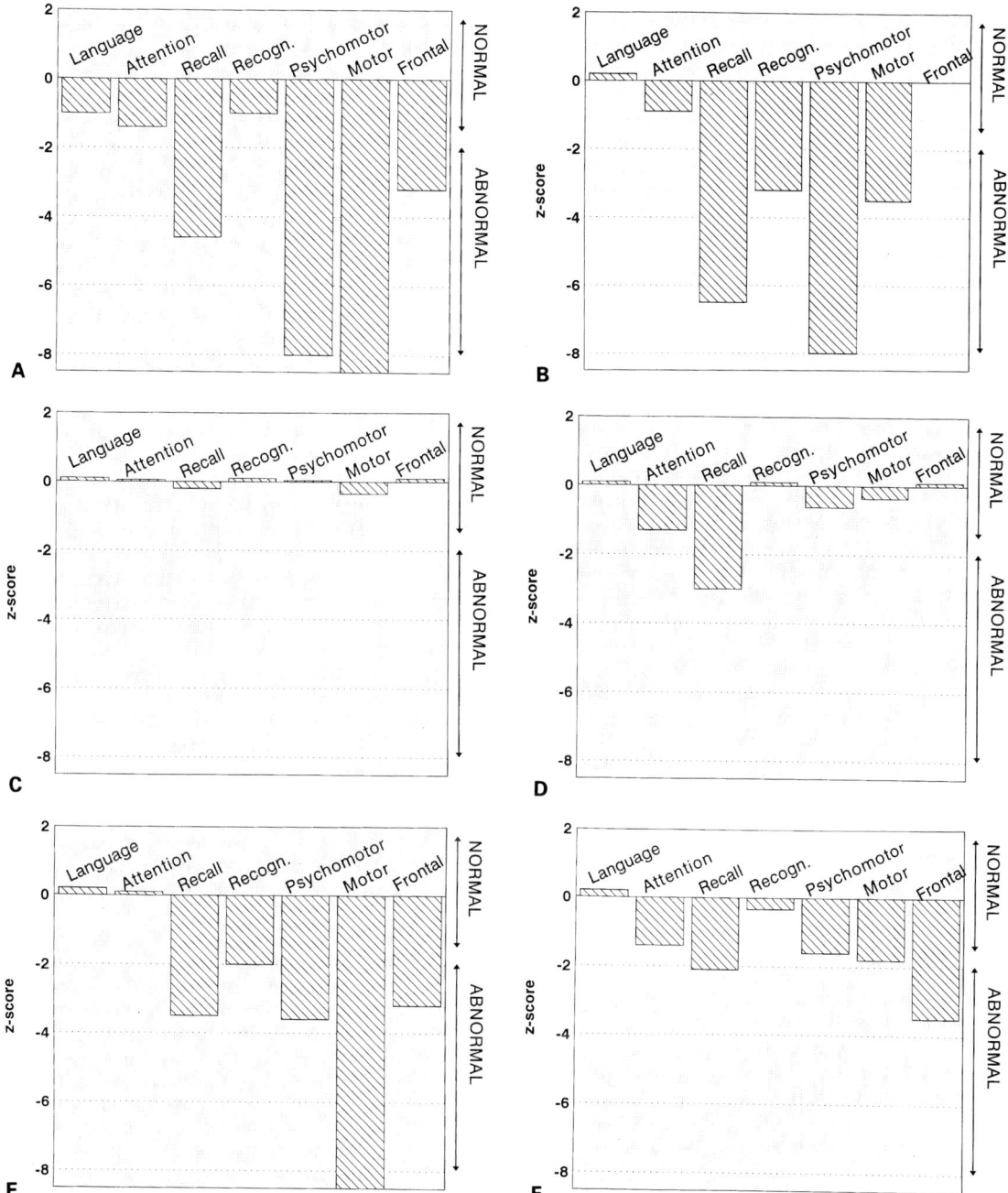

Fig. 3.7 **A** A typical neuropsychological profile from a 53-year-old homosexual man with moderate HIV dementia. Vertical axis indicates Z-score performance standard deviation units (note relatively preserved language, attention and recognition memory, but severely impaired recall memory and tests of psychomotor speed). **B** Neuropsychological profile from a 64-year-old homosexual male with HIV dementia and a history of heavy alcohol use. Note the difference in profiles with greater impairment of recognition memory than in the typical HIV dementia patient and less impairment on Grooved Pegboard. **C, D** Neuropsychological profiles from a patient with cognitive symptoms and major affective disorder before (**C**) and after (**D**) treatment. Note relative impairment of attention and concentration compared with psychomotor performance and improvement in all domains with antidepressant therapy. **E** Profile from a patient with HIV dementia. **F** Profile from a patient with HIV dementia and prominent frontal lobe dysfunction. (Prepared by Dr Ola Selnes.)

DIFFERENTIAL DIAGNOSIS

The diagnostic work-up (Table 3.7) often needs to include neuroimaging to exclude abscesses, PML and lymphomas, and examination of the cerebrospinal fluid (CSF) to exclude opportunistic infections including meningitis and neurosyphilis (Harrison & McAllister 1991). Lumbar puncture is not needed in a typical presentation of HIV without features of meningitis, because cryptococcal meningitis can be excluded by a negative serum cryptococcal antigen and neurosyphilis by a negative serum fluorescent treponemal antibody (FTA). CMV encephalitis should be considered and sought by polymerase chain reaction (PCR) in the CSF in cases of rapid deterioration, especially in the presence of CMV retinitis, hyponatraemia and evidence of periventriculitis (Holland et al 1994). In HIV dementia, the CSF often shows an increase in total protein and immunoglobulin (McArthur 1987), but pleocytosis is uncommon, occurring in 5–10%. Other routine studies do not differ from those of neurologically normal HIV-infected patients at the same stage of immunodeficiency

(see Chapter 15). In mild cases where there may be diagnostic confusion, elevation of CSF β_2-microglobulin can be useful diagnostically to distinguish progressive dementia from other causes of cognitive symptoms (McArthur et al 1992). A CSF β_2-microglobulin above 3.8 mg/l, in the absence of opportunistic infection, has a positive predictive value for dementia of 88% (McArthur et al 1992). Other markers of immune activation such as prostaglandin E_2 (Griffin et al 1993), neopterin (Brew et al 1992) and quinolinic acid levels (Heyes et al 1991) are often elevated.

Electroencephalograms (EEGs) show slowing of dominant frequencies (Fig. 3.8), a sensitive but totally non-specific finding (Parisi et al 1989). However, electroencephalography has not been systematically studied in either the diagnosis or staging of HIV dementia. In mild or moderate dementia, an EEG can be normal in up to 50% of patients (McArthur 1987). The specificity of electroencephalography in differentiating psychiatric disorders from early HIV dementia is unknown, and in general neither standard electroencephalography nor computerized spectral analysis adds much to the management of patients

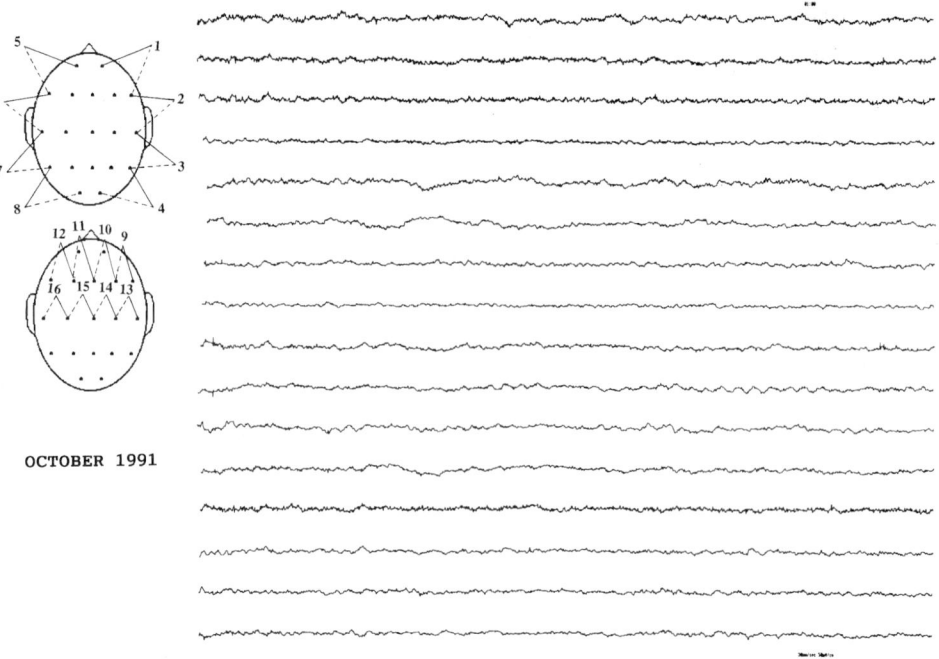

OCTOBER 1991

Fig. 3.8   EEG showing slowing of dominant rhythms in early HIV dementia.

with HIV dementia. Auditory evoked event-related potentials are delayed (Arendt et al 1993), as in other dementing diseases.

Computed tomography (CT) scans usually show atrophy and hypodensity in the white matter and are necessary to exclude rival diagnoses (Elovaara et al 1990). Progression of atrophy often parallels clinical deterioration (Fig. 3.9). Magnetic resonance imaging (MRI) is even more useful in this context (Post et al 1988). It is more sensitive than CT in detection of atrophy (Fig. 3.10) and in showing its progression (Fig. 3.11). It also more readily reveals changes in the deep white matter. These consist of hyperintensity of T2-weighted images (Fig. 3.12) of a patchy, ill-defined nature, which is difficult to detect in early stages, but which evolves to affect the deep white matter in a confluent, symmetrical pattern (Fig. 3.13). These hyperintensities are thought to represent blood–brain barrier perturbation rather than frank

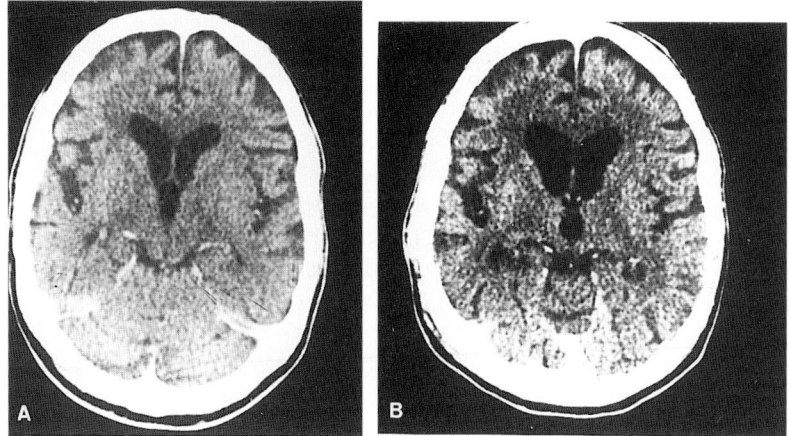

Fig. 3.9 CT scans in HIV dementia. **A** CT scan of 36-year-old intravenous drug user with AIDS-related complex and early HIV dementia. Mild fronto-temporal atrophy and ventricular enlargement are seen. **B** CT scan of same patient 3 months later with advanced dementia. Severe fronto-temporal atrophy and ventriculomegaly are noted with attenuation of the periventricular white matter.

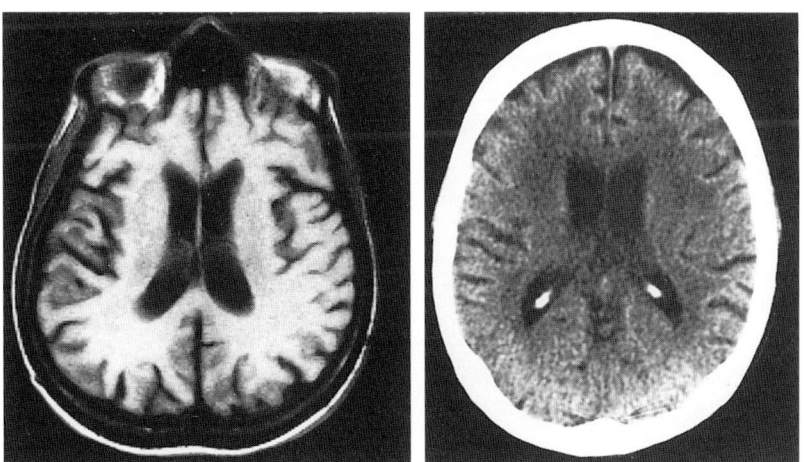

Fig. 3.10 Comparison of T1-weighted MRI scan (left) and CT scan (right) in showing atrophy in HIV dementia. MRI shows central and cortical atrophy, underestimated by CT.

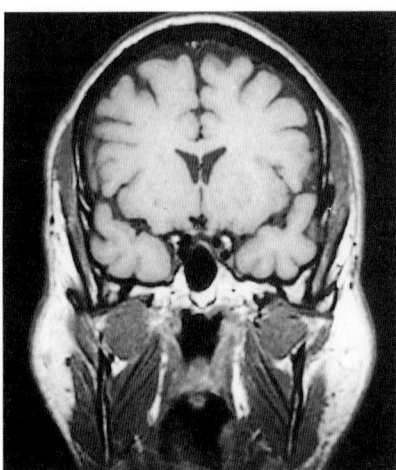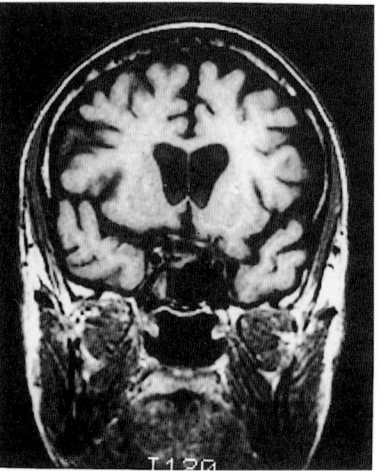

Fig. 3.11   Serial MRI T1-weighted coronal images showing evolution of atrophy in HIV dementia. Note the development of both central and cortical atrophy.

demyelination. Pathological studies have found that even in areas with prominent myelin pallor on luxol-fast blue (LFB) staining from patients with MRI white matter changes, there is no

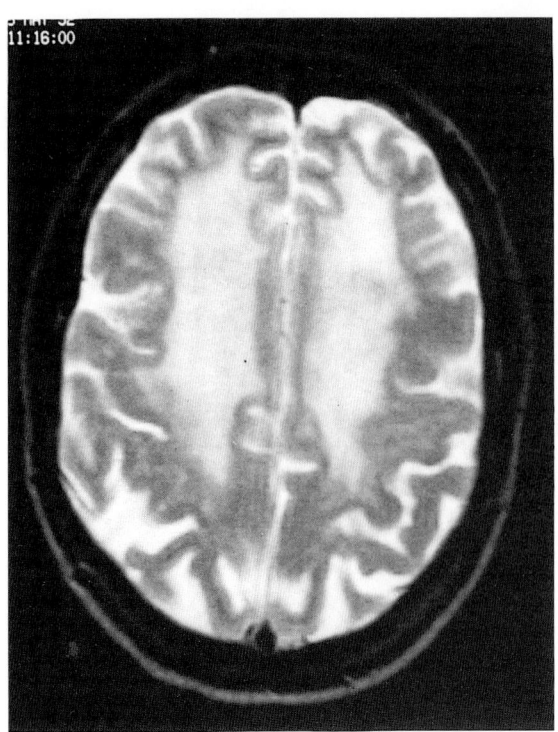

Fig. 3.12   T2-weighted MRI scan showing extensive white matter changes in a patient with HIV dementia.

evidence of myelin basic protein loss or active demyelination (Power et al 1993). Quantitative MRI reveals loss of volume in the region of the caudate (Dal Pan et al 1992) and in other basal ganglia structures (Aylward et al 1993b). There is also reduction in volume in cortical areas (Gelman & Guinto 1992, Aylward et al 1993a), and the overall pattern is one of combined central and cortical atrophy (Fig. 3.14).

Functional imaging has been used to identify CNS changes, including single positron emission computed tomography (SPECT), positron emission tomography (PET) and recently MR spectroscopy (MRS). Both SPECT and PET have been examined in small numbers of individuals with HIV dementia. Using PET, Rottenberg et al (1987) demonstrated subcortical hypermetabolism in the early stage of HIV dementia with later progression to cortical and subcortical hypometabolism. Normalization of PET abnormalities has also been shown with administration of antiretrovirals (Yarchoan et al 1987). With SPECT, abnormalities in cerebral blood flow, shown as patchy areas of hypoperfusion, have been identified both in patients with HIV dementia and in neurologically normal HIV-1 carriers, suggesting that SPECT might be a useful predictive tool (LaFrance et al 1988). Unfortunately, it appears that these findings are non-specific, because some of the changes may be mimicked by

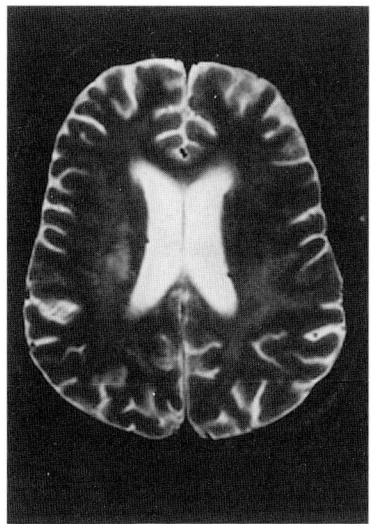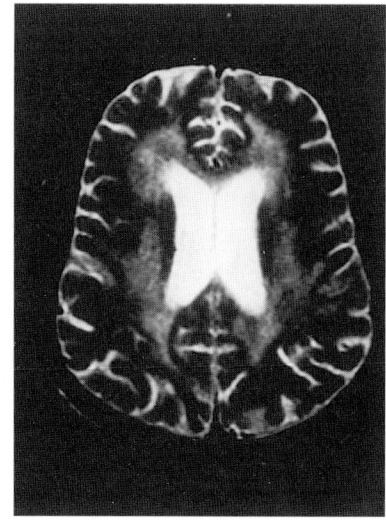

Fig. 3.13   Serial T2-weighted MRI scan revealing evolution of visible white matter changes.

the effects of cocaine (Handelsman et al 1992). MRS shows lower ratios of the neuronal marker *N*-acetyl aspartate (NAA) to choline and creatine

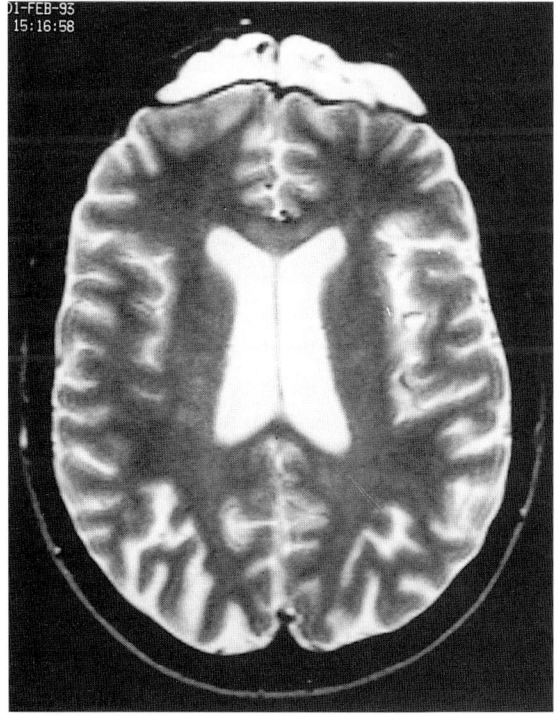

Fig. 3.14   T2 MRI scan showing central and cortical atrophy.

(Fig. 3.15 and Table 3.12) (Meyerhoff et al 1993). Loss of NAA is believed to reflect neuronal loss. There is also a reduction in high energy phosphates (Bottomley et al 1990). Again, however, the clinicopathological studies are few and this area has not been completely elucidated. Functional imaging techniques remain research tools and should not be used for diagnostic purposes at this point.

PATHOLOGY

HIV infection of brain causes distinct neuro-pathological changes termed 'HIV encephalitis' and 'HIV leucoencephalopathy' (Budka et al 1991). Other abnormalities, including astrocytic and microglial proliferation and cortical neuronal loss, have also been found in patients with AIDS and are likely to be related to productive HIV infection in the brain (Gray et al 1988, Ciardi et al 1990, Ketzler et al 1990, Budka et al 1991, Everall et al 1991, Wiley et al 1991b, Masliah et al 1992, Sinclair & Scaravilli 1992, Vazeux et al 1992). The relationship of any of these pathological changes to the clinical features of progressive dementia in AIDS remains somewhat unclear. There have only been a few studies specifically addressing clinical neuropathological correlation in HIV dementia and even fewer in which the

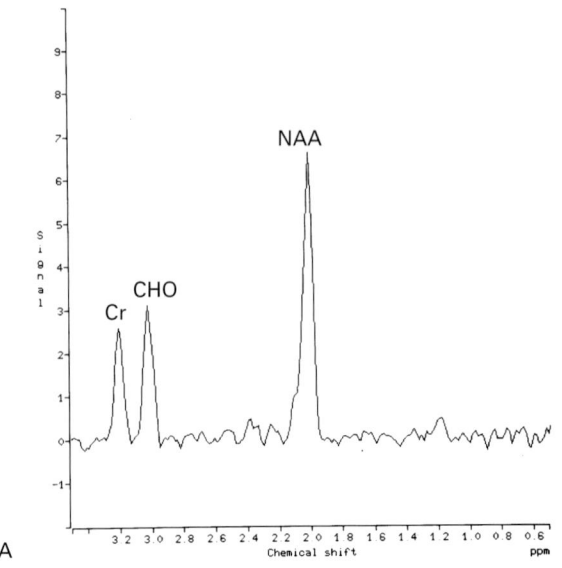
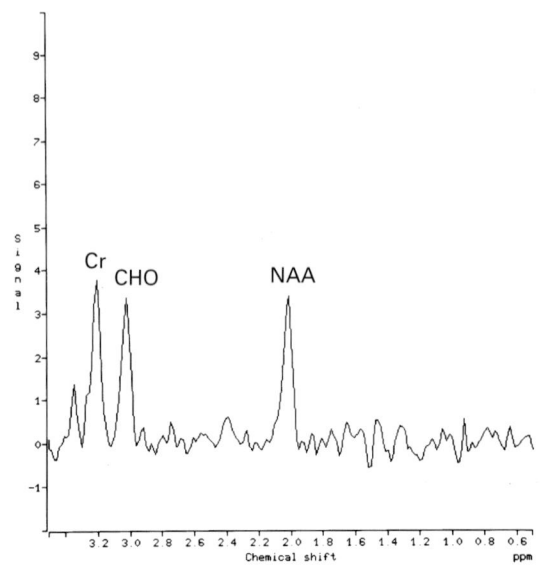

Fig. 3.15 MR spectroscopy from parieto-occipital white matter **A** in a normal with high NAA peak on the right and smaller choline (CHO) and creatine (Cr) peaks on the left and **B** in a patient with HIV dementia and white matter changes on MRI. Note the much lower NAA peak and the choline peak now lower than that of creatine.

Table 3.12 *N*-acetyl aspartate in magnetic resonance spectra (Middlesex Hospital data)

Group	*n*	Ratio
HIV -ve	24	0.55 ± 0.03
HIV +ve	22	0.52 ± 0.04
AIDS	26	$0.49 \pm 0.05\star$

$\star$ $p < 0.004$.
NAA expressed as ratio of NAA to NAA + creatine + choline.

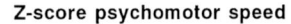
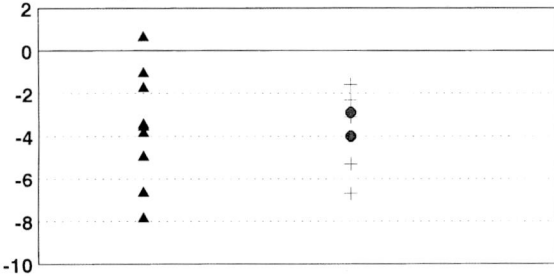

Fig. 3.16 Lack of correlation between neuropsychological abnormalities and HIV-specific neuropathological change in HIV dementia. Severity of neuropsychological deficit (vertical axis) does not correlate well with the presence of diffuse myelin pallor (DMP) (+), multinucleate giant cells and DMP (●), or the absence of either neuropathological change (▲). (Courtesy of Drs Ola Selnes and Jonathan Glass.)

clinical diagnosis of dementia was based on prospective patient identification. Further attention needs to be given to prospective studies of clinical pathological correlation to define the clinical features and course of the different pathological entities that have been defined. Some preliminary data (Fig. 3.16) suggest that the severity of neuropsychological deficit does not correlate well with the presence of multinucleated giant cells, or diffuse myelin pallor, or their combined presence.

Macroscopic changes are rare and gross examination tends to underestimate the degree of atrophy even in cases with prominent radiological atrophy. The white matter may appear softened with a grey discolouration of the centrum semi-

ovale. Gelman and Guinto (1992) measured the CSF spaces in 64 autopsied patients with AIDS compared with age-matched controls; 58% of the AIDS patients had ventricular expansion particularly in the frontal and temporal lobes. Central atrophy was greater than cortical, and those with atrophy had more evidence of encephalitis (28% multinucleated giant cells cf. 7%) and microglial nodules (53% cf. 25%), though white matter

Table 3.13   Recommended neuropathology terminology for HIV- associated CNS disease

New name	Old name	Definition
HIV encephalitis	Giant cell encephalitis, multinucleated cell encephalitis, subacute encephalitis	Multiple disseminated foci of microglia, macrophages and multinucleated giant cells (MNGCs). If MNGCs not present, HIV antigen or nucleic acids demonstrated by immunocytochemistry or in situ hybridization
HIV leucoencephalopathy	Diffuse myelin pallor, progressive diffuse leucoencephalopathy	Diffuse damage to white matter with myelin loss, reactive astrogliosis, macrophages and MNGCs or detectable HIV antigen or nucleic acids
Diffuse poliodystrophy	Subacute encephalitis	Diffuse reactive astrogliosis and microglial activation involving cerebral grey matter. Note: This term designates diffuse pathology of cortical and subcortical grey matter structures which may underlie neuronal loss, or changes in synaptic or dendritic anatomy
Vacuolar myelopathy		Multiple areas of spinal cord involved by vacuolar myelin changes with intravacuole macrophages

(After Budka et al 1991)

changes were not so closely linked (66% with atrophy, 54% without). A spectrum of microscopic changes has been described (Budka et al 1991), and was recently categorized by an international working group (Table 3.13) (see also Appendix 3).

Productive HIV infection has been detected in macrophages and microglia by a number of techniques including immunostaining, in situ hybridization, electron microscopy and in situ PCR (Shaw et al 1985, Gabuzda et al 1986, Koenig et al 1986, Wiley et al 1986, Pumarola-Sune et al 1987, Budka 1990). Neither oligodendrocytes nor neurons have shown evidence for expression of HIV transcripts, nor has proviral DNA been demonstrated in these cells. Epstein and Gendelman (1993) has recently demonstrated nef viral proteins in astrocytes from paediatric brains suggesting that cells other than macrophages and microglia may be infected. Why only nef proteins are identifiable and how frequently this occurs is unknown.

HIV encephalitis

HIV encephalitis occurs with or without leucoencephalopathy in 15–40% of AIDS brains (Budka et al 1991). In this pathological entity, there are multiple microgranulomatous foci of loosely aggregated microglia and macrophages, including multinucleated giant cells (Fig. 3.17).

If multinucleated giant cells are not seen, to meet the criteria, HIV must be demonstrated by immunostaining or in situ hybridization (Fig. 3.18). These changes tend to be perivascular in distribution and more prominent in the subcortical white matter and basal ganglia (Kure et al 1990). The most characteristic feature is the multinucleated giant cell, which was first described by Sharer et al (1986). Multinucleated giant cells (Fig. 3.19) typically contain up to 20 nuclei usually arranged around the periphery of the cell and represent syncytia of fused HIV-infected mononuclear cells. They vary in size and appearance between larger macrophage-like cells

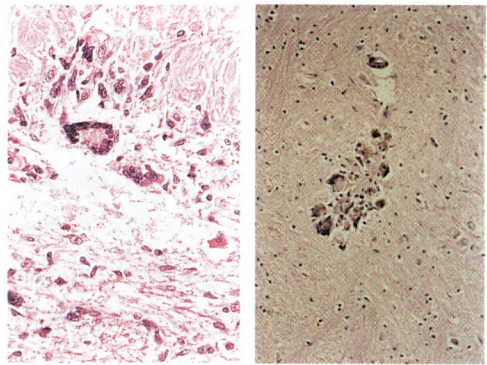

Fig. 3.17   Multinucleated giant cells in a focus of HIV encephalitis (left) and perivascular macrophage inflammation (right).

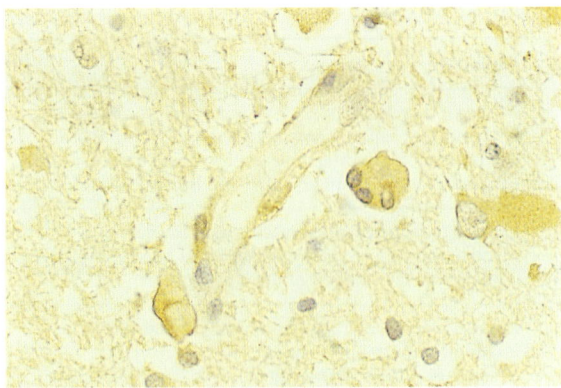

Fig. 3.18   Multinucleated giant cell stained with gp41 adjacent to a perivascular space in a case of encephalitis.

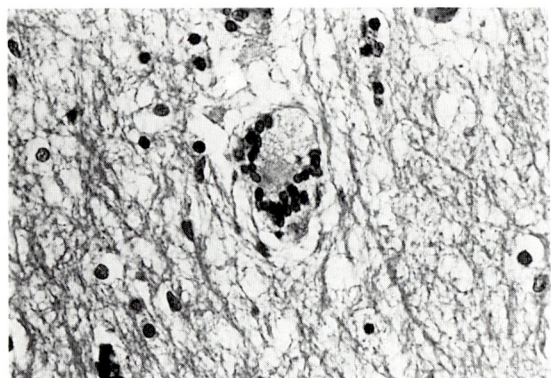

Fig. 3.19   Multinucleated giant cell from a patient with HIV encephalitis.

Table 3.14   Correlation between encephalitis and dementia complex

Histology	Clinical findings		
	Severe dementia	Moderate dementia	None
MNGCs present	10	7	0
MNGCs absent	1	8	11

MNGCs, multinucleated giant cells.
(Reproduced from Rosenblum 1990)

mostly found in the basal ganglia, subthalamic nucleus, substantia nigra, dentate nucleus and white matter (Kure et al 1990). However, using PCR techniques, HIV transcripts were more abundant in subcortical white matter than basal ganglia, cortex or deep white matter (Wesselingh et al 1993). In contrast to HIV encephalitis, CMV encephalitis does not have multinucleated giant cells and the microglial nodules are more compact and contain characteristic inclusion bodies. Both histological pictures may coincide, of course, and Wiley and Nelson (1988) found a co-occurrence of 33% in one series.

HIV leucoencephalopathy

HIV leucoencephalopathy occurred in 38% of Budka's series (Budka et al 1991) and in one-third of patients clinically diagnosed with HIV dementia (Glass et al 1993). This pathological condition is characterized by diffuse damage to the white matter with myelin pallor (diffuse myelin pallor), astrocytosis, activated macrophages (ingesting myelin debris) and some multinucleated cells. There is microglial proliferation and individual microglia show extended processes suggesting activation. As discussed above, recent studies have shown no active demyelinative process in brains with diffuse myelin pallor, and suggest that in at least some cases, myelin pallor reflects blood–brain barrier perturbation. HIV leucoencephalopathy causes symmetrical white matter pallor on whole brain slices in both the hemispheres and cerebellum. This process tends to spare the optic pathways, internal capsule, cerebellar peduncles and corpus callosum. Navia et al (1986a, b) found diffuse myelin pallor in all

and smaller microglia-like cells. With electron microscopy these cells can be seen to be shedding virions and to contain virions with intracytoplasmic vacuoles. This 'giant-cell' encephalitis affects the white matter and deep grey matter principally, but the cortical grey matter is affected, albeit to a much milder degree. Rosenblum (1990) has shown a correlation between the severity of dementia and multinucleated giant cells (Table 3.14). Widespread necrosis is rare, and there is some mild inflammatory response and prominent reactive astrocytosis. In HIV encephalitis, HIV is detectable by immunostaining for gp41 or p24 antigens, by in situ hybridization, and by PCR. The topographic localization of productive infection is still being explored. With immunostaining, HIV antigen is

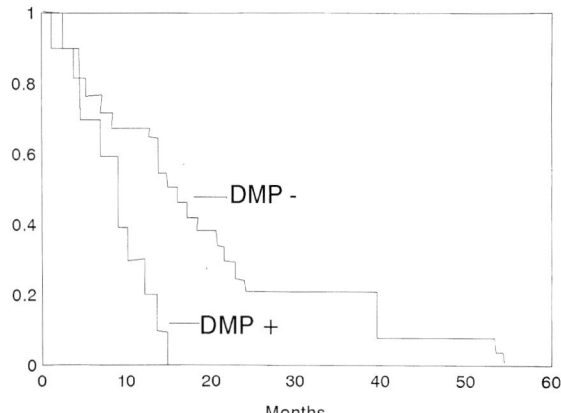

Fig. 3.20   Survival curves for demented patients with and without diffuse myelin pallor (DMP).

46 brains from patients thought to have been demented in life compared with 75% of those with no such diagnosis. Rarefaction of the white matter was only present in the brains of patients with clinical dementia, suggesting a specific association between dementia and white matter abnormalities. Schmidbauer et al (1992) found that myelin pallor, vacuolar myelin damage and angiocentric demyelinating foci correlated with severity of HIV dementia in a small series. McArthur et al (unpublished data) found that demented patients with diffuse myelin pallor had significantly shorter survival (Fig. 3.20). They also examined the correlation between neuropsychological measures and specific HIV-related neuropathological changes.

Diffuse poliodystrophy

A diffuse poliodystrophy was found in 50% of brains by Budka et al (1991), but, as with the other pathological conditions, the clinical correlates are unknown. Diffuse degenerative histological changes in the cortex, albeit mild, are quite common. Wiley et al (1991a) showed a reduced cortical thickness, and both his group and Everall et al (1991) have confirmed quantitatively that there is neuronal loss of about 30% in the frontal and parieto-occipital cortex in AIDS brains. There is also evidence of microglial proliferation and astrocytosis. Reduced levels of synaptophysin have been demonstrated in cortex and are thought to reflect reduced dendritic connections (Wiley et al 1991a, Masliah et al 1992). Recently, MRS has shown a reduced N-acetyl aspartate (NAA) peak in the parieto-occipital white matter and in other areas in AIDS patients, which is believed to reflect loss of neurones in the overlying cortex (Table 3.12). Quantitative MRI has also shown a loss of cerebral grey matter (Aylward et al 1993a). These observations, both ante- and post-mortem, suggest that we should rethink the concept of HIV dementia as a 'subcortical' process, as it is clear that cortical areas also undergo damage. The functional correlates of these cortical abnormalities are being explored in prospective studies.

Pathological evidence of immune activation

In all of the pathological conditions discussed above, including HIV encephalitis, HIV leucoencephalopathy and diffuse poliodystrophy, one common feature is the presence of inflammatory infiltrates within the brain parenchyma, usually consisting of perivascular infiltrations of monocytes, macrophages and microglia (Navia et al 1986b, Wiley et al 1986, de la Monte et al 1987, Rhodes 1987). Productive HIV expression is noted in only a minority of these cells. Tyor et al (1992) found strong evidence for widespread immune activation in the brains of patients with AIDS. Perivascular cells, consisting mainly of macrophages and occasional lymphocytes, consistently expressed MHC class II antigens. Gliosis and significant increases in the cytokines interleukin-1 (IL-1) and tumour necrosis factor-alpha (TNF-α) were present in the AIDS brains, suggesting a relative state of immune activation with production of cytokines within the brain. These studies were extended by Wesselingh et al (1993) who studied cytokine mRNA expression in brain obtained at autopsy. Levels of TNF-α mRNA were significantly higher and levels of IL-4 significantly lower in patients clinically diagnosed with HIV dementia, while levels in non-demented AIDS patients were similar to seronegative controls. TNF-α mRNA levels were highest in those with the most severe dementia and were found in numerous brain regions, not necessarily just confined to basal ganglia. The potential importance of cytokine overproduction within the CNS will be discussed below in the section on pathogenesis.

PATHOGENESIS

Invasion of the brain by HIV occurs early, as evidenced by the frequency of CSF changes (Ho et al 1985, McArthur et al 1988), by neuropathological abnormalities or the detection of HIV by PCR in HIV-positive individuals dying without AIDS (Gray et al 1993, Sinclair et al 1993). A dramatic example of the early timing of CNS infection occurred after accidental inoculation of HIV-positive blood in a patient who died shortly thereafter (Davis et al 1992). Despite the infection of the brain early in HIV infection, the development of overt dementia is delayed until severe immunodeficiency has developed. Most patients with HIV dementia have already had another AIDS-defining illness before the onset of cognitive symptoms. That the onset of dementia is rare during the asymptomatic phase of HIV infection suggests that the development of dementia requires both CNS infection with HIV and the progression of systemic HIV infection and cellular immunodeficiency. Up to now, however, it has been difficult to explain the clinical changes of HIV dementia simply as a result of HIV infection within the brain. Often, even in severely demented individuals, only relatively small amounts of HIV are identified within the brain (Gabuzda et al 1986), and infection is confined to macrophages and microglia, sparing neurones. In addition, there is frequently a discordance between the intensity of the encephalitic changes and the severity of clinical dementia (Navia et al 1986b).

Only a small fraction of cells within perivascular inflammatory cells or microglial nodules contain detectable viral antigen. Though there is a correlation between multinucleated giant cells and dementia (Table 3.14) as many as a third or even a half of brains from demented patients show little in the way of encephalitis or leucoencephalopathy. In fact Glass et al (1993), reviewing data from the Johns Hopkins brain bank, found that 50% of brains from demented patients showed neither giant cells nor leucoencephalopathy. The recent study by Everall et al (1991) has shown that whether or not AIDS patients have marked encephalitic changes they have a reduction in cortical neurones. Neuronal loss may be the critical factor in the development of neurological signs and symptoms, but its aetiology clearly differs from the direct neuronal loss with other viral encephalitides, e.g. arbo virus or herpes simplex.

Both 'host' and viral factors may be important in deciding which patients develop HIV dementia.

HIV load and dementia

Several virological measures have been used to assess HIV load, including p24 antigen in blood and CSF, limiting dilution cultures, determination of plasma viraemia and quantitative PCR to detect HIV proviral DNA or RNA transcripts. Studies of systemic viral load have demonstrated that increasing systemic HIV load, assessed either by p24 antigen (Paul et al 1987, Allain et al 1987, Lange et al 1986, Farzadegan et al 1992, MacDonell et al 1990) or by plasma viraemia (Coombs et al 1989), correlates with increasing stage of HIV infection, is associated with progression to AIDS in HIV seropositives, and generally signifies a poor prognosis. Other virological studies have demonstrated that the number of infected cells in blood and the ratio of genomic RNA to viral DNA sequences correlate with HIV disease state (Michael et al 1992). Piatak et al (1993), using quantitative competitive PCR methods, examined plasma from 66 individuals in varying stages of infection. HIV RNA ranged from 100 to nearly 22 000 000 copies/ml corresponding to 50–11 000 000 virions/ml. The quantity correlated with disease stage and CD4 count, and fell as much as 235-fold with resolution of primary infection or response to antiretroviral therapy.

To date, similar correlations of HIV load with neurological symptoms or dementia have been limited. In post-mortem brain, using Southern blot analysis, Shaw et al (1985) demonstrated more viral DNA in brain than in lymph nodes or spleen. By contrast, Vazeux et al (1992) found HIV antigen in only three of nine children with histological findings of HIV encephalitis, although all had HIV detectable by PCR within the brain. Studies of HIV load in the CSF have been equally confusing. Goswami (1991) used PCR to detect HIV sequences in CSF and found positive PCR in 95% of HIV-infected patients with neurological disease but in only 20% of patients without. By contrast, Steuler et al (1992) found proviral DNA in a higher proportion of CSF cells than in peripheral blood mononuclear cells, although there was no correlation with neurological disease. Buffet et al (1991) found that neither HIV isolation nor p24 antigen detection in CSF was associated with cognitive symptoms. Other studies of CSF p24 antigen have also shown conflicting results. In early studies, p24 antigen was detected in CSF in only about 50% of patients with dementia (Goudsmit et al 1986, Portegies et al 1989b). Using acid hydrolysis to increase the sensitivity of the assay, Royal et al (1994) detected p24 antigen in CSF in two-thirds of patients with significant dementia (MSK 2–4).

Although up to now the relationship between systemic HIV load and neurological decline has not been fully explored, evidence is beginning to appear that systemic viral load probably plays an important role in 'driving' the development of cognitive dysfunction. For example, data from the MACS have shown that neuropsychological decline is more likely to occur with lower CD4 counts, higher p24 antigen titres and higher blood lymphocyte culture yield of HIV (Dal Pan et al 1993).

Host factors and dementia

To date, epidemiological studies have not defined any specific host factors that clearly predispose to HIV dementia. In the MACS analysis (McArthur et al 1993), apart from age, no specific demographic factors correlated with an increased hazard of dementia. However, with the demonstration that there is overproduction of certain cytokines such as TNF-α within the brains of patients with HIV dementia, genetic factors may play a role in determining progression to dementia. The gene coding for TNF-α lies within the major histocompatability complex (MHC) on chromosome 6 and several studies have suggested that the level of TNF-α production (Bendtzen et al 1988) and rapid progression to AIDS (French et al 1992) are linked to the MHC. There is an association between certain haplotypes and an increased risk of progression to AIDS (Kaslow et al 1990). It is plausible that a particular haplotype might be associated with an overproduction of TNF-α or

other macrophage activating cytokines, such as IL-12 or macrophage colony-stimulating factor (MCSF).

Entry of infected monocytes into the brain appears to depend on the expression of certain adhesion molecules on the capillary endothelium. Monocytes only adhere in the presence of VCAM-1, an endothelial adhesion molecule of the immunoglobulin supergene family. Ringler et al (1993) found that VCAM-1 was only expressed in SIV-infected macaques with encephalitis, and not in those without, suggesting that expression of adhesion molecules may determine the entry of infected macrophages. The expression of the adhesion molecules may also vary among humans, thus providing another area in which host factors determine the development of neurological disease.

HIV tropism and dementia

Because not all HIV infected patients, even in the very last stages of AIDS, become demented, it has been suggested that there may be specific neurotropic or neurovirulent strains of HIV. Several aspects of the biology of HIV are important in this regard, including its neuroinvasiveness (ability to invade the nervous system), neurotropism (ability to infect cells in the brain parenchyma) and neurovirulence (ability to cause neural damage). The V3 envelope region of HIV is an important determinant of cell tropism and several groups have shown that specific sequences within this region affect tropism for lymphocytes and macrophages (Cheng-Mayer et al 1991, Westervelt et al 1991). In general, most isolates of HIV derived from brain grow more readily in cultured macrophages than lymphocytes. Watkins et al (1990) have shown that macrophage-tropic strains grow more readily in primary cultures of human microglia. Sequential studies with SIV-infected macaques have shown that lymphocyte-tropic SIV produces no brain infection. However, serial intracerebral inoculation induces envelope mutations changing the lymphocyte-tropic strain into a macrophage-tropic strain, which is capable of producing encephalitis. Desrosiers et al (1991) have shown that macrophage tropism is a prerequisite for productive infection within the brain (neurotropism), but that not all macrophage-tropic strains are equally neurotropic.

Another area of the HIV genome that may have relevance for neurotropism is the long terminal repeat (LTR). Corboy et al (1992) suggested that LTR sequences may affect tropism for specific CNS cells. Because the LTR controls transcription activity, it is possible that sequence differences in an LTR may play a role in the productivity of HIV infection within the brain and thus affect the neurovirulence of a particular HIV strain.

One hypothesis linking these observations is that specific mutations in the dominant HIV strain in an infected person may lead to the emergence of macrophage-tropic quasi-species. The emergence of macrophage-tropic strains that are also neurotropic leads to the development of productive HIV infection within the brain and subsequently to encephalitis, and dementia.

Mechanisms of neuronal damage and dysfunction

The mechanism of neuronal damage and dysfunction is probably multifactorial and not related to direct infection of neurones, astrocytes or oligodendrocytes (Table 3.15). Several reviews have summarized the experimental and clinical evidence pointing to the likelihood that indirect pathogenetic mechanisms are most likely responsible for neuronal damage and dysfunction in HIV dementia (Lipton 1992, Epstein & Gendelman 1993).

Cytopathic or neurotoxic effects of HIV

Infected monocytes in culture can cause CNS cell necrosis by cell/cell contact (Tardieu et al 1992) but cytokine-stimulated macrophages did not, suggesting a direct role for release of viral antigens. This seems unlikely to be a major factor as neuronal loss occurs in areas with few infected cells. However, some transcription products of HIV appear to be neurotoxic. Much attention has focused on the gp120 envelope protein, which is cytotoxic to neurones in cell culture (Brenneman et al 1988). It also causes myelin loss in primary cultures of rat cortex (Kimura-Kuroda et al 1993). Changes in 10 or 12 amino acid sequences in the gp120 envelope of a strain of simian immunodeficiency virus determined its macrophage and T cell tropism and cytopathogenicity (Cheng-Mayer et al 1992). Transgenic mice have been generated that contain the LTRs of two CNS-derived strains of a T cell tropic strain of

Table 3.15 Possible factors in the pathogenesis of HIV associated dementia

Direct effects of infection of neural cells	
Cytopathic	Activation of macrophages/microglia with secretion of soluble substances
Non-cytopathic	Viral proteins (gp120, nef, tat) may be neurotoxic or interfere with function
Cytokines and other macrophage products	
Toxic effects of monokines	On neurons and oligodendrocytes (TNF-α)
Astrocytic proliferation	Stimulation of further cytokine release from macrophages and production of arachidonic acid metabolites
Blood–brain barrier perturbation	Exposure of parenchymal cells to circulating systemic factors and ingress of infected monocytes
Toxic effects of other soluble factors	On neurones, astrocytes and oligodendrocytes
Increased HIV load in CNS	
Other infectious agents	CMV, JC virus stimulate transactivation of HIV
Cytokine-induced	TNF-α and other cytokines stimulate transactivation
Resistance mutations	Antiretroviral resistance permits increased HIV replication
Gp120 release from infected cells	Possible interference with 'astrocyte-derived neuronal protective factor' or other neurotrophic factors
	Possible interference with neurotransmitters, e.g. vasoactive intestinal polypeptide
Autoimmunity	Common immunological determinants between gp41 and astrocytes

(After Johnson et al 1988)

HIV. They showed widespread astrocytosis, vacuolar degeneration of dendrites and activation of microglia in the CNS, mimicking some of the effects of HIV infection in man (Toggas et al 1993). It was interesting that only mice with CNS-derived LTRs showed expression in the brain, suggesting some selective advantage for brain gene expression that may represent neuroadaptation of the strain. Expression was almost solely in neurones, which is not what is seen in man, so the precise relevance of these observations is a little unsure.

The neuronal toxicity of gp120 can be diminished by blockade of NMDA receptors and by calcium antagonists suggesting that calcium channel opening with cellular calcium overload contributes to the mechanism of cell death (Lipton 1992). Gp120 can also stimulate neurotoxin release by mononuclear phagocytes without release of glutamate (Giulian et al 1993). The identity of the neurotoxin is not yet clear, but it is heat stable and protease resistant. Another action of gp120 that is exciting interest is its ability to mediate tyrosine phosphorylation (Bhat 1993), which regulates several enzymes controlling the cell cycle. There are obvious therapeutic implications for these observations and both NMDA receptor antagonists (memantine) and calcium antagonists (nimodipine) are being tested in clinical trials.

Other viral gene products have also been incriminated. Nef protein (which has a variety of functions including down-regulation of viral expression) shares some homology with scorpion neurotoxin and is expressed more often in the brains from demented patients (Ranki et al 1991), and tat (a major protein involved in up-regulating HIV replication) is neurotoxic in tissue culture (Bahraoui et al 1991).

Products of activated macrophages

Pulliam et al (1991) and Giulian et al (1990) showed that HIV-infected macrophages produce substances that are toxic to neurones in tissue culture. Giulian's neurotoxins were heat stable and protease-resistant and their effects were blocked by NMDA antagonists, suggesting an action mediated by NMDA receptors. These observations were not confirmed in two recent reports (Bernton et al 1992, Tardieu et al 1992) and the substances have not been identified as yet. Merrill et al (1992) found that HIV-infected macrophages induced cytokine production, specifically IL-1 and TNF-α, in rodent brain cultures, an observation that is consistent with the observations of TNF-α overproduction in human autopsy tissue (Tyor et al 1992, Wesselingh et al 1993). TNF-α has numerous effects, including the induction of astrocyte proliferation (Barna et al 1990), alteration in neuronal function (Shibata & Blatteis 1992, Soliven & Albert 1992), stimulation of cytokine production by astrocytes (Aloisi et al 1992), myelin damage (Mathew & Miller 1990) and in vitro oligodendrocyte toxicity (Robbins et al 1987). In addition, TNF-α activates HIV through release of the transcription activating factor NF-kB, which binds to the LTR of HIV-1 (Duh et al 1989). Epstein and Gendelman (1993) have stressed the importance of cell-to-cell interactions in the generation of neurotoxic substances in the experimental setting. In vitro studies (Genis et al 1992, Epstein & Gendelman 1993) suggest that HIV-infected monocytes co-cultivated with neural cells produce leukotrienes and platelet activating factor (PAF), leading to neuronal injury. Again, this is consistent with the situation in vivo, where CSF levels of eicosanoids in HIV-infected patients have shown elevations in some arachidonic acid metabolites (Griffin et al 1994), although not as yet of the same leukotrienes. PAF alone or in combination with TNF-α produces neurotoxicity in vitro (Gelbard & Jett 1994). It is produced by co-cultures of HIV-infected monocytes and astrocytes but not by monocytes alone. Interactions between macrophages and astroglia appear to be involved in the production of a wide range of other potentially damaging molecules including arachidonic acid metabolites, TNF-α and IL-1b (Genis et al 1992). PAF and its structural analogues induce rises in calcium levels in cultured neurones (Kornecki & Ehrlich 1991), and enhance glutamate release (Shukla 1992, Wieraszko et al 1993). Preliminary studies have shown elevated levels of PAF in the CSF of patients with HIV dementia, which correlates with reduced NAA peaks on MRS (Gendelman H, personal communication).

Cytokines such as IL-1 and TNF-α have not only been demonstrated in vitro to stimulate replication of HIV (Merrill et al 1992), but also to stimulate astrogliosis. TNF-α and probably IL-1 are present in greater amounts in the brains of patients with AIDS and are involved in the cascade of cytokine stimulation of the immune system, which results in a large number of activated cells in the CNS. Cytokine alterations in the blood–brain barrier may also expose the brain to circulating factors contributing to neural damage (Power et al 1993). Levels of IL-4 mRNA, a T-cell-derived cytokine, decrease in brains from patients with HIV dementia presumably from a loss of TH2 lymphocytes, which are responsible for producing this cytokine (Mosmann & Coffman 1987, Clerici & Shearer 1993, Wesselingh et al 1993) IL-4 (and IL-10) are known to inhibit macrophage activation and the elaboration of other cytokines including TNF-α. With a loss of this inhibitory control late in HIV infection, macrophage activation and TNF-α production could increase with damaging effects.

Quinolinic acid, which is a breakdown product of tryptophan metabolism in macrophages, is found in elevated amounts in the CSF of patients with dementia (Heyes et al 1989, 1991). It may be more than a simple marker of macrophage activation because quinolinic acid also acts as a glutamate agonist and in vitro studies show that it is both excitotoxic and neurotoxic (Gulevich & Wiley 1991). Infections with bacteria, viruses, fungi or parasites might all be expected to produce interferonγ, which increases the activity of indoleamine 2,3, dioxygenase, the enzyme that promotes the production of l-kynurenic acid and thence quinolinic acid from l-tryptophan in macrophages. Heyes et al (1992) suggest that this may be the pathway linking various inflammatory processes, including AIDS, to neuronal dysfunction.

Another hypothesis suggests that microglial infection or activation interferes with some as yet uncharacterized physiological function essential to neuronal well-being. One candidate here is again gp120, which inhibits vasoactive peptide, which in turn enhances neuronal survival in culture (Pulliam et al 1991). Gp120 could therefore cause functional deficits by interfering with growth and maintenance of nerve cells (Levy 1993). A second candidate is nitric oxide, which Dawson et al (1993) suggested may mediate gp120 neurotoxicity.

Reconciling the many different observations and hypotheses for HIV dementia is complex and multifactorial (Table 3.15). None of the various hypotheses about the connection between virus infection and CNS dysfunction are mutually exclusive. A hypothetical schema for the neuropathogenesis of HIV dementia is shown in Table 3.16. It appears likely that with productive HIV infection within the CNS, there is an activation of macrophages and microglia with the release of cytokines into the brain parenchyma. The cytokines may play a number of roles, including the amplification of HIV replication, the stimulation of astrocytosis, and, via autocrine feedback loops, additional production of cytokines and arachidonic acid metabolites. Activated astrocytes may play a role in modulating and amplifying the release of neurotoxic substances. The NMDA receptor is the leading contender as the final common pathway for neuronal damage, and may be a target for therapeutic intervention. A synthesis is attempted in Fig. 3.21.

Nutritional and vitamin deficiencies

A relative or absolute deficiency of vitamin B_{12} has been proposed as a cofactor in the neurological impairment associated with HIV infection.

Table 3.16 Putative pathogenetic steps in HIV dementia: hypothetical mechanisms

1. HIV infection of CNS macrophages (early after primary HIV infection but controlled until later in AIDS)
2. Activation of macrophages and microglia within the CNS facilitated by systemic and CNS production of gamma-interferon
3. Expression of adhesion markers on endothelial cells and additional ingress of HIV-infected monocytes
4. Damage to blood–brain barrier with exposure of CNS macrophages to systemic elevated levels of gamma-interferon and TNF-α, with further activation
5. Reduced inhibitory control of macrophage activation by decline in down-regulatory cytokines, IL-4, IL-10
6. Macrophage products (including cytokines, quinolinic acid, nitric oxide, PAF, arachidonic acid metabolites) toxic to neurones and oligodendrocytes, and produce glial proliferation

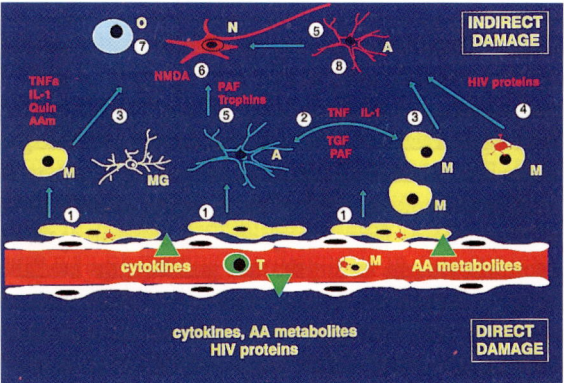

Fig. 3.21 Potential pathogenetic mechanisms in HIV-associated dementia. *Direct damage.* Through a disrupted blood–brain barrier, various factors including cytokines, arachidonic acid metabolites and HIV proteins, may damage neural elements directly. *Indirect damage.* Here a series of events may culminate in neuronal injury and loss, or neuronal dysfunction, and changes in glial cells. (1) Entry of HIV into brain may occur either by ingress of infected macrophages or via infection of endothelial cells with resulting infection of perivascular macrophages. (2) Macrophages (M) and microglia (Mg) are either infected from perivascular macrophages or become activated without productive infection. Various cytokines, including TNF-α and IL-1β, act locally on astrocytes (A) and stimulate production of astrocyte-derived substances, transforming growth factor-β (TGF-β) and platelet activating factor (PAF). These regulatory substances may regulate cytokine production from macrophages. (3) Uninfected, but activated, macrophages and microglia release a variety of substances, including TNF-α, interleukin-1 (IL-1β), quinolinic acid (Quin), and arachidonic acid metabolites (AAN), which act on neural cells, including neurones (N), astrocytes (A) and oligodendrocytes (O), to cause dysfunction, astrocytic hyperplasia and proliferation and possibly cell death. (4) Infected macrophages and microglia release HIV proteins, including gp120, tat, rev and nef, which may damage astrocytes and neurones. (5) Astrocytes stimulated by macrophage-derived cytokines may release PAF, which in turn damages neurones or other astrocytes. The production of astrocyte-derived neurotrophic factors may be reduced, affecting neuronal survival. (6) These various mechanisms may act through the final common pathway of the NMDA receptor. Stimulation of this receptor may in turn stimulate nitric oxide (NO) synthase within neurones with the local release of neurotoxic NO. (7) Oligodendrocytes may be damaged by locally produced cytokines, particularly TNF-α. (8) Astrocytes respond to locally produced cytokines, particularly TNF-α and IL-1, by activation and hyperplasia. (This figure was prepared with the assistance of Drs C. Power, J. Glass and S. Wesselingh.)

Herbert et al (1990) found that up to 50% of patients with HIV infection had subtle evidence of impaired absorption of B$_{12}$. Serum levels and Schilling tests might be normal, but low levels of serum holotranscobalamin II implied impending deficiency. The changes were attributed to gastric changes due to HIV and opportunistic infections. Beach et al (1992) found low serum B$_{12}$ in 25% of asymptomatic HIV-infected individuals and further showed some relationship between such findings and performance on some cognitive tests. The hypothesis is that poor delivery of B$_{12}$ to nervous tissue where glial cells only have receptors for holotranscobalamin leads to or aggravates cognitive dysfunction through impaired methyl group transfer and build-up of homocysteine (Herbert 1993). However, patients with HIV infection with neurological signs ($n = 18$) had normal CSF levels of methoxy mandelic acid (MMA), which is normally low in pernicious anaemia (Trimble et al 1993). There is as yet no clear indication to prescribe regular B$_{12}$ injections in the absence of pathologically low serum levels.

THERAPY OF HIV DEMENTIA

Minor HIV-associated cognitive/motor disorder

One important difference between HIV-associated dementia complex and HIV-associated minor cognitive/motor disorder (Tables 8.1 and 8.2) is in the severity of functional impairment and the impact on activities of daily living. In HIV-associated dementia complex, functioning at work and activities of daily living (ADL) such as handling money are conspicuously impaired. In the lesser HIV-related minor cognitive/motor disorder only the most taxing tasks in everyday functioning are impaired (Working Group of the American Academy of Neurology AIDS Task Force 1991). The difference is subjective and depends on clinical judgement and the use of cognitive assessments and ADL scales. Probable and possible categories reflect the level of clinical certainty and depend on the exclusion of opportunistic infections, depression, etc., and so in turn depend on the thoroughness of ancillary investigations. Patients with minor cognitive deficits should be counselled, any complicating medical or toxic factors addressed and observed carefully with serial neuropsychological tests for change. At this point

we do not know how frequently minor cognitive/
motor disorders change into frank dementia.
Mayeux et al (1993) have found that cognitive
impairment is a marker of reduced survival, but a
number of observations within prospective studies
indicate that minor cognitive/motor disorder may
remain stable for many months or years, even
without antiretroviral therapy.

Treatment of HIV-associated dementia complex

Prevention

Some existing data point to a protective effect of
zidovudine for development of HIV dementia.
For example, Portegies et al (1989a) reported that
the proportion of cases of AIDS with evidence of
AIDS dementia complex fell dramatically after
the introduction of zidovudine (doses averaging
1000–1200 mg/day) in 1987, although the MACS
data at first seemed to contradict these results and
did not show that zidovudine therapy before
AIDS was protective against the development of
dementia, but most were on 600 mg/day or less.
Two other studies suggest that a higher dose of
zidovudine is effective at preventing onset of
dementia. Hamilton et al (1992) noted that
dementia developed in six of 168 patients who
took zidovudine after opportunistic infections,
compared with none of 170 who had received it
early. The Nordic Medical Research Councils
HIV Therapy Group (1992) recorded the development of dementia in 8% of those on
400 mg/day, 6% on 800 mg/day and 3% on
1200 mg/day ($p<0.06$). These two studies suggest
a weak neuroprotective effect of zidovudine, but
only with the initiation of zidovudine before AIDS
and only for doses above 1000 mg daily. Thus,
both the timing and dose of zidovudine may be
critical with respect to prophylactic efficacy for
neurological disease. Gray et al (1991) have
advanced neuropathological data suggesting a
beneficial effect of zidovudine on HIV-related
neuropathological changes. Thus their study
suggests that multinucleated giant cells became
less frequent in autopsies when antiretroviral
treatment became widespread. Overall, the
incidence of HIV dementia does not appear to be

falling, at least based on US data from the CDC
and the MACS (Bacellar et al 1994). If zidovudine has any protective effect, it may be dose-
dependent or time-limited so that the onset of
dementia is delayed but not completely prevented.

Treatment of established dementia

Treatment of HIV dementia is focused on
antiretroviral medications as the first line of
therapy. Zidovudine, the first antiviral agent to be
used, fortunately crossed the blood–brain barrier
and the original licencing trial in patients with
advanced HIV infection reported evidence of
improved cognition in treated patients. While not
specifically a study of dementia, the short-term
effects over 16 weeks were dramatic and were
seen principally in attention and psychomotor
speed (Schmitt et al 1988). There were no
changes in affective symptoms; however, physical
symptoms diminished during the trial. No
allowance was made for the non-specific effects of
an improved sense of well-being on cognitive
performance. Children treated with open label
intravenous zidovudine showed similar impressive
improvements in neuropsychological performance, although without any clear cut dose-
response (Pizzo et al 1988). Sidtis et al (1993)
reported a small randomized placebo-controlled
trial of zidovudine for patients with HIV
dementia. Those treated with the two doses of
zidovudine (1000 or 2000 mg/day) showed more
improvement on neuropsychological tests than
those receiving placebo. Improvement was seen
both at weeks 8 and 16 of treatment. The motor
disturbances may also improve on therapy as
suggested by a study of finger tapping that showed
improvement in the zidovudine-treated group
(Arendt et al 1992). Evidence of a treatment
effect has also appeared from a pathological study
of demented patients. Glass et al (1993) found
that patients with dementia treated with antiretroviral agents for more than 12 months are less
likely to show multinucleated giant cells and/or
diffuse myelin pallor.

While the issue of optimal zidovudine dose for
treatment of HIV dementia has not yet been
determined, it is clearly not practical to treat
patients with 2000 mg per day, as was attempted

in the Sidtis placebo-controlled dementia trial. The frequency of myelosuppressive bone toxicity and other limiting side-effects is far too great at this dose. Figure 3.22 illustrates our suggested management strategies for the treatment of established HIV dementia. A trial of 'high dose' zidovudine, 1000 mg/day, remains the initial treatment of choice whether a patient has been receiving standard doses (500–600 mg/day) or has never received antiretrovirals. Haematopoietic growth factor support (erythropoietin or granulocyte colony-stimulating factor (G-CSF)) may be necessary at this dose range, and monitoring of blood count, differential and creatine phosphokinase (CPK) is necessary every 2 weeks. For anaemia, erythropoietin (recombinant human erythropoietin) is administered in doses of 50–100 units/kg two to three times a week by subcutaneous injection. Erythropoietin is recommended

only if the baseline erythropoietin serum level is less than 500 units/ml and zidovudine should be discontinued if the haemoglobin level is less than 7.5 g%. G-CSF is used for treating neutropenia in a dose of 1 mg/kg/day subcutaneously monitored with cell counts and differential twice weekly. After the white count has recovered, the G-CSF can be reduced to a maintenance dose of 0.3 mg/kg/day and the dose varied to keep the absolute neutrophil count greater than 1500/mm^3. In addition to following the clinical progress and function of the patient, we recommend monitoring treatment response with one or more neuropsychological tests. The Grooved Pegboard test or the HIV Dementia Scale, for example, provide easy methods to follow improvements. Using psychomotor speed measures as an indicator of treatment response, one can usually see evidence of improvement within 2–4 weeks.

There is very little information about the therapeutic response to dideoxyinosine (ddI) or dideoxycytidine (ddC), except for small-scale open label studies (Yarchoan et al 1990). However, in children, ddI has been shown to improve IQ scores where the plasma concentration of ddI correlated both with IQ improvement and decline in p24 antigen (Butler et al 1991). Neither ddI nor ddC penetrate the CSF as easily as zidovudine. Pharmacokinetic studies have shown a CSF:blood ratio of about 20% (Yarchoan & Broder 1989) compared with about 60% for zidovudine. Stavudine (d4T), currently undergoing clinical trials, appears to have comparable CSF penetration to zidovudine and may be a better second-choice antiretroviral than ddI or ddC for treating established dementia. It also is associated with the development of peripheral neuropathy like ddI and ddC (Dunkle et al 1992).

In treating patients with HIV dementia, one can expect the most prompt and dramatic responses in patients who are zidovudine-naive or who have only received zidovudine for a short period of time. This is presumably because the frequency of clinical resistance to zidovudine increases with duration of therapy (Richman 1993). The duration and degree of response vary widely among patients with dementia. Some patients respond very dramatically and the improvement is sustained for months or even

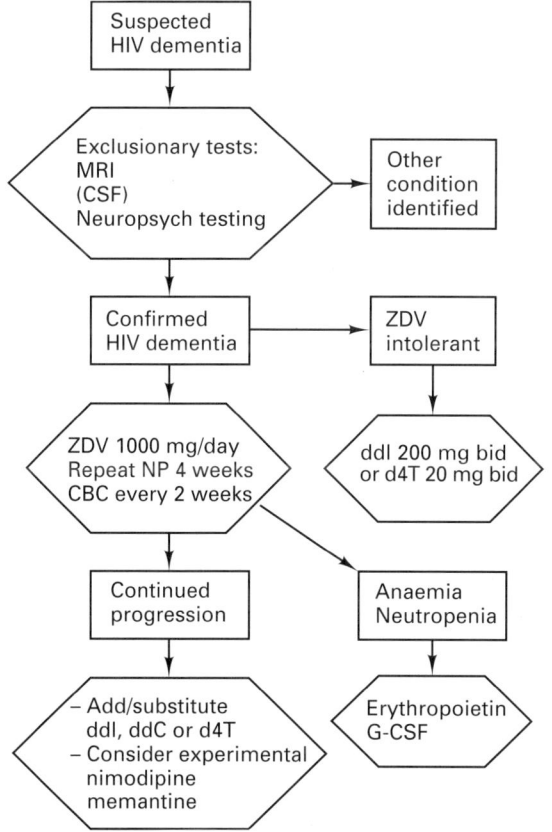

Fig. 3.22 Algorithm for management of HIV dementia. NP, neuropsychological testing; CBC, complete blood count.

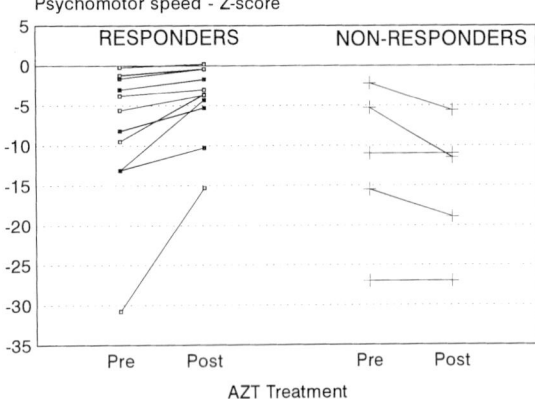

Fig. 3.23 Treatment response in established HIV dementia. Sixteen patients with established HIV dementia naive to zidovudine (AZT) were treated with doses ranging from 600 to 1000 mg daily. There was variability in response with three patients continuing to progress, two remaining stable and 11 improving after 4–8 weeks of treatment. Response measured by improvement in psychomotor speed (vertical axis represents z-score or standard deviation units) on measures of psychomotor speed before and after zidovudine treatment.

years. Others may fail to respond. The reasons underlying these differences may be multi-factorial, including the development of resistance and irreversible structural change in the brain (Fig. 3.23). Without effective treatment, survival is usually less than 6 months. An exacerbation of dementia may accompany abrupt withdrawal of zidovudine and there are reports of transient delirium developing with abrupt cessation of treatment (Pinching et al 1989).

Management

Incidental infections should be treated aggres-sively, but other psychoactive medications should be used with caution because of the sensitivity of patients with dementia to drowsiness and confu-sion. Drugs with sedating properties particularly must be used with care. Associated depression may need treatment, with imipramine, fluoxetine or amitriptyline. Doses may need to be reduced from the usual range by 50% to avoid delirium. Some physicians consider ritalin or amphetamine if apathy is the main problem; however, seizures can be precipitated. Counselling and the involve-ment of support groups is important.

Fluctuation of cognitive performance is quite common. It is important that early on the patient is informed of what is going on so that they can make informed decisions about their future, and the family can be involved if that is desired. Most will need supportive care, and advice over such matters as setting up a living will, power of attorney or testamentary capacity. A patient's wishes should be ascertained whilst they are still able to make such decisions. Hospice care may become appropriate near the end. The prognosis is variable (McArthur 1987) and while some patients progress rapidly to a mute, decerebrate or decorticate, demented state, others show an apparent plateau, maintaining a moderate level of dementia for many months before dying of opportunistic infections (McKenzie et al 1991).

Potential novel treatments for HIV dementia

As our understanding of the pathogenetic mecha-nisms underlying HIV dementia expands, so novel treatments for dementia will become more widely tested and used. For several of the mecha-nisms discussed above, agents are clinically avail-able that might be applied to the treatment of established dementia. For example, pentoxi-fylline, a substituted methylxanthine approved for treatment of intermittent claudication, has been shown to decrease TNF-α activity, both in vitro and in vivo (Dezube et al 1993).

It seems likely that the successful treatment of HIV dementia will need to reduce or block the products of macrophage activation, in addition to suppressing further viral production. Agents that might be applicable for clinical trials include drugs such as thalidomide, pentoxifylline and dexa-methasone, and the fish oil derivative omega-3 PUFA, which inhibit TNF-α production. Cell cultures of HIV-infected macrophages and human astroglial cell lines produce high levels of other potentially neurotoxic substances, including the prostaglandin precursor arachidonic acid, the leukotrienes LTB4 and LTD4, and platelet activating factor (PAF) (Genis et al 1992). Agents that decrease the production of arachidonic acid metabolites or PAF might ameliorate the neurotoxicity and improve dementia. The clinically available drugs dexamethasone and nordihydroguaiaretic acid inhibit production of arachidonic acid metabolites and decrease TNF-α production. The anxiolytics alprazolam and marinol are both PAF antagonists, and might block its neurotoxicity (Epstein L, personal communication).

Nimodipine, a calcium channel antagonist, might decrease the potential neurotoxicity of gp120 and clinical trials testing its efficacy and toxicity have been completed in the USA (Lipton 1992). Preliminary experiments with conditioned media from HIV-infected macrophages (Epstein & Gendelman 1993) suggest that their neurotoxicity could be blocked by drugs that act as antagonists at the NMDA receptor or NMDA receptor-mediated ion channels. Potentially useful agents that are clinically available include memantine, an NMDA antagonist. All of these agents are currently under trial or about to enter clinical trials for established dementia. It seems likely that an effective treatment for HIV dementia will have to include an antiretroviral with adequate brain penetrance, and agents that block some of the indirect mechanisms contributing to neural damage.

CONCLUSION

Our understanding of the pathogenesis of HIV dementia is only in its early stages. There is a clear need to better define its neuropathological substrate and clinical pathological correlations. Equally critical is the issue of antiretroviral therapy on the development and course of HIV dementia and the severity of neuropathological changes in brain. HIV dementia is uncommon during the early asymptomatic phase of HIV infection and tends to develop only after profound immunodeficiency and AIDS-defining illnesses. Its annual incidence after AIDS is about 7% and it will occur in approximately 20% of individuals with advanced HIV disease. The MACS data suggest that in a hypothetical cohort of 1000 men with AIDS, 791 would survive 6 months after AIDS, and of these, 46 would be living with dementia. By 24 months the projection is for 13 living dementia cases among 292 survivors (McArthur et al 1993a). With an estimated 1 million individuals already infected with HIV in the USA alone, we can anticipate an annual incidence of 40 000 cases of HIV dementia, approximately five times the annual incidence of multiple sclerosis. HIV dementia will likely become a leading cause of cognitive impairment in young people.

REFERENCES

Allain J P, Laurian Y, Paul D A, et al. Long-term evaluation of HIV antigen and antibodies to p24 and gp41 in patients with hemophilia. Potential clinical importance. New Engl J Med 1987; 317: 114–1121

Aloisi F, Care A, Barsellino G, et al. Production of hemolymphopoietic cytokines (IL-6, IL-8, colony-stimulating factors) by normal human astrocytes in response to IL-1 beta and tumor necrosis factor-alpha J Immunol 1992; 149: 2358–2366

Arendt G, Hefter H, Buescher L, et al. Improvement of motor performance of HIV-positive patients under AZT therapy. Neurology 1992; 42: 891–895

Arendt G, Hefter H, Jablonowski H. Acoustically evoked event-related potentials in HIV-associated dementia. EEG Clin Neurophysiol 1993; 86: 152–160

Aylward E H, Brettschneider P D, McArthur J C, et al. MRI grey matter volume reduction in HIV dementia. Am J Psychiat 1993a; submitted

Aylward E H, Henderer J D, McArthur J C, et al. Basal ganglia atrophy in HIV-1 associated dementia complex: results from quantitative neuroimaging. Neurology 1993b; 43: 2099–2104

Bacellar H, Munoz A, Miller E N, et al. Temporal trends in the incidence of HIV-Δ related neurological diseases. Multicenter AIDS cohort study 1985–1992. Neurology 1994; in press

Bahraoui E, Vives E, Mabrouk K, et al. Evidence for neurotoxic activity of Tat from human immunodeficiency virus (HIV-1). VII Int AIDS Conf Florence 1991 abstr. MB2056

Barna B P, Estes M L, Jacobs B S, et al. Human astrocytes proliferate in response to tumor necrosis factor. J Neuroimmunol 1990; 30: 239–243

Beach R S, Morgan R, Wilkie F, et al. Plasma vitamin B_{12} level as a potential cofactor in studies of human immunodeficiency virus type-1-related cognitive changes. Arch Neurol 1992; 49: 501–506

Bendtzen K, Morling N, Fomsgaard A, et al. Association between HLA-DR2 and production of tumour necrosis factor alpha and interleukin 1 by mononuclear cells activated by lipopolysaccharide. Scand J Immunol 1988; 28: 599–606

Bernton E W, Bryant H U, Decoster M A, et al. No direct neuronotoxicity by HIV-1 virions or culture fluids from HIV-1-infected T cells or monocytes. AIDS Res Hum Retroviruses 1992; 8: 495–503

Bottomley P A, Hardy C J, Cousins J P, et al. AIDS dementia complex: brain high-energy phosphate metabolite deficits. Radiology 1990; 176: 407–411

Brenneman D, Buzy J, Ruff M. Peptide T sequences prevent neuronal cell death produced by the protein gp120 of the human immunodeficiency virus. Drug Dev Res 1988; 15: 361–369

Brew B J, Bhalla R B, Paul M, et al. Cerebrospinal fluid β₂ microglobulin in patients with AIDS dementia complex: an expanded series including response to zidovudine treatment. AIDS 1992; 6: 461–465

Britton C B, Marquardt M D, Koppel B, et al. Neurological complications of the gay immunosuppressed syndrome: clinical and pathological features. Ann Neurol 1982; 12: 80

Budka H. Human immunodeficiency virus (HIV) envelope and core proteins in CNS tissues of patients with the acquired immune deficiency syndrome (AIDS). Acta Neuropathologica 1990; 79: 611–619

Budka H, Wiley C A, Kleihues P, et al. HIV-associated disease of the nervous system: review of nomenclature and proposal for neuropathology-based terminology. Brain Pathol 1991; 1: 143–152

Buffet R, Agut H, Chieze F, et al. Virological markers in the cerebrospinal fluid from HIV-1 infected individuals. AIDS 1991; 5: 1419–1424

Butler K M, Husson R N, Balis R M, et al. Dideoxyinosine in children with symptomatic human immunodeficiency virus infection. New Engl J Med 1991; 324: 137–144

Butters N, Grant I, Haxby J, et al. Assessment of AIDS related cognitive changes. Recommendations of the NIMH workshop on neuropsychological assessment approaches. J Clin Exp Neuropsychol 1990; 12: 963–978

Centers for Disease Control. Revision of the CDC surveillance case definition for acquired immunodeficiency syndrome. Morbidity and Mortality Weekly Report 1987; 36 (suppl 1S): 3S–15S

Centers for Disease Control and Prevention. HIV/AIDS Surveillance Report 1993; Feb: 1–23

Cheng-Mayer C, Shioda T, Levy J A. Host range, replicative, and cytopathic properties of human immunodeficiency virus type 1 are determined by very few amino acid changes in tat gp120. J Virol 1991; 65: 6931–6941

Cheng-Mayer C, Shioda T, Levy J A. Small regions of the env and tat genes control cellular tropism, cytopathology, and replicative properties of HIV-1. In: Rossi G B et al. Science challenging AIDS. Basel: S Karger, 1992: 188–195

Ciardi A, Sinclair E, Scaravilli F, et al. The involvement of the cerebral cortex in human immunodeficiency virus encephalopathy: a morphological and immunohistochemical study. Acta Neuropathologica 1990; 81: 51–59

Clerici M, Shearer G M. A TH1-TH2 switch is a critical step in the aetiology of HIV infection. Immunol Today 1993; 14: 107–110

Coombs R W, Collier A C, Allain J P, et al. Plasma viremia in human immunodeficiency virus infection. New Engl J Med 1989; 321: 1626–1631

Corboy J R, Buzy J M, Zink M C, et al. Expression directed from HIV long terminal repeats in the central nervous system of transgenic mice. Science 1992; 258: 1804–1808

Dal Pan G, Farzadegan H, Selnes O, et al. Systemic HIV burden and neuropsychological decline in the Multicenter AIDS Cohort Study (MACS). IX International Conference on AIDS 1993. Clin Neuropathol 1993; 12 (Suppl 1): S30 (abstr.)

Dal Pan G J, McArthur J C, Aylward E, et al. Patterns of cerebral atrophy in HIV-1-infected individuals: results of a quantitative MRI analysis. Neurology 1992; 42: 2125–2130

Davis L E, Hjelle B L, Miller V E, et al. Early viral brain invasion in iatrogenic human immunodeficiency virus infection. Neurology 1992; 42: 1736–1739

Dawson V L, Dawson T M, Uhl G R, Snyder S H. Human immunodeficiency virus type 1 core protein neurotoxicity mediated by nitric oxide in primary cortical cultures. Proc Natl Acad Sci USA 1993; 90: 3256–3259

Day J J, Grant I, Atkinson J H, et al. Incidence of AIDS dementia in a two-year follow-up of AIDS and ARC patients on an initial Phase II AZT placebo-controlled study: San Diego cohort. J Neuropsychiatr 1992; 4: 15–20

de la Monte S M, Ho D D, Schooley R T, et al. Subacute encephalomyelitis of AIDS and its relation to HTLV-III infection. Neurology 1987; 37: 562–569

Desrosiers R C, Hansen-Moosa A, Mori K, et al. Macrophage-tropic variants of SIV are associated with specific AIDS-related lesions but are not essential for the development of AIDS. Am J Pathol 1991; 139: 29–35

Dezube B J, Pardee A B, Chapman B, et al. Pentoxifylline decreases tumor necrosis factor expression and serum triglycerides in people with AIDS. J Acquired Immunodeficiency Syndromes 1993; 6: 787–794

Duh E J, Maury W J, Folks T M, et al. Tumor necrosis factor α activates human immunodeficiency virus type 1 through induction of nuclear factor binding to the NF-kB sites in the long terminal repeat. Proc Nat Acad Sci USA 1989; 86: 5974–5978

Dunkle L, Anderson R, McLaren C. Stavudine (d4T) a promising antiretroviral agent. VIII International Conference on AIDS/III STD World Congress 1992 (abstr.)

Elovaara I, Poutiainen E, Raininko R, et al. Mild brain atrophy in early HIV infection: the lack of association with cognitive deficits and HIV-specific intrathecal immune response. J Neurol Sci 1990; 99: 121–136

Epstein L G, Gendelman H E. Human immunodeficiency virus type 1 infection of the nervous system: pathogenetic mechanisms. Ann Neurol 1993; 33: 429–436

Everall I P, Luthert P J, Lantos P L. Neuronal loss in the frontal cortex in HIV infection. Lancet 1991; 337: 1119–1121

Farzadegan H, Chmiel J S, Odaka N, et al. Association of antibody to human immunodeficiency virus type 1 core protein (p24), CD4+ lymphocyte number, and AIDS-free time. J Infect Dis 1992; 166: 1217–1222

Faulstich M E. Psychiatric aspects of AIDS. Am J Psychiatr 1987; 144: 551–556

French M, Abraham L, Mallal S, et al. MHC genes and HIV. Today's Life Sci 1992; 32–36

Friedman Y, Franklin C, Freels S, Weil M H. Long-term survival of patients with AIDS, *Pneumocystis carinii* pneumonia, and respiratory failure. JAMA 1991; 266: 89–92

Fuchs D, Hausen A, Reibnegger G, et al. Immune activation and the anaemia associated with chronic inflammatory disorders. Eur J Haematol 1991; 46: 65–70

Fuchs D, Shearer G M, Boswell R N, et al. Negative correlation between blood cell counts and serum neopterin concentration in patient with HIV-1 infection. AIDS 1991; 5: 209–212

Fuchs D, Werner E R, Dierich M P, Wachter H. Cellular immune activation in the brain and human immunodeficiency virus infection (letter). Ann Neurol 1988; 24: 289

Gabuzda D H, Ho D D, de la Monte S M, et al. Immunohistochemical identification of HTLV-III antigen

in brains of patients with AIDS. Ann Neurol 1986;
20: 289–295

Gelman B B, Guinto F C. Morphometry, histopathology, and
tomography of cerebral atrophy in the acquired
immunodeficiency syndrome. Ann Neurol 1992; 32: 31–40

Genis P, Jett M, Bernton E W, et al. Cytokines and
arachidonic metabolites produced during human
immunodeficiency virus (HIV)-infected macrophage-
astroglia interactions: implications for the
neuropathogenesis of HIV disease. J Exp Med 1992;
176: 1703–1718

Giulian D, Wendt E, Vaca K, Noonan C A. Secretion of
neurotoxins in mononuclear phagocytes infected with
HIV-1. Science 1990; 250: 1593–1596

Giulian D, Wendt E, Vaca K, Noonan C A. The envelope
glycoprotein of human immunodeficiency virus type-1
stimulates release of neurotoxins from monocytes. Proc
Natl Acad Sci USA 1993; 90: 2769–2773

Glass J D, Wesselingh S L, Selnes O A, Mc Arthur J C.
Clinical-neuropathologic correlation in HIV-associated
dementia. Neurology 1993; 43: 2230–2237

Goswami K K, Miller R F, Harrison M J, et al. Expression of
HIV-1 in the cerebrospinal fluid detected by the polymerase
chain reaction and its correlation with central nervous
system disease. J Acquired Immunodeficiency Syndromes
1991; 5: 797–803

Goudsmit J, de Wolf F, Paul D A, et al. Expression of human
immunodeficiency virus antigen (HIV-Ag) in serum and
cerebrospinal fluid during acute and chronic infection.
Lancet 1986; ii: 177–180

Graham N M H, Zeger S L, Park L P, et al. The effects on
survival of early treatment of human immunodeficiency
virus infection. New Engl J Med 1992; 326: 1037–1042

Gray F, Geny C, Dournon E, et al. Neuropathological
evidence that zidovudine reduces incidence of HIV
infection of the brain. Lancet 1991; 337: 852–853

Gray F, Gherardi R, Keohane C, et al. Pathology of the
central nervous system in 40 cases of acquired immune
deficiency syndrome (AIDS). Neuropathol Appl Neurobiol
1988; 14: 365–380

Gray F, Gherardi R, Lescs M C, et al. Early brain changes in
HIV infection: neuropathologic study of 11
HIV-seropositive, non AIDS asymptomatic cases (abstr).
Neuroscience of HIV Infection: Basic and Clinical
Frontiers Clin Neuropathol 1993; 12 (suppl 1): S11

Griffin D E, Wesselingh S L, McArthur J C. Elevated central
nervous system prostaglandins in HIV-associated dementia.
Ann Neurol 1994; in press

Gulevich S J, Wiley C A. HIV infection and the brain. AIDS
1991; 5 (suppl 2): S49–S54

Gutierrez R, Atkinson J H, Grant I. Mild neurocognitive
disorder: needed addition to the nosology of cognitive
impairment (organic mental) disorders. J Neuropsychiatr
Clin Neurosci 1993; 5: 161–177

Hamilton J D, Hartigan P M, Simberkoff M S, et al. A
controlled trial of early versus late treatment with
zidovudine in symptomatic human immunodeficiency virus
infection. New Engl J Med 1992; 326: 437–443

Handelsman L, Aronson M, Maurer G, et al.
Neuropsychological and neurological manifestations of
HIV-1 dementia in drug users. J Neuropsychiatr Clin
Neurosci 1992; 4: 21–28

Harrison M J G, McAllister R H. Neurological complications
of HIV infection. In: Lambert H P, editor. Infections of the
nervous system. London: Arnold, 1991: 343–360

Herbert V. Vitamin B_{12} deficiency neuropsychiatric damage
in acquired immunodeficiency syndrome (letter). Arch
Neurol 1993; 50: 569

Herbert V, Fong W, Gulle V, Stopler T. Low
holotranscobalamin II is the earliest serum marker for
subnormal vitamin B_{12} (cobalamin) absorption in patients
with AIDS. Am J Hematol 1990; 34: 132–139

Hestad K, McArthur J H, Dal Pan G J, et al. Regional
atrophy in HIV-1 infection: association with specific
neuropsychological test performance. Acta Neurol Scand
1993; 88: 112–118

Heyes M P, Brew B J, Martin A, et al. Quinolinic acid in
cerebrospinal fluid and serum in HIV-1 infection:
relationship to clinical and neurologic status. Ann Neurol
1991; 29: 202–209

Heyes M P, Rubinow D, Lane C, Markey S P. Cerebrospinal
fluid quinolinic acid concentrations are increased in
acquired immune deficiency syndrome. Ann Neurol
1989; 26: 275–277

Heyes M P, Saito K, Crowley J S, et al. Quinolinic acid and
kynurene pathway metabolism in inflammatory and non-
inflammatory neurological disease. Brain 1992;
115: 1249–1274

Ho D D, Rota T R, Schooley R T, et al. Isolation of
HTLV-III from cerebrospinal fluid and neural tissues of
patients with neurologic syndromes related to the acquired
immunodeficiency syndrome. New Engl J Med 1985; 313:
1493–1497

Holland N R, Power C, Mathews V P, et al. CMV
encephalitis in acquired immunodeficiency syndrome
(AIDS): clinical features and course. Neurology 1994;
44: 507–514

Horowitz S L, Benson D F, Gottlieb M S, et al. Neurological
complications of gay-related immunodeficiency disorder.
Ann Neurol 1982; 12: 80

Janssen R S. New faces of the HIV epidemic. Clin
Neuropathol 1993; 12 (suppl 1): S3

Janssen R S, Cornblath D R, Epstein L G, et al.
Nomenclature and research case definitions for
neurological manifestations of human immunodeficiency
virus type-1 (HIV-1) infection. Report of a Working Group
of the American Academy of Neurology AIDS Task Force.
Neurology 1991; 41: 778–785

Janssen R S, Nwanyanwu O C, Selik R M, Stehr-Green J K.
Epidemiology of human immunodeficiency virus
encephalopathy in the United States. Neurology 1992;
42: 1472–1476

Johnson R T, McArthur J C, Narayan O. The neurobiology of
human immunodeficiency virus infections. FASEB J 1988;
2: 2970–2981

Kaslow R, Duquesnoy R, VanRaden M, et al. A1, Cw7, B8,
DR3 HLA antigen combination associated with rapid
decline of T-helper lymphocytes in HIV-1 infection. A
report from the Multicenter AIDS Cohort Study. Lancet
1990; 335: 927–930

Ketzler S, Weis S, Haug H, Budka H. Loss of neurons in the
frontal cortex in AIDS brains. Acta Neuropathologica
1990; 80: 92–94

Kimura-Kuroda J, Nagashima K, Yasui K. HIV-1 g120
causes demyelination in a primary culture of rat cerebral
cortex. Clin Neuropathol 1993; 12 (suppl 1): S3

Koenig S, Gendelman H E, Orenstein J M, et al. Detection of
AIDS virus in macrophages in brain tissue from AIDS
patients with encephalopathy. Science 1986;
233: 1089–1093

Kornecki E, Ehrlich Y H. Calcium ion mobilisation in neuronal cells induced by PAF. Lipids 1991; 26: 1243–1246

Kure K, Weidenheim K M, Lyman W D, Dickson D W. Morphology and distribution of HIV-1 gp41-positive microglia in subacute AIDS encephalitis. Pattern of involvement resembling a multisystem degeneration. Acta Neuropathologica 1990; 80: 393–400

LaFrance N, Pearlson G D, Schaerf F W, et al. I-123 IMP-SPECT in HIV-related dementia. Adv Funct Imaging 1988; 1: 9–15

Lange J M, Paul D A, Huisman H G, et al. Persistent HIV antigenaemia and decline of HIV core antibodies associated with transition to AIDS. Br Med J 1986; 293: 1459–1462

Levy J. Pathogenesis of human immunodeficiency virus infection. Microbiol Rev 1993; 57: 183–289

Levy R M, Bredesen D E, Rosenblum M L. Neurological manifestations of the acquired immune deficiency syndrome (AIDS): experience at UCSF and review of the literature. J Neurosurg 1985; 62: 475–495

Lipton S A. HIV-related neurotoxicity. Brain Path 1991; 1: 193–199

Lipton S A. Models of neuronal injury in AIDS: another role for the NMDA receptor? TINS 1992; 15: 75–79

MacDonell K B, Chmiel J S, Poggensee L, et al. Predicting progression to AIDS: combined usefulness of CD4 lymphocyte counts and p24 antigenemia. Am J Med 1990; 89: 706–712

Maj M, Janssen R, Satz P, et al. The World Health Organization's cross-cultural study on neuropsychiatric aspects of infection with the human immunodeficiency virus 1 (HIV-1). Br J Psychiatr 1991; 159: 351–356

Masliah E, Ge N, Morey M, et al. Cortical dendritic pathology in human immunodeficiency virus encephalitis. Lab Invest 1992; 66: 285–291

Mathew T C, Miller F D. Increased expression of T alpha 1 alpha-tubulin mRNA during collateral and NGF-induced sprouting of sympathetic neurons. Dev Biol 1990; 141: 84–92

Matsuyama T, Kobayashi N, Yamamoto N. Cytokines and HIV infection: is AIDS a tumor necrosis factor disease? AIDS 1991; 5: 1405–1417

Mayeux R, Stern Y, Tang M X, et al. Mortality risks in gay men with human immunodeficiency virus infection and cognitive impairment. Neurology 1993; 43: 176–182

McAllister R H, Herns M V, Harrison M J G, et al. Neurological and neuropsychological performance in HIV seropositive asymptomatic individuals. J Neurol Neurosurg Psychiatr 1992; 55: 143–148

McArthur J C. Neurologic manifestations of AIDS. Medicine (Baltimore) 1987; 66: 407–437

McArthur J C, Cohen B A, Farzedegan H, et al. Cerebrospinal fluid abnormalities in homosexual men with and without neuropsychiatric findings. Ann Neurol 1988; 23: S34–S37

McArthur J C, Hoover D R, Bacellar H, et al. Dementia in AIDS patients: incidence and risk factors. Neurology 1993; 43: 2245–2252

McArthur J C, Nance-Sproson T E, Griffin D E, et al. The diagnostic utility of elevation in cerebrospinal fluid β_2 microglobulin in HIV-1 dementia. Neurology 1992; 42: 1707–1712

McKenzie R, Travis W D, Dolan S A, et al. The causes of death in patients with HIV infection: a clinical and pathological study with emphasis on the role of pulmonary disease. Medicine 1991; 70: 326–343

Merrill J E, Chen I. HIV-1, macrophages, glial cells, and cytokines in AIDS nervous system disease. FASEB J 1991; 5: 2391–2397

Merrill J E, Koyanagi Y, Zack J, et al. Induction of interleukin-1 and tumour necrosis factor alpha in brain cultures by human immunodeficiency virus type 1. J Virol 1992; 66: 2217–2225

Merrill P T, Paige G D, Abrams R A, et al. Ocular motor abnormalities in human immunodeficiency virus infection. Ann Neurol 1991; 30: 130–138

Meyerhoff D J, MacKay S, Bachman L, et al. Reduced brain N-acetyl aspartate suggests neuronal loss in cognitively impaired human immunodeficiency virus-seropositive individuals. Neurology 1993; 43: 509–515

Michael N L, Vahey M, Burke D S, Redfield R R. Viral DNA and mRNA expression correlate with the stage of human immunodeficiency virus (HIV) type 1 infection in humans: evidence for viral replication in all stages of HIV disease. J Virol 1992; 66: 310–316

Moore R D, Hidalgo J, Sugland B W, Chaisson R E. Zidovudine and the natural history of the acquired immunodeficiency syndrome. New Engl J Med 1991; 324: 1412–1416

Mosmann T R, Coffman R L. Two types of mouse helper T cell clones. Immunol Today 1987; 8: 223–227

Navia B A, Cho E S, Petito C K, Price R W. The AIDS dementia complex: II. Neuropathology. Ann Neurol 1986a; 19: 525–535

Navia B A, Jordan B D, Price R W. The AIDS dementia complex: I. Clinical features. Ann Neurol 1986b; 19: 517–524

Nordic Medical Research Councils HIV Therapy Group. Double blind dose-response study of zidovudine in AIDS and advanced HIV infection. Br Med J 1992; 304: 13–17

Parisi A, Perri G D, Strosselli M, et al. Usefulness of computerised electroencephalography in diagnosing, staging and monitoring AIDS dementia complex. AIDS 1989; 3: 209–213

Paul D A, Falk L A, Kessler H A, et al. Correlation of serum HIV antigen and antibody with clinical status in HIV-infected patients. J Med Virol 1987; 22: 357–363

Piatak M, Saag M S, Yang L C, et al. High levels of HIV-1 in plasma during all stages of infection determined by competitive PCR. Science 1993; 259: 1749–1754

Piette J, Mor V, Fleishman J. Patterns of survival with AIDS in the United States. Health Services Res 1991; 26: 75–95

Pinching A J, Helbert M, Peddle B, et al. Clinical experience with zidovudine for patients with acquired immune deficiency syndrome and acquired immune deficiency syndrome-related complex. J Infect 1989; 18 (suppl I): 33–40

Pizzo P A, Eddy J, Falloon J, et al. Effect of continuous intravenous infusion of zidovudine (AZT) in children with symptomatic HIV infection. New Engl J Med 1988; 319: 889–896

Portegies P, de Gans J, Lange J M, et al. Declining incidence of AIDS dementia complex after introduction of zidovudine treatment (published erratum appears in BMJ 1989 Nov 4; 299 (6708): 1141). Br Med J 1989a; 299: 819–821

Portegies P, Epstein L G, Hung S T, et al. Human immunodeficiency virus type 1 antigen in cerebrospinal fluid. Correlation with clinical neurologic status. Arch Neurol 1989b; 46: 261–264

Post M J, Tate R M, Quencer G T, et al. CT, MR, and pathology in HIV encephalitis and meningitis. AM J Radiol 1988; 151: 373–380

Power C, Kong P A, Crawford T O, et al. Cerebral white matter changes in HIV dementia: alterations in the blood–brain barrier. Ann Neurol 1993; 34: 339–350

Power C, Selnes O A, Grim J M, McArthur J C. The HIV Dementia Scale: a rapid screening test. J AIDS 1994; in press

Price R W, Brew B J. The AIDS dementia complex. J Infect Dis 1988; 158: 1079–1083

Pulliam L, Herndier B G, Tang N M, McGrath M S. Human immunodeficiency virus-infected macrophages produce soluble factors that cause histological and neurochemical alterations in cultured human brains. J Clin Invest 1991; 87: 503–512

Pumarola-Sune T, Navia B A, Cordon-Cardo C, et al. HIV antigen in the brains of patients with the AIDS dementia complex. Ann Neurol 1987; 21: 490–496

Ranki A, Ovod V, Haitia M, et al. High expression of NEF protein in HIV-infected brain astrocytes associated with rapidly progressing CNS disease. VII International AIDS Conference, Florence 1991; abstr. TuAA100

Reardon J, Singleton J, Wilson M J, Alderete E. Epidemiology of HIV encephalopathy (HIV-E): reported frequencies in California, 1988–1991. VIII International Conference on AIDS/III STD World Congress 1992; POC 4009 (abstr.)

Rhodes R H. Histopathology of the central nervous system in the acquired immunodeficiency syndrome. Hum Pathol 1987; 18: 636–643

Richman D D. HIV drug resistance. Ann Rev Pharmacol Toxicol 1993; 33: 149–164

Ringler D, Sasseville V, Mori K, et al. Viral and host parameters involved in the development of SIV encephalitis. Clin Neuropathol 1993; 12 (suppl): S6–7

Robbins D S, Shirazi Y, Drysdale B E, et al. Production of cytotoxic factor for oligodendrocytes by stimulated astrocytes. J Immunol 1987; 139: 2593–2597

Rosenblum M K. Infection of the central nervous system by the human immunodeficiency virus type 1: morphology and relation to syndromes of progressive encephalopathy and myelopathy in patients with AIDS. In: Rosen P P, Fechner R E, editors. Pathology Annual, part 1. Connecticut: Appleton & Lange, 1990: 117–169

Rottenberg D A, Moeller J R, Strother S C, et al. The metabolic pathology of the AIDS dementia complex. Ann Neurol 1987; 22: 700–706

Royal W, Selnes O A, Concha M, et al. Cerebrospinal fluid HIV-1 p24 antigen levels in HIV-1 related dementia. Ann Neurol 1994; in press

Scaravilli F, Sinclair E, Gray F, Ciardi A. Detection of HIV proviral DNA in HIV-positive non-AIDS drug users and its relationship to pathology of the cerebral cortex. Neuroscience of HIV Infection: Basic and Clinical Frontiers. Clin Neuropathol 1993; 12 (suppl 1) (abstr.)

Schmidbauer M, Huemer M, Cristina S, et al. Morphological spectrum, distribution and clinical correlation of white matter lesions in AIDS brains. Neuropathol Appl Neurobiol 1992; 18: 489–501

Schmitt F A, Bigley J W, McKinnis R, et al. Neuropsychological outcome of zidovudine (AZT) treatment of patients with AIDS and AIDS-related complex. New Engl J Med 1988; 319: 1573–1578

Selmaj K W, Raine C S. Tumor necrosis factor mediates myelin and oligodendrocyte damage in vitro. Ann Neurol 1988; 23: 339–346

Selnes O A, Jacobson L, Machado A M, et al. Normative data for a brief neuropsychological screening battery. Percept Mot Skills 1991a; 73: 539–550

Selnes O A, McArthur J C, Gordon B, et al. Patterns of cognitive decline in incidence of HIV dementia: longitudinal observations from the Multicentre AIDS Cohort Study. Neurology 1991b; 41: 252 (abstr.)

Selnes O A, Miller E, McArthur J C, et al. HIV-1 infection: no evidence of cognitive decline during the asymptomatic stages. Neurology 1990; 40: 204–208

Sharer L R, Epstein L G, Cho E-S, et al. Pathological features of AIDS encephalopathy in children: evidence for LAV/HTLV-III infection in brain. Hum Pathol 1986; 17: 271–284

Shaw G M, Harper M E, Hahn B H, et al. HTLV-III infection in brains of children and adults with AIDS encephalopathy. Science 1985; 227: 177–182

Shibata M, Blatteis C M. Differential effects of cytokines on thermosensitive neurons in guinea pig preoptic area slices. Am J Physiol 1991; 261: R1096–R1103

Shukla S D. Platelet-activating factor receptor and signal transduction mechanisms. FASEB J 1992; 42: 2296–2301

Sidtis J L, Gatsonis C, Price R W, et al. Zidovudine treatment of the AIDS dementia complex: results of a placebo-controlled trial. Ann Neurol 1993; 33: 343–349

Sinclair E, Scaravilli F. Detection of HIV proviral DNA in cortex and white matter of AIDS brains by non-isotopic polymerase chain reaction: correlation with diffuse poliodystrophy. AIDS 1992; 6: 925–932

Snider W D, Simpson D M, Nielsen S, et al. Neurological complications of acquired immune deficiency syndrome: analysis of 50 patients. Ann Neurol 1983; 14: 403–418

Soliven B, Albert J. Tumor necrosis factor modulates Ca^{2+} currents in cultured sympathetic neurons. J Neurosci 1992; 12: 2665–2671

Steuler H, Munzinger S, Wildemann B, Storch-Hagenlocher B. Quantitation of HIV-1 proviral DNA in cells from cerebrospinal fluid. J Acquired Immunodeficiency Syndromes 1992; 5: 405–408

Tardieu M, Hery C, Peudenier S, et al. Human immunodeficiency virus type 1-infected monocytic cells can destroy human neural cells after cell-to-cell adhesion. Ann Neurol 1992; 32: 11–17

Toggas S, Masliah E, Rockenstein E, Mucke L. Neurotoxicity of viral proteins – HIV-1 gp120 effects in transgenic mice. Clin Neuropathol 1993; 12 (suppl 1): S4–5

Trimble K C, Goggins M G, Molloy A M, et al. Vitamin B_{12} deficiency is not a cause of HIV-associated neuropathy. AIDS 1993; 7: 1132–1133

Tross S, Price R W, Navia B, et al. Neuropsychological characterization of the AIDS dementia complex: a preliminary report. AIDS 1988; 2: 81–88

Tyor W R, Glass J D, Griffin J W, et al. Cytokine expression in the brain during AIDS. Ann Neurol 1992; 31: 349–360

Van Gorp W G, Miller E N, Satz P, Visscher B. Neuropsychological performance in HIV-1 immunocompromised patients: a preliminary report. J Clin Exp Neuropsychol 1989; 11: 763–773

Vazeux R, Lacroix-Ciaudo C, Blanche S, et al. Low levels of human immunodeficiency virus replication in the brain tissue of children with severe acquired immunodeficiency syndrome encephalopathy. Am J Pathol 1992; 140: 137–144

Watkins B A, Dorn H H, Kelly W B, et al. Specific tropism of

HIV-1 for microglial cells in primary human brain cultures. Science 1990; 249: 549–553

Wesselingh S L, Power C, Glass J, et al. Intracerebral cytokine messenger RNA expression in acquired immunodeficiency syndrome dementia. Ann Neurol 1993; 33: 576–582

Westervelt P, Gendelman H E, Ratner L. Identification of a determinant within the human immunodeficiency virus 1 surface envelope glycoprotein critical for productive infection of primary monocytes. Proc Nat Acad Sci USA 1991; 88: 3097–3101

Wieraszko A, Li G, Kornecki E, et al. Long term potentiation in the hippocampus induced by platelet activating factor. Neuron 1993; 10: 553–557

Wiley C A, Nelson J A. Role of human immunodeficiency virus and cytomegalovirus in AIDS encephalitis. Am J Pathol 1988; 133: 73–81

Wiley C A, Ge N, Morey M, et al. Golgi impregnation studies of dendritic pathology in HIV encephalitis. J Neuropathol Exp Neurol 1991a; 50: 324

Wiley C A, Masliah E, Morey M, et al. Neocortical damage during HIV infection. Ann Neurol 1991b; 29: 651–657

Wiley C A, Schrier R D, Nelson J A, et al. Cellular localization of human immunodeficiency virus infection within the brains of acquired immune deficiency syndrome patients. Proc Nat Acad Sci USA 1986; 83: 7089–7093

Working Group of the American Academy of Neurology AIDS Task Force. Nomenclature and research case definitions for neurologic manifestations of human immunodeficiency virus-type 1 (HIV-1) infection. Neurology 1991; 41: 778–785

Yarchoan R, Broder S. Anti-retroviral therapy of AIDS and related disorders: general principles and specific development of dideoxynucleosides. Pharmacol Theru 1989; 40: 329–348

Yarchoan R, Berg G, Brouwers P, et al. Response of human immunodeficiency-virus-associated neurological disease to 3'-azido-3'-deoxythymidine. Lancet 1987; i: 132–135

Yarchoan R, Pluda J M, Thomas R V, et al. Long-term toxicity/activity profile of 2',3'-dideoxyinosine in AIDS and AIDS-related complex. Lancet 1990; 336: 526–529

4. HIV infection in children

INTRODUCTION

The impact of HIV infection among infants and children is increasing dramatically in all geographic areas, with huge increases anticipated in the numbers of infected children and of paediatric AIDS cases. Table 4.1 illustrates projections of paediatric HIV infections and AIDS cases from 1992 through 1995 by geographic area. The cumulative number of HIV-infected children from 1992 to 1995 is expected to double (Mann et al 1992), a projection significantly higher than that of the World Health Organization. The increase in the numbers of HIV-infected children results from a parallel increase in the numbers of HIV-infected mothers. Both in the USA and Western Europe, the majority of paediatric HIV infection is acquired vertically from perinatal transmission by mothers infected from injection drug use or from sexual contact with injection drug users (IDUs). In Africa, the major risk factor in mothers is heterosexual sex. Since the introduction of systematic serological screening in many countries, the proportion of paediatric cases with transmission of HIV from contaminated blood is continuing to fall. Fig. 4.1 illustrates the mode of transmission, race and age of paediatric AIDS cases in the USA. In the USA, most paediatric AIDS cases are seen in urban areas with high frequency of injection drug use: New York, Newark, Miami, Los Angeles and Houston. Of 3577 paediatric AIDS cases recorded in Europe up to September 1992, most came from Rumania where the major cause had been the use of unsterilized needles and syringes. With these removed, 80% were born to infected mothers. These numbers can only be the tip of an iceberg. A survey of 443 474 maternal blood samples in the south of England revealed a seroprevalence rate of 0.5 per thousand (Peckham & Giaquinto 1993). Only one in five of these cases came to light by routine reporting. In addition to cases in infants and young children, there appears to be a high and rising rate of HIV infection among adolescents, both from sexual transmission and injection drug use.

Table 4.1 Cumulative paediatric HIV infections by geographic area of affinity

Geographic area of affinity	AIDS cases 1 Jan 1992	AIDS cases 1995 estimate	HIV infections 1 Jan 1992, estimate	HIV infections 1995 estimate	Infections % increase 1992–1995
North America	9000	21 000	16 000	29 000	81
Western Europe	4000	12 000	8000	19 500	144
Latin America	21 500	56 000	40 500	84 000	107
Sub-Saharan Africa	520 500	1 338 500	969 500	20 30 500	109
Caribbean	8000	23 500	16 000	37 500	134
Southeast Asia	9500	40 500	24 000	72 500	202
Total	573 500	1 494 900	1 076 450	2 279 500	112

(After Mann et al 1992)

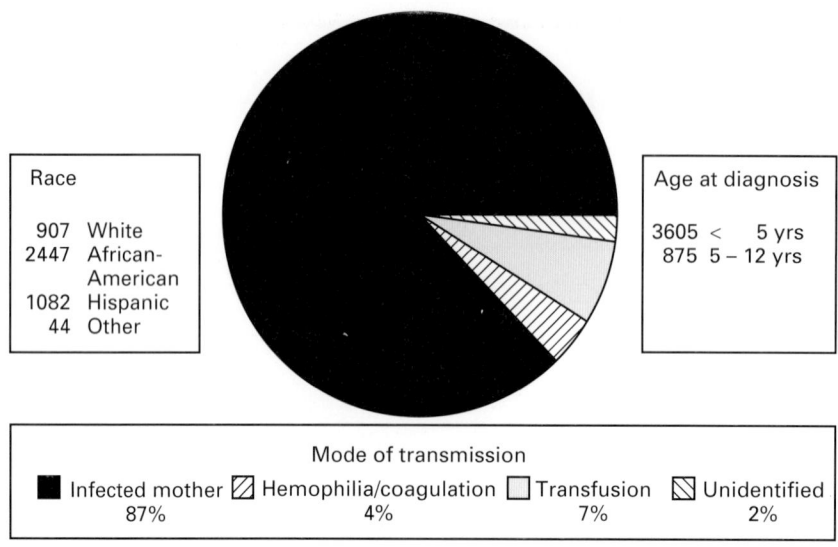

Race

907 White
2447 African-
      American
1082 Hispanic
44 Other

Age at diagnosis

3605 <   5 yrs
875 5 – 12 yrs

Mode of transmission
■ Infected mother ▨ Hemophilia/coagulation ▢ Transfusion ◩ Unidentified
       87%   4%   7%   2%

Fig. 4.1   Mode of transmission, age and sex of paediatric AIDS cases in the USA. (Source: Centers for Disease Control and Prevention. HIV/AIDS Surveillance Report 5: 3–19 (1993)

Evidence exists that HIV may be vertically transmitted intrauterine, intrapartum or during the post-partum period. While it is unclear which of these is the predominant mode of infection, analogies exist with the well-documented intra-partum transmission of hepatitis B. It is believed that at least half of maternal–infant transmission of HIV occurs in the late intrapartum period. Factors influential in perinatal transmission include the mother's stage of HIV infection, with higher rates among women with symptomatic HIV infection, and the co-occurrence of other genital ulcerative diseases. Despite the potential risks of transmission through breast feeding, breast feeding is currently not discouraged in developing countries. Where safe alternatives exist in developed countries, breast feeding is discouraged. Current studies suggest that approximately one-third of infants born to an HIV-infected mother will become infected. ELISA and Western blot assays are not diagnostic in infants younger than 15 months of age because maternal IgG crosses the placenta. There is no reliable IgM response in infancy; however, IgA antibodies may appear as early as 6 months of age (Quinn et al 1991). Some uninfected infants who are seropositive at birth (because of maternal IgG) revert to seronegative during the first year of life. Viral cultures of cord blood or measurement of circulating p24 antigen

are relatively insensitive, but recently polymerase chain reaction (PCR) has been used to detect HIV proviral sequences and detection of HIV proviral DNA or transcribed RNA confirms paediatric infection. In one study PCR was used to detect HIV proviral sequences from blood obtained during the neonatal period. PCR was positive in five of seven infants in whom AIDS later developed, but negative in neonatal samples from nine infants who remained well (Rogers et al 1989). After 18 months of age, antibody status is reliable.

CLINICAL FEATURES OF HIV INFECTION IN CHILDREN

Cellular immunity is impaired in HIV-infected children as in adults; however, the wide range of CD4 counts in infants and children means that symptoms can develop at higher levels of CD4 than in adults. For the same reason, the CD4 count is not as useful prognostically as in adults. Immune activation markers are, however, useful prognostic markers (Siller et al 1993). Elevated dysfunctional immunoglobulins are almost universal and children are predisposed to recurrent bacterial infections with encapsulated organisms (e.g. *Streptococcus pneumoniae*, *Haemophilus influenzae*). The incubation period for perinatally infected children is short with a median age of onset of symptoms around 9 months. In general, children with perinatally acquired HIV infection have a dismal prognosis, most becoming symptomatic before 1 year of age (Scott et al 1989). In one series of 172 children with perinatally acquired HIV infection, symptomatic disease presented at a median age of 8 months and only 21% presented after the age of 2 years.

One major difference between HIV-infected children and adults is in the lower frequency of opportunistic infections such as toxoplasmosis, cryptococcal meningitis, cytomegalovirus (CMV) and progressive multifocal leucoencephalopathy (PML). All of these are common in adults, but are unusual in children, presumably because children have not yet been exposed to these opportunistic organisms. Both CMV retinitis and Kaposi's sarcoma are extremely rare in children, and neoplastic processes, such as systemic lymphoma and primary central nervous system (CNS) lymphoma, are also unusual. By contrast, recurrent bacterial infections and lymphocytic interstitial pneumonitis (LIP) are much more common in children, occurring in 30–60%. Table 4.2 is a summary of the September 1987 surveillance case definition for paediatric HIV infection (less than 13 years of age), and Table 4.3 is the CDC classification system for HIV infection in children. Table 4.4 lists the frequency of paediatric AIDS-defining illnesses in one large series. Progressive encephalopathy, the childhood equivalent of HIV dementia, is one of the most common manifestations of HIV infection in children and in one series progressive encephalopathy developed in

Table 4.2 Summary of the definition of HIV infection in children

Infants and children under 15 months of age with perinatal infection
1. Virus in blood or tissues
   or
2. HIV antibody
   and
   evidence of both cellular and humoral immune deficiency
   and
   one or more categories in Class P-2 (Table 4.3)
3. Symptoms meeting CDC case definition of AIDS

(Reproduced from Center for Disease Control Morbidity and Mortality Weekly Report 1987)

Table 4.3 CDC classification system of HIV in children

Class P-0.   Indeterminate infection
Infants < 15 months born to infected mothers but without definitive evidence of HIV infection or AIDS

Class P-1.   Asymptomatic infection
Subclass A: Normal immune function
Subclass B: Abnormal immune function
Subclass C: Immune function not tested

Class P-2.   Symptomatic infection
Subclass A: Non-specific findings – fever, failure to thrive, generalized lymphadenopathy, hepatomegaly, splenomegaly, enlarged parotid glands, persistent or recurrent diarrhoea
Subclass B: Progressive neurological disease
Subclass C: Lymphoid interstitial pneumonitis
Subclass D: Secondary infectious diseases
   Category D-1: Opportunistic infections in the CDC case definition – bacterial, fungal, parasitic and viral
   Category D-2: Unexplained, recurrent serious bacterial infections
   Category D-3: Other specified secondary infectious diseases
Subclass E: Secondary cancers
   Category E-1: Cancers in the AIDS case definition
   Category E-2: Other malignancies possibly associated with HIV
Subclass F: Other conditions possibly due to HIV infection – hepatitis, cardiomyopathy, nephropathy, haematological disorders

(Reproduced from Center for Disease Control Morbidity and Mortality Weekly Report 1987)

Table 4.4 Most frequent AIDS-indicator diseases in children aged less than 13 years old (1991, USA)[a]

Disease	%
Pneumocystis carinii pneumonia[b]	32
Lymphoid interstitial pneumonia[b]	21
Bacterial infections, multiple or recurrent	18
HIV encephalopathy	14
Candidiasis of oesophagus[b]	14
HIV wasting syndrome	12
Candidiasis of bronchi, trachea or lungs	5
CMV disease (other than retinitis)	5
Mycobacterium avium intracellulare[b]	3
Mycobacterium tuberculosis (disseminated or extrapulmonary)	1
Toxoplasmosis	1
Systemic lymphoma	1
Progressive multifocal leucoencephalopathy	0?
Cryptococcosis (extrapulmonary)	0[c]
Kaposi's sarcoma[b]	0[d]
Primary CNS lymphoma	0[d]

[a] 683 paediatric cases were reported to CDC in 1991;
[b] definite plus presumptive cases; [c] three cases; [d] two cases.

12% as the first AIDS-indicator illness and in 16% at any time (Scott et al 1989).

Common systemic manifestations in children

Lymphocytic interstitial pneumonia

Lymphocytic interstitial pneumonitis (LIP) occurs in about half of children with AIDS. Children develop progressive bilateral diffuse reticular nodular infiltrates, sometimes with hilar adenopathy and hypoxaemia. LIP is generally distinguished from *Pneumocystis carinii* pneumonia (PCP) because the latter is typically more acute in onset with fever, dyspnoea and cough. The prognosis for children with LIP is better than for those who present with opportunistic infections (Janssen et al 1989), with a median survival in one series of 72 months.

Pneumocystis carinii pneumonia

This is the most common opportunistic infection in children and occurs in over 50% of children, usually presenting as an acute interstitial pneumonia. It is usually diagnosed by bronchoscopy with broncho-alveolar lavage with or without transbronchial biopsy. Trimethoprim sulphamethoxazole, as in adults, is used for treatment, but can cause leucopenia, thrombocytopenia, rash and fever.

Other important infections

Other important opportunistic infections in children include disseminated *Mycobacterium avium intracellulare* infection, which is frequently associated with severe weight loss, chronic fevers and debilitation. Candidal oesophagitis, cardiomyopathy, cryptosporidiosis, nephropathy and chronic herpes simplex virus infection are all relatively commonly encountered (Scott et al 1989). Recurrent bacterial infections accounted for 10% of all AIDS indicator diseases in this series and were associated with a median survival of 50 months, substantially longer than encephalopathy.

Neurological manifestations (see Appendix 4 for criteria)

Progressive encephalopathy

In 1985, four children with paediatric AIDS were reported with a progressive encephalopathy with loss of motor milestones or intellectual abilities and weakness with pyramidal tract signs (Epstein et al 1985). Other features included ataxia, acquired microcephaly and myoclonic jerks. Computed tomographic (CT) scans showed severe cerebral atrophy and hydrocephalus ex vacuo, changes that progressed in parallel with neurological decline. Longitudinal developmental assessment of these children showed that many attained early developmental milestones at appropriate ages, but development delay subsequently developed in all (Belman et al 1985) (Fig. 4.2). The syndrome of progressive encephalopathy now appears to be one of the more common manifestations of paediatric AIDS with a dismal mortality: median survival of 11 months in one series (Scott et al 1989). Recent statistics from the CDC show that 13% of children under 15 years of age had encephalopathy as their first AIDS-defining illness (Janssen et al 1992) (Fig. 4.3). The high frequency of neurological involvement developing during symptomatic HIV infection is evident from one prospective study in 68 infants and children, of which 61 (90%) had CNS dysfunction (Belman et al 1988). The most frequent manifestations included acquired microcephaly, cognitive impairment and bilateral pyramidal tract signs (Table 4.5). However, the timing and course of encephalopathy varied and distinct patterns were evident: rapidly progressive, slowly progressive, plateau with later deterioration, and static (Fig. 4.4) (Belman et al 1988). Progressive encephalopathy developed in 42 of 68 (62%) of the children, either as a rapidly or slowly progressive encephalopathy. Figs 4.2 and 4.4 and Table 4.6 demonstrate the course and manifestations of the different patterns of encephalopathy. In this series, 17 children had non-progressive courses with a static encephalopathy, either with cognitive and motor deficits or stable mental retardation. It is unclear whether these children with static deficits will go on later to develop progressive encephalopathy or whether their encephalopathy is from a different aetiology than HIV.

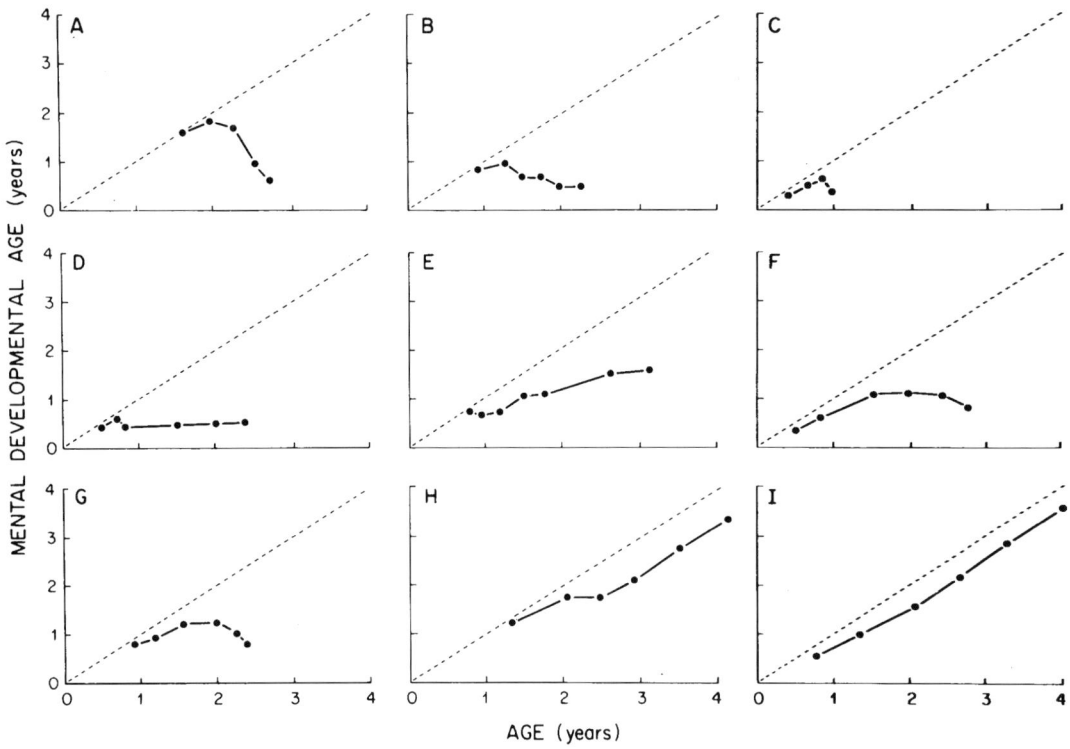

Fig. 4.2 Encephalopathic course of nine patients. Dashed line, 'normal' mental development; dotted line, patient's mental developmental age. (Reproduced from Belman et al 1990.)

Several prospective studies have been completed or are in progress. In one study of HIV-infected infants with perinatal infection, Aylward et al

(1992), using the Bayley Scales of Infant Development, compared 96 infants between 5.5 and 24 months of age (12 seropositive, 45 seroneg-

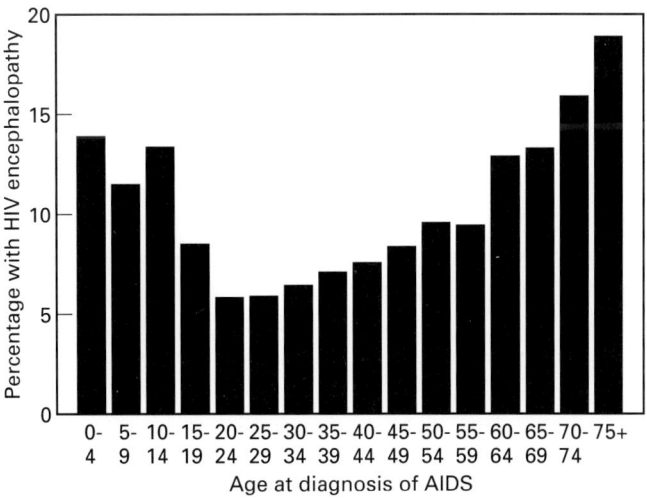

Fig. 4.3 Age distribution of patients reported as having evidence of HIV 'encephalopathy'. (Reproduced from Janssen et al 1992.)

Table 4.5 Clinical features of progressive encephalopathy

Infants and young children	School-age children
Developmental delay	Apathy
Loss of developmental milestones	Social withdrawal
Acquired microcephaly	Increased emotional lability
Progressive motor dysfunction	Attention deficit disorders
Spastic quadriparesis ± pseudobulbar signs	Psychomotor slowing
	Motor involvement
Cerebellar signs	Progressive spastic quadriparesis
Hypomimia	
Mutism	Movement disorders
Extrapyramidal signs	Cerebellar signs
Rigidity	Declining IQ
Dystonic posturing	
Tremor	
Opisthotonos	

Adolescents – Little information available, probably similar to adults

(After Belman 1993)

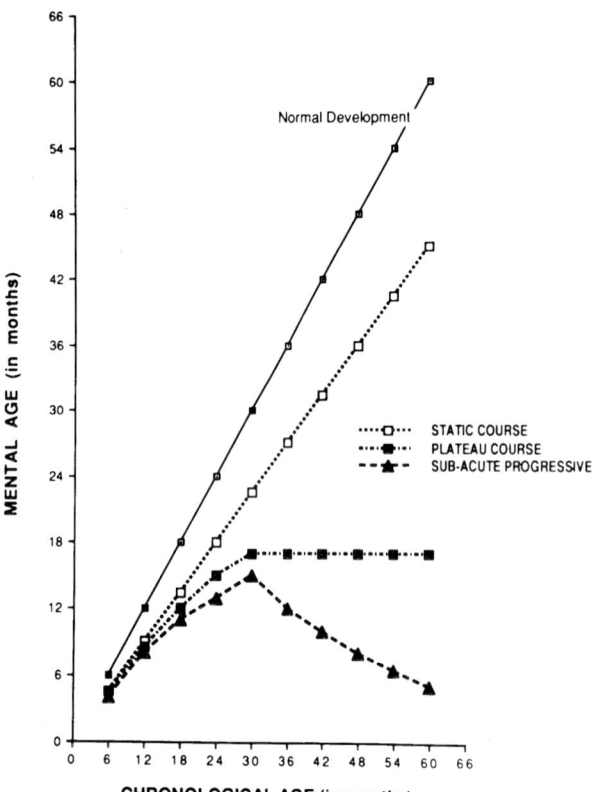

Fig. 4.4 Different encephalopathic courses. (Reproduced from Brouwers et al 1990a.)

ative, 39 seroreverters). The seropositive infants had significantly reduced mental development and psychomotor development compared with the non-infected groups. Interestingly, as in adults, significant motor and cognitive delays due to HIV infection were not apparent in children with relatively few systemic symptoms. The results from this study are in agreement with an earlier study of vertically infected children (Diamond et al 1987). A similar study of children infected via neonatal blood transfusion showed small, but significant, differences in motor speed, visual scanning and cognitive flexibility, but not in overall IQ test scores in infected children (Cohen et al 1991). Other studies have documented a range of neurocognitive abnormalities in severely symptomatic children with paediatric AIDS, including delays in perceptuomotor skills and visuospatial perceptual functioning with relatively preserved verbal skills (Diamond et al 1987, Ultmann et al 1987, Belman et al 1988). In many cases it is difficult to separate the CNS effects of HIV infection from its systemic effects and the systemic effects of chronic illness, cachexia, debilitation, and from those children exposed to drugs in utero or born prematurely (Brouwers et al 1990a).

Laboratory studies in progressive encephalopathy

CT scans of infants and children with HIV-associated progressive encephalopathy (Mintz & Epstein 1992) show variable degrees of generalized cerebral atrophy (85%) and white matter abnormalities. Progressive calcification of basal ganglia or frontal white matter occurs less commonly (15%) (Fig. 4.5). Magnetic resonance imaging (MRI) also shows generalized atrophy with abnormal signal intensity in the white matter and deep grey structures (low signal with calcification). Studies of cerebrospinal fluid (CSF) show non-specific abnormalities as in adults with HIV dementia and, as yet, no predictive markers for subsequent neurological deterioration have been found. P24 antigen is frequently elevated in the CSF of children with progressive encephalopathy (Epstein et al 1987). The pattern of immune activation markers, such as

Table 4.6   Neurological course and manifestations in paediatric HIV infection

	Course (no. of patients)				
	Progressive		Static		
	Progressive (n = 11)	Plateau, progressive (n = 13)	Plateau (n = 18)	Cognitive + motor deficits (n = 10)	Cognitive deficits (n = 7)
Acquired Microcephaly (< 2%)	6	11	14	3	0
Early developmental history					
Normal	5	9	9	1	2
Mild delays	3	1	5	4	3
Moderate to severe delays	1	3	3	5	2
Cognitive deficits					
Profound	10	12	9	0	0
Mild to moderate	NA	NA	2	5	3
Borderline	NA	NA	3	4	4
Pyramidal tract signs					
Mild	1	1	4	6	0
Moderate	2	4	7	4	0
Severe	8	8	5	0	0
Movement disorders	1	4	1	0	0
Ataxia	2	3	1	0	0
Mortality (%)	9 (82)	14 (100)	10 (55)	0	0

(After Belman et al 1988)

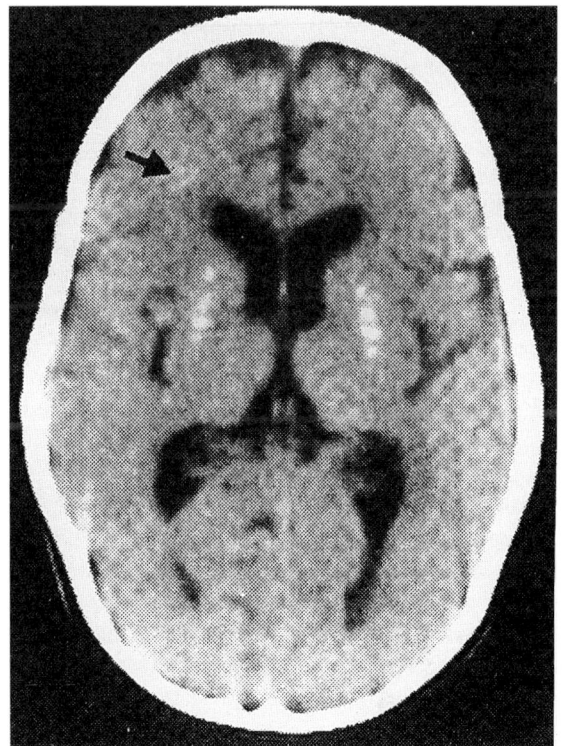

Fig. 4.5   CT scan of child with AIDS showing calcification in the basal ganglia and frontal white matter. (Reproduced from Kendall 1993 with permission of Springer-Verlag.)

β_2-microglobulin and neopterin, or cytokines in CSF have not been as well studied as in adults. Serum tumour necrosis factor correlates with the presence of progressive encephalopathy, although CSF levels in general do not (Mintz et al 1989).

Therapy of progressive encephalopathy

Antiretroviral therapy is the major treatment option in infants and children with progressive encephalopathy. Consistent and dramatic improvement in neurocognitive performance was seen in 13 children treated with continuous intravenous infusion of zidovudine (Pizzo et al 1988) (Fig. 4.6). The doses used in the study ranged from 12 mg/kg/day to 21.6 mg/kg/day and steady-state CSF levels averaged 24% of plasma levels. Improvements in CT-documented atrophy and in regional glucose metabolism were also seen in some children. The clinical improvement occurred within 3–4 weeks, the same time course as in adults (Yarchoan et al 1987) and was sustained during treatment. Neurocognitive improvement was noted at all dosing levels (the

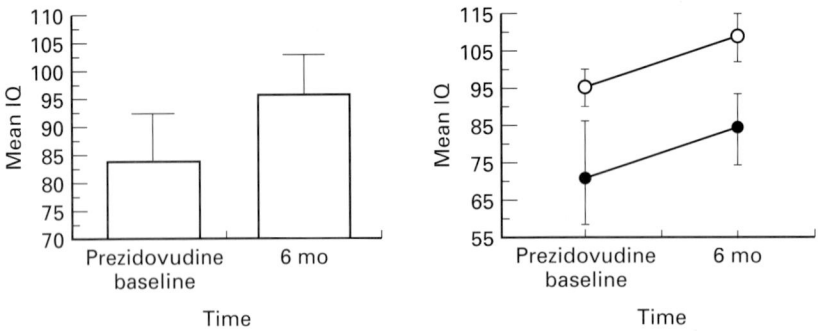

Fig. 4.6 Changes in IQ score pre-zidovudine and after 6 months' treatment. (After Brouwers et al 1990b.)

lowest dosing level was approximately equivalent to an adult oral dose of 1000 mg/day). Unfortunately, the experience with oral zidovudine for treatment of progressive encephalopathy in children has been less encouraging, with the same problems of bone marrow suppression and the development of resistance to zidovudine as in adults. Experience with ddI for treatment of encephalopathy is limited. In one phase I/II study, 43 children with symptomatic HIV infection received oral ddI in varying doses (from 60 to 540 mg/m^2). Peripheral neuropathy was not observed in any of the children. Follow-up neuropsychological testing was available for 34 of 35 children who completed 24 weeks of treatment. There was no change in the mean IQ score after 24 weeks; however, almost one-third (11 of 34) of the children had encephalopathy at baseline with a mean full-scale IQ of 64.6. The IQ score improved in two of the 11 patients with encephalopathy and in four of 14 patients with baseline IQ scores in the normal range. No change was detected in the nine children with IQs above 110 at baseline. A significant correlation was found between the plasma concentration of ddI and the change in IQ score, particularly in those children with normal IQ at baseline (Butler et al 1991). Borrowing from the adult experience, at this point the first-line treatment of progressive encephalopathy in children is high-dose zidovudine (15 mg/kg/day). The standard dosing of ddI for children is based on surface area (200 mg/m^2/day).

MYELOPATHY, NEUROPATHY AND MYOPATHY

Vacuolar myelopathy appears to be very uncommon in children and is rarely, if ever, recognized clinically. As mentioned above, there have been only very infrequent reports of pathologically documented vacuolar myelopathy. One child's cord lesion proved to be due to measles virus infection (Mintz & Epstein 1992). Similarly, peripheral neuropathy, either HIV-associated sensory neuropathy or toxic effects of treatment with dideoxynucleosides, has not been documented in infants or young children. Clearly, the difficulties of assessing peripheral nerve function in children clinically or electrophysiologically have made it difficult to detect subclinical peripheral neuropathy. Nonetheless, it does appear that sensory neuropathies are far less common than in adults. One reason for the difference in incidence in sensory neuropathy could relate to the proposed mechanism in adults. A relatively minor insult such as toxic exposure, e.g. alcohol or solvents, might set the stage for a macrophage-induced damage. In children, the exposure to toxins would be less or perhaps the nerves are less susceptible to this damage. There have been occasional case reports of inflammatory demyelinating polyneuropathy in AIDS, but whether the incidence is truly higher in HIV-infected individuals is unclear (Raphael et al 1991). As in adults, a toxic myopathy with zidovudine has been reported in children (Walter et al 1991).

NEUROPATHOLOGY IN PAEDIATRIC AIDS

The most common neuropathological findings are basal ganglia calcification and the changes of HIV encephalitis (Sharer & Mintz 1993). Basal ganglia calcification occurs more commonly and is more obvious than in adults. In many children it can be shown to develop progressively on serial CT scans (Dickson et al 1989), and is associated with brain atrophy and diffuse myelin pallor. Calcification tends to develop in association with HIV encephalitis and is more common in older children. Occasionally calcification is seen in the neuropil. The mineral deposits are largely due to calcium and iron. They are vascular or perivascular in site and are most common in the globus pallidus, putamen and frontal white matter; the caudate is spared. Histologically, it is detectable in almost all cases (Sharer & Mintz 1993). The HIV encephalitis is similar to that occurring in adults with perivascular infiltrates of macrophages, microglial nodules, multinucleated giant cells, gliosis and diffuse myelin pallor. HIV immunostaining localizes productive HIV infection to the perivascular macrophages or multinucleated giant cells. As in adults, the presence of multinucleated giant cells correlates with the progressive encephalopathy. The similarity with the pathology of HIV-associated dementia motor complex in adults suggests that coinfection is unlikely to be critical to the shared pathology because infections are rare in children. In the spinal cord, the most common finding is corticospinal tract degeneration with myelin pallor in the lateral corticospinal tracts. Vacuolar myelopathy is rare, being absent in one series (Dickson et al 1989) and present in only two of 20 children in another series (Sharer et al 1990). Table 4.7 summarizes the major neuropathological findings.

Cerebrovascular pathology may be more common in children than adults and was noted in nine of 24 cases in one series (Dickson et al 1989). Review of these cases showed that one infant had an intracranial haemorrhage associated with immune thrombocytopenia, two children had smaller haemorrhages, and six had non-haemorrhagic infarctions. Two children had large vessel arteriopathies, one probably associated with

Table 4.7 Neuropathological findings in paediatric HIV infection

Feature	Frequency
Basal ganglia calcification	21/24
HIV encephalitis	15/24
Corticospinal tract degeneration	15/20
Basal ganglia astrogliosis	9/14
White matter astrogliosis	14/14
gp41 immunostaining	4/14

(Reproduced from Dickson et al 1989)

Herpes zoster infection, with eosinophilic intranuclear inclusions resembling Cowdry type II inclusions. The second child had multinucleated cells in the vessel wall associated with focal destruction of the elastic lamina.

CNS OPPORTUNISTIC INFECTIONS

Compared with adults, the frequency of CNS opportunistic processes is relatively low. In contrast to adults, the most common cause of an intracranial mass lesion in infants and young children is primary CNS lymphoma rather than toxoplasmosis. This usually presents with subacute onset of focal neurological signs or seizures (Epstein et al 1988). Radiological features are similar to those occurring in adults with single or multiple contrast-enhancing mass lesions, often with a periventricular location. The common adult infections (toxoplasmosis, cryptococcal meningitis and tuberculous meningitis) are infrequent. CMV encephalitis does occur, although less frequently than in adults, and in one series was identified in two of 24 autopsied paediatric cases (Dickson et al 1989). This contrasts with a frequency in adult autopsies of 20–35% (Cornford et al 1992).

When acute infection with *Toxoplasma gondii* occurs during pregnancy, the parasite can infect the fetus and in the first trimester may cause severe neurological lesions. In a large French study of 746 cases of maternal toxoplasma infection, infection was diagnosed antenatally in 39 of 42 fetuses by fetal blood sampling and amniocentesis. All mothers were treated with spiramycin throughout pregnancy and if fetal infection was demonstrated, pyrimethamine and either sulphadoxine or sulphadiazine were added. Of 15 fetuses with congenital toxoplasmosis who were carried to term, all remained well except for two who had chorioretinitis. Toxoplasmosis is far less common in the USA, but if maternal toxoplasmosis develops during pregnancy, empirical treatment with pyrimethamine and sulphadiazine should be initiated and prenatal diagnosis considered with fetal blood sampling and amniocentesis. Ultrasound can be performed every 2 weeks to monitor fetal development. Long-acting sulphonamides such as sulphadoxine should be avoided because of the risk of toxic epidermal necrolysis (Daffos et al 1988).

The possibility of *Candida*, CMV or PCP should always be considered as treatment is available. Nutritional support may be needed. Steroids may be appropriate for LIP and thrombocytopenia. Immunoglobulin may be prescribed because despite the children's hyperglobulinaemia, they 'look' like children with hypogammaglobulinaemia, with the attendant vulnerability to bacterial infections. Routine immunizations should be given, but not BCG, and only inactivated polio vaccine should be used in the family.

REFERENCES

Aylward E H, Mutz A M, Hutton N, et al. Cognitive and motor development in infants at risk for human immunodeficiency virus. Am J Dis Child 1992; 146: 218–222

Belman A L. AIDS and paediatric neurology. Neurology Clinics 1990; 8: 571–603

Belman A L. HIV-1 related CNS disease in infants and children. American Academy of Neurology 1993.

Belman A L. Diamond G, Dickson D, et al. Pediatric acquired immunodeficiency syndrome. Neurologic syndromes (published erratum appears in Am J Dis Child 1988 May; 142(5): 507). Am J Dis Child 1988; 142: 29–35

Belman A L, Ultmann M H, Horoupian D, et al. Neurological complications in infants and children with acquired immune deficiency syndrome. Ann Neurol 1985; 18: 560–566

Brouwers P, Belman A L, Epstein L. Central nervous system involvement: manifestations and evaluation. In: Pizzo P A, Wilfert C M, editors. Pediatric AIDS: The challenge of HIV infection in infants, children, and adolescents. Baltimore: Williams & Wilkins, 1990a: 318–335

Brouwers P, Moss H, Wolters P, et al. Effect of continuous-infusion zidovudine therapy on neuropsychological functioning in children with symptomatic human immunodeficiency virus infection. J Pediatr 1990b; 117: 980–985

Butler K M, Husson R N, Balis R M, et al. Dideoxyinosine in children with symptomatic human immunodeficiency virus infection. N Engl J Med 1991; 324: 137–144

Centers for Disease Control Morbidity and Mortality Weekly Report. Classification system for human immunodeficiency virus (HIV) infection in children under 13 years of age. MMWR 1987; 36: 225–236

Cohen S E, Mundy T, Karassik B, et al. Neuropsychological functioning in human immunodeficiency virus type 1 seropositive children infected through neonatal blood transfusion. Pediatrics 1991; 88: 58–68

Cornford M E, Holden J K, Boyd M C, et al. Neuropathology of the acquired immune deficiency syndrome (AIDS): report of 39 autopsies from Vancouver, British Columbia. Can J Neurol Sci 1992; 19: 442–452

Daffos F, Forestier F, Capella-Pavlovsky M, et al. Prenatal management of 746 pregnancies at risk for congenital toxoplasmosis. N Engl J Med 1988; 318: 271–275

Diamond G, Kaufman J, Belman A, et al. Characterization of cognitive functioning in a subgroup of children with congenital HIV infection. Arch Clin Neuropsychol 1987; 2: 245–256

Dickson D W, Belman A L, Park Y D, et al. Central nervous system pathology in pediatric AIDS: an autopsy study. APMIS Suppl 1989; 8: 40–57

Epstein L G, DiCarlo F J, Joshi V V, et al. Primary lymphoma of the central nervous system in children with acquired immunodeficiency syndrome. Pediatrics 1988; 82: 355–363

Epstein L G, Goudsmit J, Paul D A, et al. Expression of human immunodeficiency virus in cerebrospinal fluid of children with progressive encephalopathy. Ann Neurol 1987; 21: 397–401

Epstein L G, Sharer L R, Joshi V V, et al. Progressive encephalopathy in children with acquired immune deficiency syndrome. Ann Neurol 1985; 17: 488–496

Janssen R S, Nwanyanwu O C, Selik R M, Stehr-Green J K. Epidemiology of human immunodeficiency virus encephalopathy in the United States. Neurology 1992; 42: 1472–1476

Janssen R S, Saykin A J, Cannon L, et al. Neurological and neuropsychological manifestations of HIV-1 infection: association with AIDS-related complex but not asymptomatic HIV-1 infection. Ann Neurol 1989; 26: 592–600

Kendall B E. In: Scaravilli F, editor. Neuropathology of HIV infection. London: Springer-Verlag, 1993

Mann J M, Tarantola D J M, Netter T W. AIDS in the world. Cambridge, MA: Harvard University Press, 1992

Mintz M, Epstein L G. Neurologic manifestations of paediatric acquired immunodeficiency syndrome: clinical features and therapeutic approaches. Sem Neurol 1992; 12: 51–56

Mintz M, Rapaport R, Oleske J M, et al. Elevated serum levels of tumor necrosis factor are associated with progressive encephalopathy in children with acquired immunodeficiency syndrome. Am J Dis Child 1989; 143: 771–774

Peckham C, Giaquinto C. HIV infection in children. In: Adler M W, editor. ABC of AIDS, 3rd Edn. London: BMJ Publishing Group, 1993: 57–62

Pizzo P A, Eddy J, Falloon J, et al. Effect of continuous intravenous infusion of zidovudine (AZT) in children with symptomatic HIV infection. N Engl J Med 1988; 319: 889–896

Quinn T C, Kline R L, Halsey N, et al. Early diagnosis of perinatal HIV infection by detection of viral-specific IgA antibodies. JAMA 1991; 266: 3439–3442

Raphael S A, Price M L, Lischner H W, et al. Inflammatory demyelinating polyneuropathy in AIDS. J Pediatr 1991; 118: 242–245

Rogers M F, Ou C-Y, Rayfield M, et al. Use of the polymerase chain reaction for early detection of the proviral sequences of human immunodeficiency virus in infants born to seropositive mothers. N Engl J Med 1989; 320: 1649–1654

Scott G B, Hutto C, Makuch R W, et al. Survival in children with perinatally acquired human immunodeficiency virus type 1 infection. N Engl J Med 1989; 321: 1791–1796

Sharer L R, Dowling P C, Michaels J, et al. Spinal cord disease in children with HIV-1 infection: a combined molecular biological and neuropathological study. Neuropathol Appl Neurobiol 1990; 16: 317–331

Sharer L R, Mintz M. Neuropathology of AIDS in children. In: Scaravilli F, editor. The neuropathology of AIDS. Berlin: Springer-Verlag, 1993: 201–214

Siller L, Martin N L, Kostuchenko P, et al. Serum levels of soluble CD8, neopterin, beta-2-microglobulin and P24 antigen as indicators of disease progression in children with AIDS on zidovudine therapy. AIDS 1993; 7: 369–373

Ultmann M H, Diamond G W, Ruff H A, et al. Developmental abnormalities in children with acquired immunodeficiency syndrome (AIDS): a follow-up study. Int J Neurosci 1987; 32: 661–667

Walter E B, Drucker R P, McKinney R E, Wilfert C M. Myopathy in human immunodeficiency virus-infected children receiving long-term zidovudine therapy. Pediatrics 1991; 119: 152–155

Yarchoan R, Berg G, Brouwers P, et al. Response of human immunodeficiency virus associated neurological disease to 3'-azido-3'-deoxy-thymidine. Lancet 1987; 1: 132–135

5. Spinal cord disease

INTRODUCTION

It is difficult to obtain accurate figures for the frequency of spinal cord disease during HIV infection. Nonetheless, several clinical series have demonstrated that it is frequent enough and its causes sufficiently varied to warrant separate discussion. Spinal cord disease is commonly found at autopsy. Petito found histological abnormalities in 50% of 178 cords (Table 5.1) (Petito et al 1985, Petito 1993), but clinical manifestations are unusual. For example, McArthur (1987) diagnosed a cord lesion in only 13 of 186 (7%) referred patients. Several different causes of myelopathy need to be considered as summarized in Table 5.2.

HIV-ASSOCIATED MYELITIS

A subacute self-limiting myelitis may complicate seroconversion (Denning et al 1987), the patient developing a temporary paraparesis. This resembles other acute viral myelitides, and is only diagnosed if HIV antigenaemia and viraemia are sought, because HIV antibodies may be negative. Antiviral therapy should probably be instituted, but the prognosis appears good, as for other seroconversion-related neurological conditions (Chapter 2). In the one case described, no details of pathological involvement are given, but perhaps this is analogous to the transient encephalopathy that sometimes accompanies HIV seroconversion.

HERPES GROUP MYELITIDES

The differential diagnosis of such a myelitis when it occurs at a later stage includes opportunistic herpes viruses (Herpes zoster, cytomegalovirus (CMV), Herpes simplex), which may all be responsible for a spinal cord syndrome (Britton et al 1985, Tucker et al 1985). Reactivation of varicella zoster virus (VZV), for example, is common in AIDS and usually produces the typical dermatomal vesicular rash of herpes zoster (shingles). Rarely, a myelitis follows 1–3 weeks later. This has also been described in the pre-AIDS era in elderly or immunosuppressed

Table 5.1 Main types of spinal cord disease in 178 patients with AIDS

	No. of patients
Vacuolar myelopathy	51
Microglial nodule myelitis	26
Herpes myelitis	14
Other infections	11
Lymphoma	4

(Reproduced from Petito 1993 with permission of Springer Verlag, London Ltd.)

Table 5.2 Differential diagnosis of myelopathy in AIDS

Primary HIV	Seroconversion illness
	Vacuolar myelopathy
Other infections	Epidural abscess
	Intraspinal bacterial
	Syphilis
	HTLV-I
	M. tuberculosis
	Herpes group
Vitamin deficiency	B_{12} (subacute combined)
	E
Structural	Spondylotic disease
	Herniated disc
	Epidural haemorrhage
	Intramedullary haemorrhage

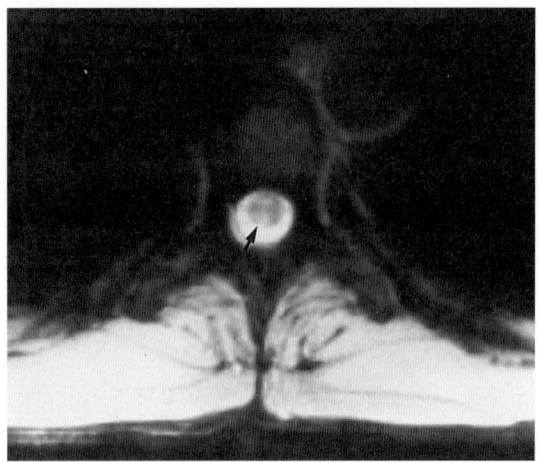

Fig. 5.1 High signal in the spinal cord in the high cervical region on T2-weighted MRI in a case of herpes zoster myelitis. (Reproduced from Grant et al 1993.)

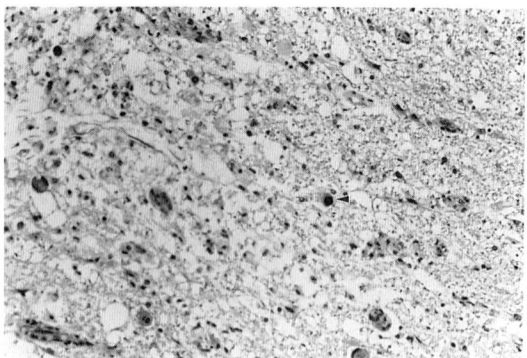

Fig. 5.2 Histological appearance of CMV myelitis with cytomegalic cell arrowed.

patients. The neurological deficit is said to begin with ipsilateral motor signs followed by spinothalamic and inconstantly posterior column damage (Devinsky et al 1991). Most patients end up with paraplegia, or in a personal case with quadriplegia (Fig. 5.1). The pathology combines inflammation and vasculitic infarction, which may be haemorrhagic, with local infection of oligodendroglia and local demyelination, and necrosis. Petito found signs of zoster myelitis in two of 178 spinal cords. Acyclovir is used for treatment of presumptive herpes simplex or zoster myelitis in the same doses as used for treatment of herpes simplex encephalitis: 30 mg/kg/day intravenously for 10–14 days. The response is variable and depends on whether haemorrhagic infarction has occurred. The diagnosis is based on identification of existing or previous skin lesions, signs of inflammation in the cord from cerebrospinal fluid (CSF) and on magnetic resonance imaging (MRI), and demonstration of herpes simplex or zoster in CSF or cord tissue by culture, polymerase chain reaction (PCR), serology (intrathecal synthesis) or immunostaining.

CMV myelitis (Fig. 5.2) generally occurs only in patients with advanced HIV infection with CD4 counts less than 50. CMV myelitis (Tucker et al 1985) should be suspected in patients with viraemia or retinitis and a rapidly progressive ascending myelopathy. Clues to its recognition

and distinction from vacuolar myelopathy are the frequently inflammatory CSF with pleocytosis and positive CMV cultures. Not infrequently, radiculitis and myelitis occur together. MRI may show enhancement of nerve roots and features of inflammation in the cord (Fig. 5.3). These patients have a necrotizing myelitis with foci of demyelination, and may show signs of a vasculitis. Microglial nodules due to CMV infection may be a coincidental autopsy finding in the cord, as in the brain, in patients with no related clinical problem. Herpes simplex virus (HSV) can cause the same presentation, and again be detected in the CSF, which may show little in the way of pleocytosis. HSV in the cord is usually a co-infection with CMV (Petito 1993). Necrosis and Cowdry type A inclusions suggest the HSV is causative. In situations where CMV and/or HSV could be implicated, acyclovir or ganciclovir should be prescribed in the hope that the neurological deficit can be limited.

OTHER INFECTIONS

A rare cause of myelitis is syphilis. One published patient developed a subacute paraplegia with a thoracic 'level'. The CSF showed a mild pleocytosis and positive fluorescent treponemal antibody test (FTA). The leg weakness recovered dramatically on penicillin (Berger 1992).

Another possible cause for a progressive paraparesis is co-infection with HTLV-I. Antibodies to this virus were detected in a large number of patients in Martinique who were suffering from

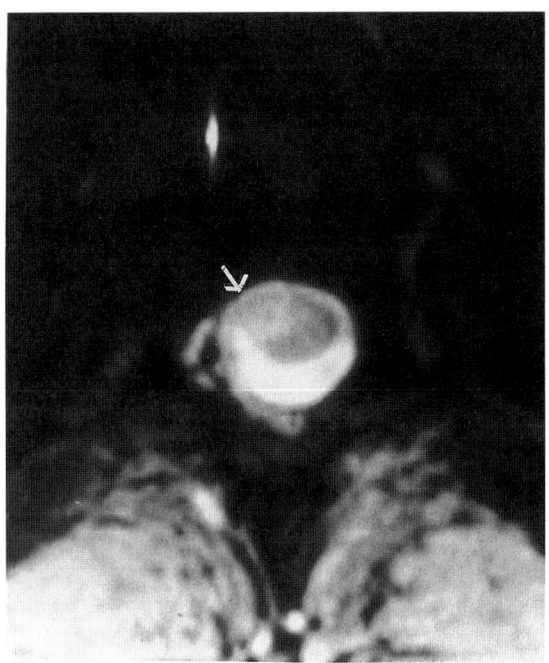

Fig. 5.3 High signal in the cord on T2-weighted MRI in a patient with myelitis attributed to CMV.

tropical spastic paraparesis (Gessain et al 1985), and its causative role was confirmed by virus detection in the CSF and circulating lymphocytes. In the tropics the clinical picture is usually of a slowly evolving spastic paraplegia, with back pain, paraesthesiae and sphincter disturbance. In the USA, pain and paraesthesiae are not prominent and the rate of progression can be more aggressive (Sheremata et al 1992). The modes of transmission include mother to child, either across the placenta or via breast milk, by blood transfusion, intravenous drug use or by sexual contact. Although the clinical picture highlights cord damage, MRI shows some white matter involvement in the hemispheres, and nerve conduction studies show a subclinical peripheral neuropathy. The neuropathological features are of an inflammatory necrotic myelitis. Several cases of dual infection have been described (Berger et al 1991), including one in whom steroids produced a clinical response (McArthur et al 1990). HTLV-I antibodies should be sought in HIV-infected individuals who develop a paraparesis of unknown cause, especially if spasticity and pain are clinically prominent and the patient has no dementia

and is not immunosuppressed. The clinical spectrum of illness accompanying HTLV-I infection in places like Martinique and the Caribbean in non-HIV-infected patients includes peripheral and radicular syndromes and myositis, so HTLV-I should perhaps be considered as a co-pathogen in a wider context than just a myelopathy (Cruickshank et al 1992).

OTHER SPINAL CORD PRESENTATIONS

More acute spinal cord presentations, for example with a sudden painless paraplegia, will be suggestive of cord infarction, which has been described in patients with vasculitis. Recovery would not be expected (Gray & Gherardi 1990).

Pain may accompany any of the viral myelitides, but should always be considered a possible indication of cord compression. Compressive lesions are most likely to be lymphomas (Jordan et al 1985), but plasmacytoma (Snider et al 1983), glioma (Weill et al 1987), central disc prolapse and epidural abscesses due to bacteria, fungi or mycobacteria (Doll et al 1987) are all possible. Intramedullary toxoplasmosis (Herskovitz et al 1989) and tuberculosis (Woolsey et al 1988) have also been described. Investigation by MRI or myelography is needed to reveal treatable options such as lymphoma, tuberculous (Fig. 5.4) or toxoplasma abscesses. Surgery may be needed before the precise diagnosis is clear.

The incidence of spinal epidural abscess seems to be rising, at least in intravenous drug users (IVDU) (Koppel et al 1988), though there is no direct evidence that HIV infection is responsible. Darouiche et al (1992) reviewed 43 cases from 1981 to 1991, and found only one with HIV infection. The classical clinical presentation (Danner & Hartman 1987) is of a febrile patient with back pain and radicular pain who develops a paraparesis over 48–72 hours, though a subacute course over a month or so is also encountered. The examination may reveal spinal tenderness in a patient with systemic illness. The diagnostic procedure of choice is a gadolinium-enhanced MR examination, although plain radiographs and computed tomography (CT) may reveal osteomyelitis and paravertebral masses. In the presence

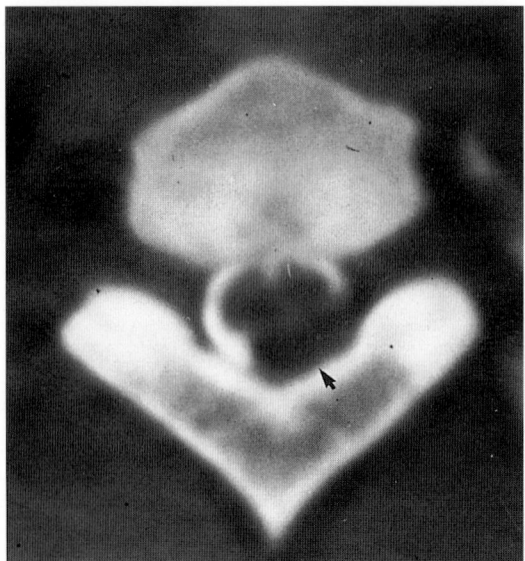

Fig. 5.4   Tuberculoma causing paraparesis in a patient with tuberculomatous meningitis.

of meningitis, CT myelography may be more discriminatory (Teman 1992). CSF examination may be hazardous if the abscess lies in the path of the needle, and the findings of an elevated protein and pleocytosis are not definitive. Positive cultures from the CSF are only obtained in some 20% according to Darouiche et al (1992). The abscess usually extends over three or four vertebrae. The most common organism is *Staphylococcus* of haematogenous spread. Gram-negative organisms such as *Mycobacterium tuberculosis* and *Nocardia* (Siao et al 1989) are all possible, especially in the context of IVDU. Surgical drainage is usually needed, though patients with little or no neurological deficit can be treated conservatively (with intravenous antibiotics) with close clinical and MRI monitoring. Antibiotic regimens are initially chosen to cover staphylococci and gram-negative organisms until blood and/or needle biopsy or surgical cultures are available. An algorithm for management is advanced by Koppel et al (1988). Steroids may be relatively contraindicated because Danner and Hartman (1987) noted a poor outcome in their presence. The prognosis for neurological recovery is critically dependent on the severity at presentation and the rapidity of institution of definitive therapy. Unless drainage is obtained whilst there is no more than moderate deficit, recovery is unlikely.

There is anecdotal evidence that patients with AIDS do particularly badly.

Relapsing and remitting cord disease with associated optic neuritis has been described with evidence that the pathological process was probably akin to multiple sclerosis occurring in a patient shortly after seroconversion (Berger et al 1992) (see also discussion in Chapter 2, p. 22).

VACUOLAR MYELOPATHY (Table 5.3)

Vacuolar myelopathy was initially recognized in 1985 by Petito et al and has been included as part of the AIDS dementia complex by some because dementia and vacuolar myelopathy frequently co-exist. In fact, it appears that vacuolar myelopathy is a discrete disorder that may present without dementia, and whose course does not always parallel cognitive decline. While rare as an initial presentation of AIDS, several patients have developed vacuolar myelopathy as their initial AIDS-defining illness. More typically, as with dementia, the myelopathy develops after AIDS, and has been estimated to clinically affect 5–10% of AIDS patients (McArthur 1987). The clinical expression of vacuolar myelopathy clearly underestimates its frequency because vacuolar myelopathy is present at autopsy in up to 47% of adult AIDS patients (3% in children).

The appropriate clinical syndrome is thus much rarer than the pathological lesion at autopsy, although Petito (1993) has suggested that some related clinical findings occur in as many as 60% of those with an autopsy diagnosis of vacuolar myelopathy. It is possible that the clinical signs are being missed in terminal patients or are being misinterpreted as signs of the encephalopathy that the patient also has.

Table 5.3   Definition of HIV-related myelopathy

1. Acquired abnormality in lower limbs (weakness, incoordination) out of proportion to upper limbs confirmed by examination (weakness, ataxia, hyperreflexia, extensor plantars, ± sensory changes) ± sphincter problem
2. Severe enough to need at least unilateral support for walking
3. Any cognitive impairment is mild and does not affect activities of daily living
4. No other cause after laboratory investigation

(From Janssen et al 1991)

Symptomatic patients (Table 5.4) develop a progressive paraparesis with sensory ataxia and sphincter impairment over the course of a few weeks or months. Typically, the onset of the myelopathy is much slower than CMV myelitis. The examination reveals spasticity and hyperreflexia in the lower limbs particularly. The patient's ataxia is usually related to overt joint position sense loss. A sensory neuropathy (see Chapter 6) frequently accompanies vacuolar myelopathy. When the weakness is mild there is a real problem in determining whether the long tract signs are due to spinal cord or cerebral pathology. This is especially true in the presence of dementia and hyperreflexia including primitive cranial reflexes such as the pout and palmomental reflexes. A telltale sensory level is unusual.

Neurological evaluation within 3 months of death in 56 patients with pathologically confirmed vacuolar myelopathy and 48 control patients without vacuolar myelopathy has been reported by Dal Pan et al (1992). Signs and symptoms of a myelopathy were detected in 15 of 56 patients with vacuolar myelopathy. The most frequent clinical features included lower limb weakness in all 15 (100%), lower limb spasticity in 53%, sensory ataxia in 20%, gait spasticity in 60% and knee hyperreflexia in 93%. Other frequent findings were distal sensory neuropathy in eight patients, with ankle areflexia or hyporeflexia. A discrete sensory level was found only in two patients and only one had bowel and bladder incontinence. Onset of symptoms ranged from 3 to 16 weeks before diagnosis of myelopathy. Thoracic spine MRI was normal in four individuals in whom it was performed. Symptomatic myelopathy was present in none of the patients with grade I vacuolar myelopathy, 5 of 26 with grade II and 10 of 13 with grade III. HIV dementia, as well as other AIDS-related infections

and neoplastic nervous system disorders, occurred with equal frequency; however, distal sensory neuropathy was more frequent among patients with vacuolar myelopathy.

The gross appearance of the cord at autopsy is unremarkable, or shows a little pallor on myelin stains. The histological picture (see Appendix 3 for criteria) is striking, however, and shows spongy degeneration and intramyelin vacuolation affecting principally the dorsal and lateral parts of the cord (Fig. 5.5). The gracile tract is particularly affected. The vacuoles contain lipid-laden macrophages (Fig. 5.6), and this feature is necessary to exclude artefactual vacuolation. Tyor et al (1993) have demonstrated intense macrophage infiltration and evidence of activation, and cytokine levels are elevated. At the ultrastructural level the vacuoles can be seen to be an expansion of periaxonal spaces. The damage is limited to myelin of central origin with an abrupt change where central and peripheral myelin meet at the root entry zone. Axons are only affected in late stages, or in areas of severe damage. There is a variable amount of macrophage infiltration and some reactive astrocytosis dependent on the severity. Macrophages are frequently intravacuolar. Many macrophages express both class I and class II MHC antigens and are interleukin-1 (IL-1) and tumour necrosis factor-alpha (TNF-α) positive suggesting immune activation with cytokine elaboration. Electron microscopy reveals the presence of macrophage/ microglial processes intercalated between the axons and myelin

Table 5.4 Clinical features of vacuolar myelopathy

- 10–20% of AIDS patients clinically affected
- Usually advanced immune deficiency
- Can be presenting manifestation
- Hyperreflexia in legs, spastic weakness, slowed rapid alternating movements
- Sensory ataxia, no sensory level
- Accompanying neuropathy and dementia

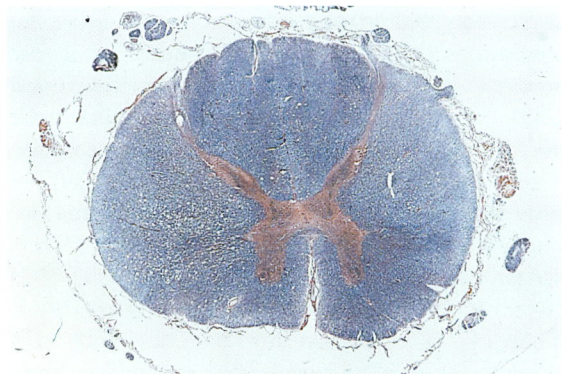

Fig. 5.5 Vacuolation (particularly of lateral columns) in a case of vacuolar myelopathy.

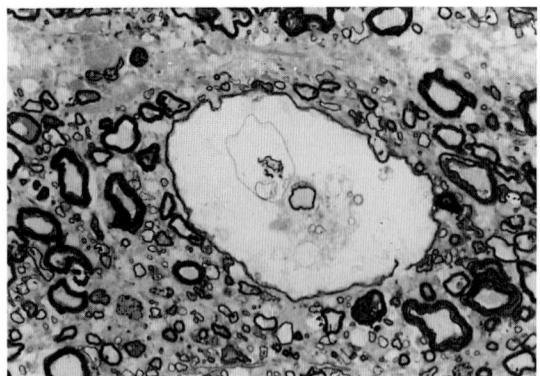

Fig. 5.6   Histological appearances of the spinal cord affected by vacuolar myelopathy. A large vacuole contains a macrophage proving that the cavity is not post-mortem artefact.

sheaths (Baumrind N, unpublished observations). Such activated macrophages are found in patients without pathological evidence of vacuolar myelopathy, suggesting their activation precedes the development of vacuoles and may therefore be primarily involved in the pathogenesis of the disease. Both ascending and descending tracts are involved. The early changes are symmetrical, but later it is not unusual to see quite marked asymmetry of the pathology in the lateral columns. Some reports have noted that the major changes are in the mid to lower thoracic cord (Petito et al 1985). A thoracic predilection has also been noted for Simian immunodeficiency virus infection in the macaque and for HTLV-I.

The condition has been called HIV-associated myelopathy as no opportunistic pathogen has been identified in affected cases, and HIV can sometimes (but not always) be detected in the sections (Ho et al 1985). Multinucleated giant cells, characteristic of HIV encephalitis, are occasionally detectable; micronodules are rare. The search for HIV by PCR in the cord has often proved negative (Petito 1993), or only macrophage infection has been detectable; HIV RNA is sometimes detected in macrophages in the cord (Rosenblum et al 1989, Weisner et al 1990). There is a tendency for patients with this myelopathy to have peripheral neuropathy; however, dementia seems to occur as a separate disorder (Dal Pan et al 1993). Rare individuals

have the same histological changes in the cerebral white matter.

The role of HIV in this syndrome is thus a little uncertain. Kamin and Petito (1991) in a survey of over 3000 autopsies found a few examples of vacuolar myelopathy in non-AIDS cases. Some of the related conditions such as systemic lupus erythematosus, leukaemia, cancer and renal transplantation might suggest an immunological basis. Toxins such as triethyl tin can also produce vacuolation. Intramyelin sheath swelling is also seen in vitamin B_1, B_{12} and folate deficiency. Sharer et al (1986), noting its rareness in children, suggested that an opportunistic infection might be responsible. Other retroviruses also cause myelopathies, e.g. murine retrovirus (Gardner 1985) and HTLV-I is responsible for human tropical spastic paraplegia (Bhigjee et al 1991). However, the pathology of the cord in tropical spastic paraplegia (Table 5.5) differs, with prominent inflammation, necrosis and demyelination in grey and white matter, and serological evidence makes it highly unlikely that HTLV-I is responsible for vacuolar myelopathy in AIDS (Brew et al 1989).

The pattern of cord changes in AIDS, by contrast, closely resembles that of subacute combined degeneration of the cord due to vitamin B_{12} deficiency. However, vitamin B_{12} levels are usually normal, though some are at the lower limit, and occasionally the patient has frank B_{12} deficiency (Harriman et al 1989) perhaps due to malabsorption, for example due to cryptosporidiosis (Ho et al 1985). Harriman's data suggested

Table 5.5   Comparison of TSP/HAM and vacuolar myelopathy

TSP/HAM	Vacuolar myelopathy
Spastic paraparesis	Spastic paraparesis
Course: years	Course: months
No dementia	Associated dementia: 60%
Normal/high CD4	Low CD4/immune suppression
CSF: pleocytosis 20–100	CSF: normal/slight pleocytosis
Intrathecal synthesis of anti-HTLV-I	Intrathecal synthesis of anti-HIV
Pathology: inflammatory myelitis	Pathology: spongiform change periaxonal vacuolation

TSP/HAM, tropical spastic paraplegia/HTLV-I associated myelopathy.

that 7% of HIV-infected subjects and 15% of those with AIDS had low serum B_{12} levels, and Kieburtz et al (1991) found low levels or an abnormal Schilling test in 10 of 49 patients in a HIV neurology clinic. They thought that some had malabsorption, but in others this was not the explanation. Others have suggested that HIV infection in some way disturbs methyl group metabolism mimicking the metabolic lesion of B_{12} deficiency, so B_{12} levels would not necessarily be crucial to the development of clinical abnormality. Surtees et al (1990) suggested that there may be a disturbance of methylation in the HIV-infected nervous system of children. Their data (Table 5.6) show abnormal levels of methylation products in the CSF of children with neurological manifestations of AIDS. Keating et al (1991) measured S-adenosylmethionine (SAM) and S-adenosylhomocysteine (SAH) in the CSF of 20 HIV-seropositive and 30 HIV-negative subjects. The ratio reflects the activity of methionine synthase activity, which is inhibited by folate and B_{12} deficiency, and a low ratio would be expected to lead to hypomethylation of myelin components. The SAM/SAH ratio was indeed lower in the HIV+ group (2.7 ± 1.0 vs. 7.6 ± 3.4, $p < 0.001$) and is also low in B_{12} deficiency. The role of B_{12} in the methylation pathway suggests a possible link-up with the histological findings. However, a recent study of cobalamin metabolites in serum from patients with pathologically confirmed vacuolar myelopathy showed no differences in cobalamin or folate metabolites. This suggests that alterations or deficiencies in cobalamin are not directly implicated in the development of vacuolar myelopathy (Dal Pan et al 1993).

Generally, investigations can be limited, especially if the development of the myelopathy is

slow and there are no indications of a sensory level or of herpes group infection. Standard spine MRI is usually normal and does not need to be performed except where the onset of features is atypical. Recently, using surface coils and specialized acquisition parameters, Santosh et al (1993) have been able to demonstrate tract changes in vacuolar myelopathy (Fig. 5.7) and eventually, with further refinements in MRI technology, the diagnosis may be confirmed radiologically. Vitamin B_{12} and folate levels should be obtained and serologies for syphilis and HTLV-I checked. CSF studies have been similar to those in HIV dementia, usually showing non-specific abnormalities of protein and immunoglobulin elevation with little or no pleocytosis. Again, in a typical or mild case, CSF examination is not mandatory. Evoked potentials yield non-specific abnormalities that can be difficult to interpret in the presence of coincidental peripheral neuropathy or disease of the cerebral white matter. They are more helpful in assessing patients with symptoms suspicious of a myelopathy in whom there are indefinite clinical signs and the organic nature of their complaints is in doubt.

Patients with this type of cord disease generally have advanced HIV infection so antiviral treatment is likely to have already been started. If not, it is indicated, though there are no formal studies of the response of spinal cord signs and symptoms. Vitamin B_{12} may be given, especially if

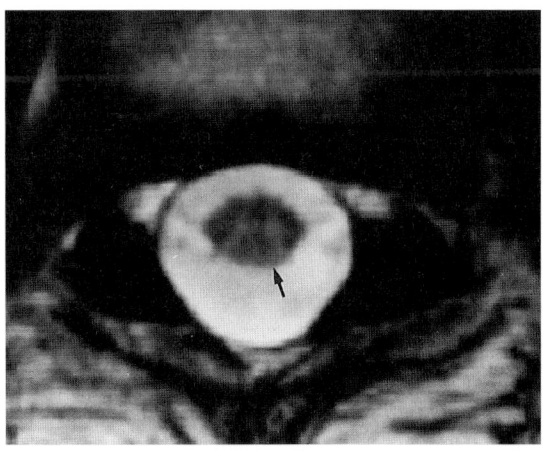

Fig. 5.7 T2-weighted MRI showing abnormal signal from the gracile tracts in an AIDS patient.

Table 5.6 Levels of 5-methyltetrahydrofolate (MTHF), methionine (METH) and S-adenosyl methionine (SAM) in the CSF

	HIV	Control	p value
SAM (nmol/l)	118 ± 36	247 ± 14	<0.001
METH (μmol/l)	2.9 ± 1.1	4.4 ± 0.3	<0.1
MTHF (nmol/l)	26 ± 7	90 ± 5	<0.001

(Reproduced from Surtees et al 1990)

serum levels are at the low end of the normal range. Physiotherapy and medication for spasticity are important in maintaining mobility, but the prognosis seems to be poor with progressive paralysis.

Children are rarely affected. Their cords at autopsy may show delayed myelination, which may contribute to the pyramidal signs often encountered in paediatric AIDS (Dickson et al 1989).

MANAGEMENT PLAN

The finding of a spastic paraplegia requires spinal imaging to exclude epidural abscesses, tuberculosis and lymphoma. In their absence the CSF must be examined for evidence of herpes virus and syphilis. Vitamin B_{12} and folate levels in the blood should be requested and serology for HTLV-I considered. If vacuolar myelopathy looks likely, MRI of the brain and neurophysiological studies of subclinical neuropathy may provide some support for the diagnosis. In the absence of treatable pathology, antiretrovirals and B_{12} should supplement symptomatic management of spasticity and sphincter impairment.

REFERENCES

Berger J R. Spinal cord syphilis associated with human immunodeficiency virus infection: a treatable myelopathy. Am J Med 1992; 92: 101–103

Berger J R, Raffanti S, Svenningsson A, et al. The role of HTLV in HIV-1 neurologic disease. Neurology 1991; 41: 197–202

Berger J R, Tornatore C, Major E O, et al. Relapsing and remitting human immunodeficiency virus-associated leukoencephalopathy. Ann Neurol 1992; 31: 34–38

Bhigjee A I, Wiley C A, Wachsman W, et al. HTLV-I-associated myelopathy: clinicopathological correlation with localisation of provirus to spinal cord. Neurology 1991; 41: 1990–1992

Brew B J, Hardy W, Zuckerman E, et al. AIDS related vacuolar myelopathy is not associated with coinfection by human T-lymphotropic virus type 1. Ann Neurol 1989; 26: 679–681

Britton D B, Mesa-Tejada R, Fenoglio C M, et al. A new complication of AIDS: thoracic myelitis caused by herpes simplex virus. Neurology 1985; 35: 1071–1074

Cruickshank J K, Corbin D O C, Bucher B, Vernant J C. HTLV-1 and neurological disease. Baillière's Clin Neurol 1992; 1: 61–81

Dal Pan G, Glass J, Zeidman S, McArthur J. Atypical HIV-associated myelopathy: diagnosis by cord biopsy (abstract). Neurology 1992; 42 (suppl): 257

Dal Pan G J, Allen R H, Glass J D, et al. Cobalamin (vitamin B_{12}) dependent metabolism is not altered in HIV-1-associated vacuolar myelopathy. Am Nerv Ass Oct 18–20, 1993, Boston

Danner R L, Hartman B J. Update of spinal epidural abscess: 35 cases and review of the literature. Rev Infect Dis 1987; 9: 265–274

Darouiche R O, Hamill R J, Greenberg S B, et al. Bacterial spinal epidural abscess: review of 43 cases and literature survey. Medicine 1992; 71: 369–385

Denning D W, Anderson J, Rudge P, Smith H. Acute myelopathy associated with primary infection with human immunodeficiency virus. Br Med J 1987; 294: 143–144

Devinsky O, Cho E-S, Petito C K, Price R W. Herpes zoster myelitis. Brain 1991; 114: 1181–1196

Dickson D W, Belman A L, Park Y D, et al. Central nervous system pathology in pediatric AIDS: an autopsy study. APMIS 1989; S8: 40–57

Doll D C, Yarbro J W, Phillips K, et al. Mycobacterial spinal cord abscess with an ascending polyneuropathy. Ann Intern Med 1987; 106: 333–334

Gardner M B. Retroviral spongiform polioencephalomyelpathy. Rev Infect Dis 1985; 7: 99–110

Gessain A, Vernant J A, Maurs L, et al. Antibodies to HTLV-1 in patients with tropical spastic paraparesis. Lancet 1985; ii: 407–409

Grant A D, Fox J D, Brink N S, Miller R F. Detection of varicella-zoster virus DNA using the polymerase chain reaction in an immunocompromised patient with transverse myelitis secondary to herpes zoster. Genitourin Med 1993; 69: 273–275

Gray F, Gherardi R. Lesions of the spinal cord and spinal roots in the acquired immunodeficiency syndrome. Rev Neurol 1990; 146: 655–664

Harriman G R, Smith P D, Horne M K, et al. Vitamin B_{12} malabsorption in patients with acquired immunodeficiency syndrome. Arch Intern Med 1989; 149: 2039–2041

Herskovitz S, Siegel S E, Schneider A T, et al. Spinal cord toxoplasmosis in AIDS. Neurology 1989; 39: 1552–1553

Ho D D, Rota M A, Schooley R T, et al. Isolation of HTLV-III from cerebrospinal fluid and neural tissues of patients with neurological syndromes related to acquired immunodeficiency syndrome. N Engl J Med 1985; 313: 1493–1497

Janssen R S, Cornblath D R, Epstein L G, et al. Nomenclature and research case definitions for neurological manifestations of human immunodeficiency virus type-1 (HIV-1) infection. Report of a Working Group of the American Academy of Neurology AIDS Task Force. Neurology 1991; 41: 778–785

Jordan B D, Navia B A, Petito C, et al. Neurological syndromes complicating AIDS. Front Radiat Ther Oncol 1985; 19: 82–87

Kamin S S, Petito C K. Idiopathic myelopathies with white matter vacuolation in non-acquired immunodeficiency syndrome patients. Hum Pathol 1991; 22: 816–824

Keating J N, Trimble K C, Mulcahy F, et al. Evidence of brain methyltransferase inhibition and early brain involvement in HIV-positive patients. Lancet 1991; 337: 935–939

Kieburtz K D, Giang D W, Schiffer R B, Vakil M. Abnormal vitamin B_{12} metabolism in human immunodeficiency infection. Association with neurologic dysfunction. Arch Neurol 1991; 48: 312–314

Koppel B S, Tuchman A J, Mangiardi J R, et al. Epidural spinal infection in intravenous drug abusers. Arch Neurol 1988; 45: 1331–1337

Koppel B S, Tuchman A J, Mangiardi J R, et al. Epidural spinal infection in intravenous drug abusers. Arch Neurol 1992; 45: 1331–1337

McArthur J C. Neurological manifestations of AIDS. Medicine 1987; 66: 407–437

McArthur J C, Griffin J W, Cornblath D R, et al. Steroid responsive myeloneuropathy in a man dually infected with HIV-1 and HTLV-1. Neurology 1990; 40: 938–944

Petito C K. Myelopathies. In: Scaravilli F, editor. The neuropathology of HIV infection. London: Springer-Verlag, 1993: 187–199

Petito C K, Navia B A, Cho E S, et al. Vacuolar myelopathy pathologically resembling subacute combined degeneration in patients with acquired immune deficiency syndrome. N Engl J Med 1985; 312: 874–879

Rosenblum M, Scheck A C, Cronin K, et al. Dissociation of AIDS related vacuolar myelopathy and productive HIV infection of the spinal cord. Neurology 1989; 39: 892–896

Santosh C G, Bell J E, Best I J K. Abnormalities of the spinal tracts in AIDS: correlation of postmortem MR findings with neuropathology. Clin Neuropathol 1993; 12: S23

Sharer L R, Epstein L G, Cho E S, et al. HTLV-III and vacuolar myelopathy. N Engl J Med 1986; 315: 62–63

Sheramata W A, Berer J R, Harrington W J, et al. Human T lymphotrophic virus type 1-associated myelopathy. A report of 10 patients born in the United States. Arch Neurol 1992; 49: 1113–1118

Siao P, McCabe P, Yagnik P. Nocardial spinal epidural abscess. Neurology 1989; 39: 996

Snider W D, Simpson D M, Nielsen S, et al. Neurological complications of the acquired immunodeficiency syndrome: analysis of 50 patients. Ann Neurol 1983; 14: 403–418

Surtees R, Hyland K, Smith I. Central nervous system methyl group metabolism in children with neurological complications of HIV infection. Lancet 1990; i: 619–621

Teman A J. Spinal epidural abscess early detection with gadolinium magnetic resonance imaging. Arch Neurol 1992; 49: 743–746

Tucker T, Dix R D, Katzen C, et al. Cytomegalovirus and herpes simplex virus ascending myelitis in a patient with acquired immune deficiency syndrome. Ann Neurol 1985; 18: 74–79

Tyor W R, Glass J D, Baumrind N, et al. Cytokine expression in macrophages in HIV-1 associated vacuolar myelopathy. Neurology 1993; 43: 1002–1009

Weill O, Finaud M, Bille F, et al. Gliome malin medullaire: une nouvelle complication de l'infection par le HIV? Presse Med 1987; 16: 1977

Weisner B, Peress N, LaNeve D, et al. Human immunodeficiency virus type 1 expression in the central nervous system correlates directly with extent of disease. Proc Natl Acad Sci USA 1990; 87: 3997–4001

Woolsey R M, Chambers T J, Chung H K, et al. Mycobacterial meningomyelitis associated with human immunodeficiency virus infection. Arch Neurol 1988; 45: 691–693

6. Peripheral nerve disease

PERIPHERAL NEUROPATHY

Although the CNS complications of HIV-1 infection constitute the most significant neurological disorders with respect to morbidity and mortality, the peripheral nervous system can also be involved in diverse ways (see Appendix 5 for criteria). Not only do novel and distinct clinical syndromes exist, but the frequency and timing of onset varies (Table 6.1), suggesting that diverse pathogenetic mechanisms may produce the different peripheral neuropathies (Cornblath et al 1987, Parry 1988).

The incidence of neuropathy increases with advancing immune suppression and onset of symptomatic HIV disease, and the incidence of sensory neuropathies has been increasing steeply over the last 3 years (Fig. 6.1). Rarely, peripheral or cranial neuropathies will develop with HIV-1 seroconversion, usually together with an acute aseptic meningitis (Vendrell et al 1987, Belec et al 1989, Wechsler & Ho 1989). The incidence of symptomatic peripheral neuropathy is very low among HIV carriers, however, but up to 10% may have electrophysiological abnormalities suggesting early involvement of peripheral nerves (Chavanet et al 1988). Careful examination and electrophysiological testing have documented evidence of neuropathy in the majority of patients with AIDS (So et al 1988, Gastaut et al 1989, Jakobsen et al 1989), and almost all biopsies are abnormal with fibre loss (Raphael et al 1991). The neuropathy is usually of a sensory type and can be clinically silent.

HIV-associated sensory neuropathy

Snider's review of the neurological complications of AIDS made it clear that peripheral neuropathy was going to be a common clinical feature. The first form of neuropathy identified early in the epidemic was a predominantly sensory axonal neuropathy. Subclinical signs of mild neuropathy

Table 6.1 Peripheral nerve syndromes

Syndrome	Stage
AIDP	Asymptomatic > AIDS
CIDP	Asymptomatic > AIDS
Mononeuritis multiplex	AIDS
Autonomic neuropathy	AIDS
Isolated nerve lesions	Any stage
Distal sensory neuropathy	AIDS
Ataxic sensory neuropathy	Seroconversion
Lumbar polyradiculopathy	AIDS
Lymphomatous neuropathy	AIDS
Iatrogenic neuropathy	Any stage

AIDP, acute inflammatory demyelinating neuropathy; CIDP, chronic inflammatory demyelinating neuropathy.

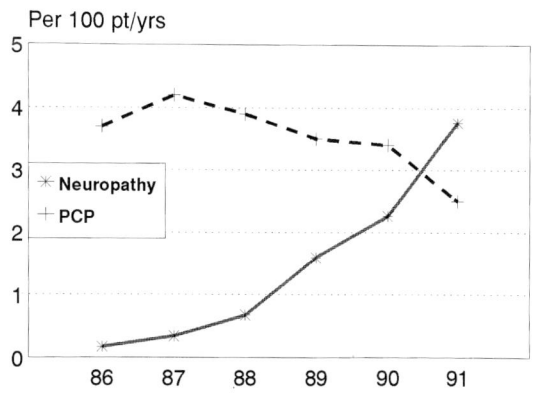

Fig. 6.1 Incidence of sensory neuropathy compared with that of *Pneumocystis carinii* pneumonia (PCP) in the Multicentre AIDS cohort study. (Courtesy of Helena Bacellar.)

Table 6.2 Definitional criteria for HIV-1 associated predominantly sensory polyneuropathy

Probable (must have each of the following):
1. Distal limb sensory symptoms (feet > hands) of a peripheral nerve nature (e.g. numbness, burning, or pain)
2. Neurological examination confirming a distal, relatively symmetrical polyneuropathy in which sensory abnormalities predominate
3. Electrodiagnostic studies indicative of a polyneuropathy with features of both axonal loss and demyelination*
4. Normal CSF cell count and only minimal, if any, elevation of protein, with negative VDRL*
5. No other aetiology (including toxic exposure to didanosine or dideoxycytidine). Nerve biopsy may be indicated to rule out certain aetiologies such as amyloid, but is not a requirement

Possible (must have one of the following):
1. Other potential aetiology present (must have each of the following):
   (a) As above (see Probable) criteria 1, 2 and 3
   (b) Other potential aetiology is present and the cause is uncertain
2. Incomplete clinical evaluation (must have each of the following):
   (a) As above (see Probable) criteria 1 and 2
   (b) Aetiology cannot be determined (appropriate laboratory investigations not performed)

(Reproduced from Janssen et al 1991)
*In our opinion, not essential for definite diagnosis

Table 6.3 Signs and symptoms of predominantly sensory neuropathy (expressed as percentage)

Symptoms	
Pain on soles of feet	62
Paraesthesias	38
Signs	
Absent ankle jerks	50
Reduced ankle jerks	46
Knee jerks brisk compared with ankle jerks	46
Elevated pain and vibration thresholds	85
Intrinsic foot weakness	31

(After Cornblath et al 1988)

are common in patients with symptomatic HIV infection or AIDS (Fuller et al 1991, McAllister et al 1992), and some (Gastaut 1989) but not all (McAllister et al 1992, Barohn et al 1993) studies have claimed signs of a neuropathy may precede immune dysfunction. Up to 30% of patients with AIDS develop a neuropathy characterized by painful sensory symptoms in the feet (Snider et al 1983, Cornblath & McArthur 1988, So et al 1988), usually late in the course of HIV-1 infection and in association with systemic opportunistic infections and profound immunodeficiency. Table 6.2 contains the AAN definitional criteria which we would modify by not requiring electrophysiological or CSF confirmation. This disorder can be recognized by characteristic complaints of shooting pains, paraesthesias and dysaesthesias and contact hypersensitivity in the feet with reduced or absent ankle reflexes and elevated sensory thresholds. The typical presentation is with the development over a few weeks of burning or aching in the toes and forefeet, usually symmetrically with the development of numbness

or dysaesthesias. Many patients describe their symptoms as being 'like frostbite' or 'like walking on broken glass'. In about one-third of patients with sensory symptoms, pain is functionally limiting. Table 6.3 illustrates the frequency of symptoms and signs. Distal muscle weakness occurs in one-third of patients, although it is not a prominent feature. The fingers and hands are usually spared. Walking or standing for prolonged periods may be affected and many patients avoid wearing tight shoes or socks. Children apparently do not develop sensory neuropathy. However, very few systematic studies have been completed, so it is possible that a mild neuropathy might exist.

Course

Because most patients who develop symptomatic sensory neuropathy have advanced HIV infection and survive less than 12 months, there has been little opportunity to study its long-term course. Occasionally, in patients who have lived with a sensory neuropathy for several months, symptoms will advance above the ankles or begin to affect fingers and hands. However, most patients' symptoms remain confined to the feet. With time, in a proportion of patients, painful sensory complaints subside as if the neuropathy 'burns out' and spontaneous pain diminishes, to be replaced by residual symptoms of numbness and contact hypersensitivity. Proprioceptive and thermal sensitivity are not greatly affected, at least in terms of symptomatic involvement, although quantitative testing does show abnormalities in thresholds to warm and cold (Winer et al 1992) or vibration. Up to now, zidovudine treatment has had little beneficial effect, but is not associated with a toxic sensory neuropathy. Alternative nucleoside antiretrovirals such as dideoxyinosine (ddI) and dideoxycytidine (ddC) are frequently associated with the production of a toxic sensory neuropathy, which is discussed in a later section.

Evaluation of sensory neuropathy

In evaluating patients with sensory neuropathy, consideration should also be given to nutritional and toxic causes such as alcohol, diabetes, pyridoxine excess and vitamin B_{12} deficiency. Neurotoxic drugs to be considered include isoniazid for mycobacterial infections (although this neuropathy should always have been prevented by the concurrent prescribing of pyridoxine), vincristine for Kaposi's sarcoma (KS) or systemic lymphoma, or an antiviral agent such as ddI or ddC. A predominantly sensory neuropathy with loss of the ankle jerks but with no weakness is more likely to be HIV related than due to vincristine, for example, because the latter causes early weakness, particularly of finger extension, and is more likely to be associated with loss of all reflexes. DdI and ddC neuropathy is also axonal in type and can be painful, and is more difficult to distinguish from HIV-associated sensory neuropathy. The onset of symptoms, after starting treatment, especially in someone with asymptomatic HIV infection, would favour neurotoxicity. However, neuropathy usually only develops after several weeks of treatment with the neurotoxic antiretrovirals and is dose-dependent. If stopping all potentially neurotoxic therapy and a 'drug holiday' fails to affect the neuropathic symptoms, it is reasonable to conclude that the patient's peripheral neuropathy is HIV related.

When symptoms and signs are restricted to the legs a spinal cord or cauda equina lesion may be suspected. Cytomegalovirus (CMV) radiculitis is another possibility in patients with CD4 counts <100 and complaints of weakness, back pain or sphincter disturbance. It is unusual for peripheral neuropathy to cause sensory change as high as mid thigh so such a finding would impune the cord or roots and call for myelography or magnetic resonance imaging (MRI). Nerve conduction studies and somatosensory evoked potentials can be helpful in distinguishing between peripheral neuropathy and a cord or root problem as the cause of sensory symptoms when there are no simple clinical pointers. Extensor plantar responses may coincide with a peripheral neuropathy due to HIV-associated myelopathy or dementia, adding to the confusion. AIDS has to be added to the list of causes (much beloved of examiners) of the combination of absent ankle jerks and positive Babinski responses.

Neurodiagnostic testing

The cerebrospinal fluid (CSF) usually shows a normal or slightly elevated protein and a few cells (5–10), but does not differ from the 'typical' CSF profile of advanced HIV infection. The presence of polymorphs would raise the possibility of CMV radiculopathy.

Nerve conduction studies show small or absent sensory action potentials, normal or small muscle action potentials recorded with surface electrodes and only slight slowing of motor conduction velocity. Muscle sampling reveals normal-appearing motor units or shows signs of denervation with spontaneous fibrillation potentials. These electrophysiological characteristics are consistent with a length-dependent or dying back axonopathy (Cornblath & McArthur 1988, Simpson & Wolfe 1991, Winer et al 1992). Nerve conduction studies have not proved practical for screening or for serial determinations, however, because they are costly and do not assess the function of small myelinated or unmyelinated fibres. Quantitative sensory testing (QST) has become a reliable and repeatable method of assessing both large and small fibre nerve function (Asbury & Porte 1992). Abnormalities of both vibratory (large fibres) and thermal thresholds (small fibres) have been identified in sensory neuropathy and ddC-induced toxic neuropathy (Hall et al 1991, Winer et al 1992, Blum et al 1993). Because QST is now more widely available and is less invasive than conventional electrophysiological techniques, it may provide a simple, reproducible and repeatable measure of the function of both myelinated and unmyelinated nerve fibres. It can be performed serially and correlated with pain characteristics and neuro-

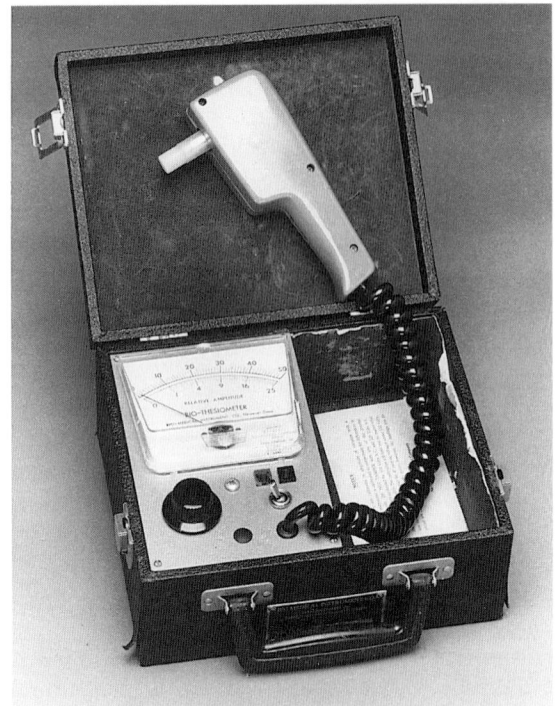

Fig. 6.2 Quantitative sensory testing: the 'biothesiometer' for vibration threshold measurements.

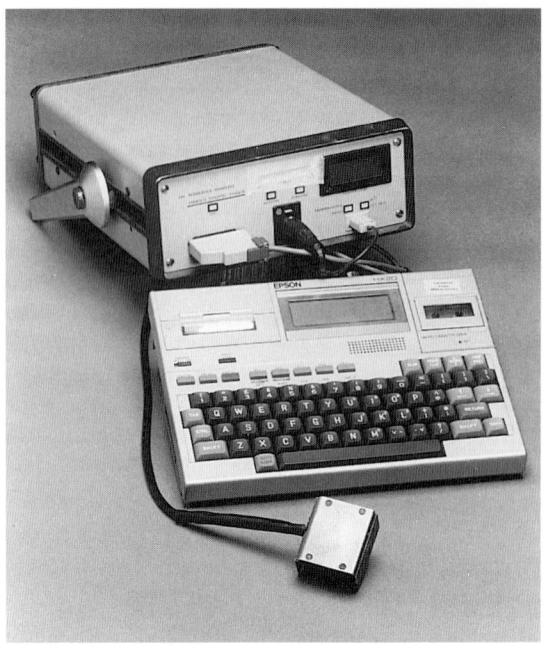

Fig. 6.3 Quantitative sensory testing: Middlesex Hospital Thermal Testing system.

pathological features. The devices available (Fig 6.2 and 6.3), unlike nerve conduction velocities, rely on a patient's description of whether a stimulus is felt or not. However, forced choice paradigms have been developed that make the test more precise, although they may not be reliable in a demented patient. Several commercially available devices are available to measure vibration threshold (Fig. 6.2), thermal thresholds (Fig. 6.3) and non-physiological modalities such as current perception thresholds. Because the pathological features of the HIV-associated sensory neuropathy suggest a predominance of small fibre involvement, at least early on, thermal thresholds may be the most useful in screening for sensory neuropathy. In fact, a recent study showed that thermal thresholds were abnormal in 14 of 15 patients with clinical and electrophysiological evidence of neuropathy, three of six symptomatic patients with normal nerve conduction studies and three of 10 patients with no neuropathic symptoms or signs (Winer et al 1992). The Middlesex Hospital data also show the relative sensitivity of electrophysiological and QST techniques in the examination of seropositive patients (Table 6.4).

Pathology

Severe sensory neuropathy is associated with degeneration of the rostral gracile tracts (Rance et al 1988), a well-recognized pattern of distal axonal degeneration of the primary sensory neurone (Fig. 6.4) (Chaunu et al 1989). Nerve biopsies show predominantly axonal neuropathy with loss of axons and varying degrees of (secondary) demyelination and inflammation. The inflammation is not in a vasculitic pattern and may not be appreciated unless specific immunostaining for T cells or macrophages is performed. The majority of infiltrating cells are macrophages with associated CD8$^+$ lymphocytes (reflecting the depletion of CD4 cells in the peripheral blood) (Cornblath et al 1990). Macrophage infiltration is also found in the dorsal root ganglia (DRG) and rostral gracile tracts. Immunohistochemical studies of peripheral nerve obtained at biopsy or autopsy have shown that most

Table 6.4   Comparison of QST and electrophysiological screening for peripheral neuropathy

	Cold (°C)	Warm (°C)	Vibration (units)	Sural SAP (μV)	DML TIB. (ms)	MCV TIB. (m/s)	SSEP TIB. (ms)	F wave (ms)
Seronegative (n = 21)	0.48 ± 0.43	1.5 ± 2.2	7.3 ± 3.5	12.9 ± 5.9	4.3 ± 0.74	43.9 ± 4.0	23.7 ± 1.5	52.7 ± 5.2
Seropositive (n = 36)	0.50 ± 0.37	1.7 ± 1.7	8.5 ± 5.1	10.4 ± 4.2	4.4 ± 0.75	42.9 ± 4.1	24.3 ± 1.9	54.8 ± 7.4
Symptomatic (n = 29)	0.70 ± 0.8	2.9 ± 2.9*	8.4 ± 5.0	9.3 ± 5.9**	4.7 ± 0.73**	43.8 ± 4.5	25.1 ± 2***	54.5 ± 3.9

Data expressed as mean ± SD.
* $p = 0.04$;   ** $p = 0.03$;   *** $p = 0.01$; symptomatic (CDC stage C) vs. seronegative controls. (Middlesex Hospital data)

infiltrating macrophages are activated and express MHC class II antigens on their surface, as well as cytokines including tumour necrosis factor-alpha (TNF-α), interleukin (IL)-6 and interferon γ. In a careful morphometric analysis of peripheral nerve obtained at autopsy, Griffin et al (1994a) compared the densities of myelinated and unmyelinated fibres in sural nerves between AIDS patients with and without clinically recognized sensory neuropathies and HIV-seronegative individuals with comparable sensory neuropathies. Wallerian degeneration of myelinated fibres was found in the distal sural nerves of all AIDS patients, even those without neuropathic symptoms, with a median reduction in myelinated fibre density of 27% compared with controls (Fig. 6.5). The degree of fibre loss was independent of

whether the sensory neuropathy was symptomatic before death or not. The unmyelinated fibre loss was more severe in the AIDS patients than in the other groups, including the HIV-seronegative patients with comparable severity of sensory neuropathy. The peripheral fibre loss was more severe distally than proximally, consistent with a

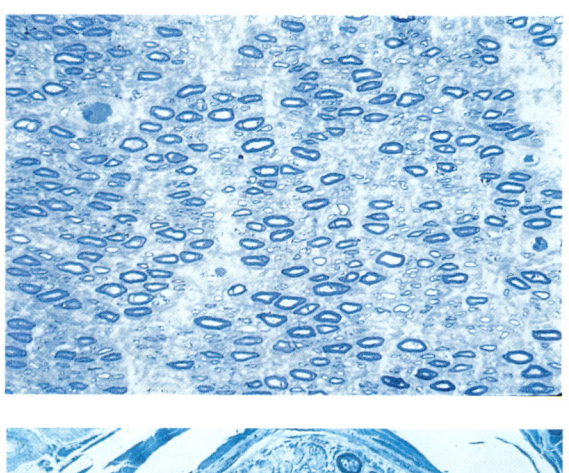

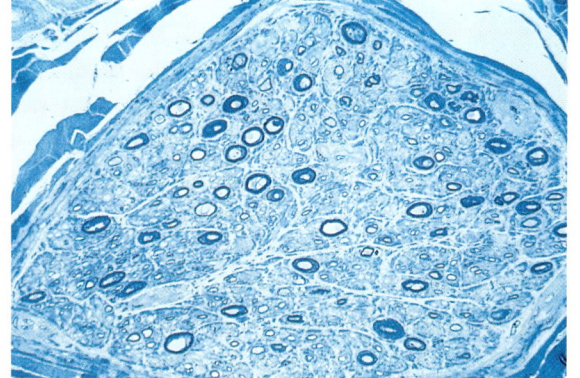

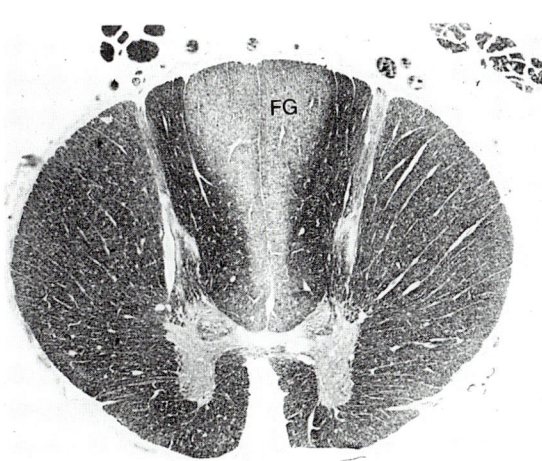

Fig. 6.4   Transverse section through the thoracic cord showing discrete and severe loss of myelin in the fasciculus gracilis (FG) in a case of sensory neuropathy. (Reproduced from Rance et al 1988 with permission of *Neurology*.)

Fig. 6.5   Sural nerve biopsies showing more fibre loss in the distal section of the nerve due to 'dying back' axonal neuropathy. **A**, proximal part of nerve in calf, **B**, section at ankle (×56).

distal axonal degeneration or 'dying back' process. The striking unmyelinated fibre loss with C fibre degeneration may underlie the neuropathic pain so common in HIV-associated sensory neuropathy. In diabetic neuropathy, some have proposed that pain arises from regenerating nerve fibres (Asbury & Fields 1984). This mechanism seems unlikely in HIV-associated sensory neuropathy because no regenerating fibres have yet been found.

Pathogenesis (Table 6.5)

The pathogenesis of HIV-associated sensory neuropathy remains unclear. A number of hypotheses have been considered. Because the sensory neuropathy was recognized early as a feature of late-stage HIV infection, and was commonly seen in patients with marked wasting, the concept was advanced that this was a nutritional neuropathy. So et al (1988) in a clinical and electrophysiological survey of patients with AIDS found weight loss to be more common in those with detectable neuropathy. Other studies, including those by Griffin et al (1994a), have not reproduced these findings and there is no clear-cut association between the degree or rapidity of wasting or specific nutritional deficiencies and the severity of sensory neuropathy (Fuller et al 1991). It remains possible that a deficiency in specific nutrients or vitamins plays a role. However, both the clinical features and the neuropathology are different from typical nutritional neuropathies.

Another possibility is that CMV plays a pathogenic role. Fuller et al (1989, 1993) reported an association between symptoms of sensory neuropathy and CMV infection and suggested that CMV infection of, and damage to, the DRG

Table 6.5   Potential steps in pathogenesis of sensory neuropathy

1. Development of mild distal axonal degeneration during HIV infection as a result of nutritional deficiencies, alcohol exposure or neurotoxic medications
2. Recruitment of hyperresponsive macrophages into the distal peripheral nerves
3. Activation of infiltrating macrophages with elaboration of neurotoxic cytokines, TNF-α, IL-1
4. Production of nerve growth factor may be reduced preventing nerve regeneration

might lead to distal axonal degeneration. CMV is a frequent disseminated infection in the late stages of HIV infection when the CD4 count is less than 100 and has been associated with a progressive radiculomyelitis (Eidelberg et al 1986, Behar et al 1987, Miller et al 1990). Nearly 40% of patients with AIDS have CMV viraemia. In a recent autopsy series, CMV was found in the peripheral nervous system, usually in endothelial cells, in 26% of patients dying with AIDS and in 46% of those who had lived for 2 or more years after their AIDS-defining illness (Cornford et al 1992b). In contrast, data from the MACS show that the mean CD4 count within 9 months of onset of sensory neuropathy is 203 compared with 110 for CMV retinitis. This suggests that neuropathy predates CMV end organ disease and suggests that CMV is not the primary cause of sensory neuropathy. In another series of 123 individuals with CMV retinitis, sensory neuropathy was identified in 17% compared with 21% without CMV retinitis (Jabs, personal communication 1992). These data contrast with the association that Fuller et al (1989) noted between CMV disease and neuropathy. Furthermore, although CMV has been identified in peripheral nerve, definitive evidence of CMV in DRG is usually absent (Griffin et al 1994a, Scaravilli et al 1992). While disseminated CMV infection may contribute to peripheral nerve damage, possibly through an effect on endothelial cells and the microvasculature, it does not appear to be the prime cause of this form of neuropathy.

Identifiable productive HIV replication is even less frequent than in the brain or spinal cord (Griffin et al 1994b). Recent studies using in situ polymerase chain reaction (PCR) have failed to show any evidence of transcribed HIV RNA (Wesselingh S, personal communication). The prominence of infiltration with activated macrophages led to a search for cytokines within the peripheral nerve. Macrophages in the peripheral nerves of AIDS patients express activation markers and produce TNF-α. The TNF-α positive macrophages are usually found in association with degenerating nerve fibres. Other cytokines, including IL-1 and IL-6, are also found, although the density of staining is less. High levels of TNF-α mRNA have been found using RNA

PCR (Wesselingh S, unpublished data). The stimulus for macrophage entry and activation is uncertain. If in fact macrophages are 'hyper-responsive' in AIDS, as has been suggested, a minor degree of neuropathy might cause the selective recruitment of activated macrophages into peripheral nerve with the release of neuro-toxic cytokines and induction of the clinical features of sensory neuropathy. A minor degree of nutritional or ethanol related damage might serve as this initial trigger for the hyper-responsive macrophage response.

Treatment of sensory neuropathy

The management of neuropathic symptoms either from HIV-associated sensory neuropathy or toxic neuropathy associated with antiretroviral use involves similar strategies (Fig. 6.6). We do not have restorative treatments for sensory neuro-pathy at this point; however, the potential exists for stimulating the regeneration of damaged nerve fibres with neurotrophic factors such as nerve growth factor (NGF). Small nerve fibres, a population severely affected in HIV sensory neuropathies, are NGF responsive, providing a rationale for its use in these neuropathies (Apfel et al 1991). Currently, human NGF is under-going toxicity trials in humans and it is hoped that efficacy trials for HIV sensory neuropathy will begin within the next 2 years.

One of the difficulties in treating neuropathic pain is in the assessment of treatment response. Frequently, the severity of neuropathic pain fluctuates from day to day or even hour to hour. The psychological state of the patient, other physical symptoms and the effects of fever and fatigue may all exacerbate the emotional impact of neuropathic pain on functional activities. Despite this, it is important to attempt to quantify neuro-pathic pain symptoms to enable rational adjust-ments in treatments to be made. A number of instruments exist for quantifying neuropathic pain. Some, like the Graceley and McGill Pain Questionnaire, are predominantly qualitative, relying on a patient's choice of pain descriptors.

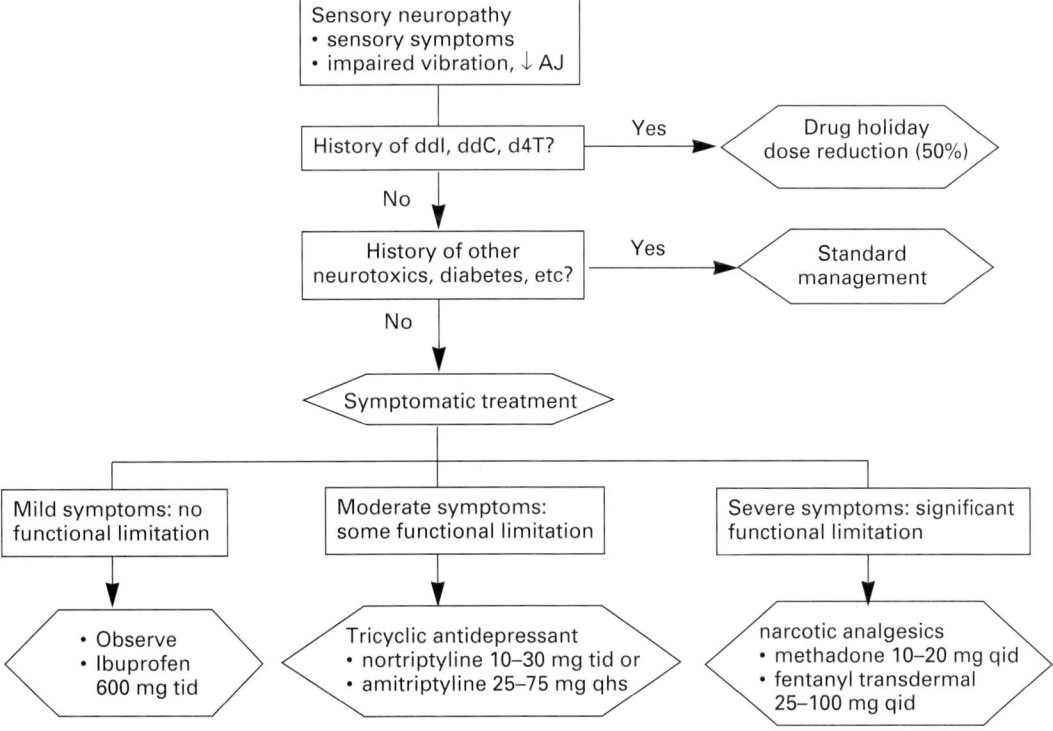

Fig. 6.6 Scheme for management of sensory neuropathy.

The simplest tool to use is a visual analogue scale (VAS) in which the patient indicates the severity of pain by placing a point on a line of a certain length. The position of that point provides a continuous measure of pain severity. An even simpler version of the VAS is to use rated responses (0–10) where 0 corresponds to no pain and 10 to the worst pain. In practice, one can have the patient maintain a daily 'pain diary' where the patient is asked to record on a daily basis the graded severity of the 'worst' pain.

Symptomatic treatment is started for sensory neuropathies depending on the patient's level of symptoms and functional impairment (Casey 1988). Thus, mild neuropathic symptoms, with only distal paraesthesias, may be tolerated by many patients without the need for medications (see algorithm). Patients may develop physical 'tricks' that are helpful in relieving the pressure on hypersensitive feet: for example, avoiding tight footwear, walking only short distances, avoiding standing for long periods, or soaking the feet in ice water periodically during the day. It was originally hoped that the topical agent, capsaicin, might be useful for treatment of neuropathic symptoms. Capsaicin, an extract of red pepper, depletes C fibres of substance P, the pain neurotransmitter. Capsaicin creams (0.025% or 0.075%) have been shown to be useful for treatment of post-herpetic neuralgia and diabetic neuropathy. Unfortunately, in our experience in attempting to use them for HIV sensory neuropathy, they are not well tolerated. Their application to the skin often induces an initial intensification of pain and many patients discontinue them after only 2 or 3 days before an adequate trial has been completed. In one uncontrolled study of 23 HIV-positive patients with sensory neuropathy, 13 dropped out immediately because of initial burning pain (Cotton 1990). It remains possible that if treatment were to be continued for 10–14 days, a benefit might be seen. Another topical agent that is sometimes used, particularly in a patient who cannot tolerate systemic medications, is a high concentration of lidocaine cream (20–30%) in a lecithin base applied directly to the toes and feet with an occlusive dressing. A newly developed combination cream containing lidocaine 2–5% and prilocaine 2–5% (EMLA) may be as effective. These lidocaine creams induce numbness, obviously, but this sensation may be preferred by some patients over the neuropathic symptoms. The use of TENS (transdermal electrical nerve stimulation) or MENS (microcurrent electrical nerve stimulation) devices has been tried for pain associated with HIV sensory neuropathies, but neither has produced any consistent results.

Unfortunately the selection of systemic symptomatic treatments is empirical and, in our experience, it has not been possible to select agents based on the type of neuropathic symptoms. Thus, while some have advocated the use of tricyclic antidepressant for constant burning dysaesthetic pain, and membrane-stabilizing drugs or anticonvulsants for lancinating or sharp shooting pains, we have not found this distinction helpful. As the algorithm illustrates, mild symptoms that are not functionally limiting may be tolerated without medications or with non-steroidal anti-inflammatory drugs (NSAIDs), e.g. ibuprofen 600–800 mg t.i.d. The rationale for their use is their well-demonstrated analgesic effect. Controlled trials of NSAIDs in neuropathic pain are very limited, but anecdotal experience suggests that they may provide some relief, for example if used before walking or at night.

More limiting symptoms that affect a patient's ability to walk and stand usually require the pain-modifying effect of tricyclic antidepressants. The efficacy of tricyclic antidepressants has been proven in many chronic pain states and painful neuropathies. Amitriptyline is effective for painful diabetic neuropathy and post-herpetic neuralgia (Max et al 1992). Desipramine and nortriptyline have also been proven effective for several types of neuropathic pain. The tricyclic antidepressants probably affect the monoamine-dependent pain modulating systems, including the serotonergic and noradrenergic tracts between the medulla and the dorsal horns in the spinal cord. To date, no controlled trials of tricyclic antidepressants have been completed for HIV sensory neuropathies, although several are planned. The tricyclic antidepressants have been shown to control painful symptoms in diabetic neuropathy better than fluoxetine (Max et al 1992). The choice of agents depends in part on when the symptoms are worse.

Thus, for night time pain, wakening the patient from sleep frequently, a sedating tricyclic antidepressant such as amitriptyline is most useful. To reduce excessive anticholinergic effects or delirium in a patient with cognitive impairment, amitriptyline is started at a low dose of 10–25 mg q.d.s. and gradually increased up to 75 mg q.d.s. If day-time neuropathic discomfort is the major concern, nortriptyline, which is less anticholinergic and sedating, is used beginning with 10 mg t.i.d. and increasing as needed to 30 mg t.i.d. Tricyclic antidepressants are not always well tolerated, particularly if the initial dosage is too high. They should, of course, be avoided in patients with conductive block, prostatism and narrow angle glaucoma. Some patients find the anticholinergic effects of dry mouth and mental 'fuzziness' intolerable, and in a demented patient, delirium can be precipitated at relatively small doses. Other useful tricyclic antidepressants include doxepin, imipramine and desipramine. Symptomatic relief usually takes 1–3 weeks to achieve, depending on how quickly the dose can be built up. Plasma concentrations of tricyclic antidepressants do not correlate well with analgesic efficacy, but may be useful to check compliance or absorption. Unfortunately, not all patients respond to the first tricyclic antidepressant used. If one tricyclic antidepressant is not effective or is associated with limiting side-effects, it is worth trying a second before giving up.

If a patient cannot tolerate tricyclic antidepressants, the next choice for a second-line agent would be the oral local anaesthetic mexiletine. The initial dose is 150 mg/day, increasing to 600–900 mg/day. Mexiletine should be administered with food or antacids. The most frequent adverse reactions were upper gastrointestinal distress, lightheadedness, tremor and incoordination difficulties, which were usually dose-related or limited by taking the drug with food or antacid. Blood levels should be monitored to keep concentrations between 0.5 μg/ml and 2.0 μg/ml. Other agents, including baclofen, phenytoin, carbamazepine and clonazepam, have all been tried in individual patients, but again have not yet been subjected to clinical trial in AIDS. Experience with them in HIV infection has generally been unfavourable despite their proven efficacy for some forms of neuropathic pain.

For the patient with severe neuropathic symptoms that are limiting function and inhibiting walking, narcotic analgesics may be required. While there is of course a concern of causing addiction by using narcotic analgesics, a number of studies have shown that overall the proportion of patients who *develop* substance abuse problems with carefully prescribed narcotics is relatively low. The potential for abuse and addiction is of course much higher among patients with a previous history of substance abuse. Nonetheless, many patients with advanced HIV infection, with only a few months of life left, may be incapacitated by neuropathic symptoms and it seems reasonable in this situation, which is analogous to treating cancer pain, to use narcotic analgesics when needed. There are a number of narcotic analgesics that are useful and a nomogram is included to allow calculation of equivalent dosages in switching from one drug to another (Fig. 6.7). There are two strategies for initiating narcotics. The first, generally used only for those few patients with very severe, incapacitating pain, requires inpatient hospitalization. Parenteral morphine is used either by regular injection or through 'patient controlled analgesia' and the daily dose of morphine adequate to control pain is calculated. Maintenance doses of morphine or methadone (calculated from the nomogram) can then be commenced to keep the neuropathic pain in check. As with the treatment of cancer pain, regular dosing of analgesics is far more effective than intermittent 'prn' dosing. A second strategy for patients with less intense pain in an outpatient setting is to begin a narcotic analgesic and gradually increase the dose over a few days until pain control is achieved. Useful choices for oral narcotics include methadone (which requires t.i.d. dosing for pain control), sustained release morphine, and recently introduced transdermal preparations of fentanyl. Average daily doses of narcotics for severe neuropathic pain are methadone 60–80 mg/day (given as 20 mg t.i.d. or q.i.d.) or transdermal fentanyl 25–100μg every other day.

There are several practical points that will assist in successful use of narcotic analgesics (Table 6.6).

HIGH POTENCY NARCOTICS

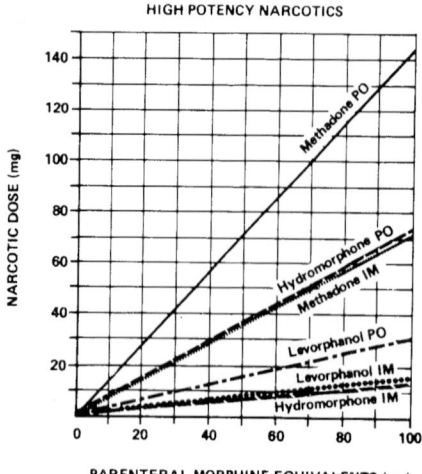

LOW POTENCY NARCOTICS

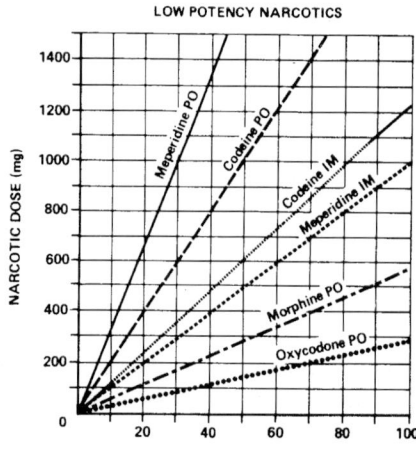

Fig. 6.7 Narcotic conversion nomogram. Because of individual differences in absorption, renal and hepatic function, dose equivalencies can only be approximate. Thus 20 mg or parenteral morphine is about equivalent to 27 mg of oral methadone, 50 mg of oral oxycodone and 650 mg of oral meperidine. If a patient requires 20 mg of parenteral morphine to control pain in severe sensory neuropathy, the equivalent dose of oral morphine is likely to be 400 mg/day (Marks & Sachar 1973, Grossman & Sheidler 1987). (Reproduced from Grossman & Sheidler 1987 with permission of WHO.)

First, prn dosing should be avoided and patients should be evaluated frequently for side-effects or failure of symptom control. Second, tricyclic antidepressants may be used in combination and allow for lower doses of narcotics to be used. Third, the rapid development of tolerance should be anticipated in patients with a history of

Table 6.6   Guidelines for narcotic therapy in HIV neuropathy

- Use only after non-narcotic therapies have failed
- Anticipate rapid tolerance and drug-seeking behaviour with previous history of substance abuse
- Prescribing patterns:
    Single practitioner prescribes medications
    'Lost' prescriptions are not refilled
    Narcotic prescriptions should be carefully rationed
    Medications should be prescribed regularly, not given prn
- For intermittent inadequate control, patients may take a set number (e.g. 4–6) of 'rescue doses' during the month
- Patients should be seen monthly for assessment of symptom control, side-effects and prescription renewals
- Drug hoarding, selling medications, uncontrolled dose escalation or acquiring drugs from other physicians should be managed by discontinuation of narcotics

(After Portenoy 1993)

substance abuse. Fourth, clear guidelines should be set for prescribing patterns with the patient and record all prescription amounts and dates. Narcotic prescriptions should not be rewritten if a prescription has been 'lost' or 'stolen'. Useful guidelines to the use of narcotic analgesics for neuropathic pain and the risks of addiction are provided in Portenoy (1991, 1994) and Portenoy & Foley (1986).

Opioid withdrawal is characterized by typical signs (Table 6.7) beginning within 4–6 hours, peaking between 2 and 3 days, and lasting up to 7–12 days. Unlike withdrawal from alcohol and benzodiazepines, opioid withdrawal is not commonly lethal or associated with seizures or delirium.

Table 6.7   Signs and symptoms of opioid withdrawal

General
Anxiety, opioid craving
Vital signs
Hypertension, tachycardia, fever
Nervous system
Restlessness, irritability, tremor, chills, insomnia, muscle cramps, yawning
Skin
Perspiration, piloerection (goose flesh), eyes, nose, throat, pupillary dilatation, lachrymation, rhinorrhoea
Gastrointestinal
Anorexia, nausea, vomiting, hyperactive bowel sounds, diarrhoea

(Reproduced from Selwyn & O'Connor 1992 with permission of W B Saunders Company)

TOXIC NEUROPATHIES

Toxic neuropathies are not associated with zidovudine therapy, but two nucleoside antiretrovirals, 2',3'-dideoxycytidine (ddC) and dideoxyinosine (ddI), can produce a painful sensory neuropathy. D4T has also been linked with the development of sensory neuropathy; however, its frequency with this drug is still uncertain. In these cases, the neuropathy is consistent with a toxic neuropathy with the onset of neuropathic symptoms after several weeks of therapy and usually only with high doses (e.g. > 750 mg/day of ddI or >2.25 mg/day of ddC). At currently recommended doses, toxic neuropathy occurs more frequently with ddC than ddI. In a large community-based trial of ddI and ddC in 467 patients who were zidovudine intolerant, peripheral neuropathy developed in 29% of ddC recipients compared with 13% using ddI (Blum et al 1993). Symptoms of ddI/ddC toxic neuropathy include foot pain, shooting pains, dysaesthesias and contact hypersensitivity. Patients develop paraesthesiae and pain and contact hypersensitivity in the feet in a way that closely mimics HIV-associated sensory neuropathy in untreated patients. The onset may be explosive with a crescendo of intense paraesthesiae and patients may be off their feet within 2 weeks because of severe pain. More typically, symptoms begin with an aching in the forefoot, which evolves over a few weeks into paraesthesias, pain and contact hypersensitivity. The fingers are more frequently affected than HIV-associated sensory neuropathy. Both ddI and ddC neuropathies are clearly dose related. For example, Lambert et al (1990) recorded neuropathy in seven out of 22 patients given >12 mg/kg ddI, but in only one of 15 patients given lower doses. Schaumberg et al (1990) showed a similar effect with ddC, which caused neuropathy in all subjects who received >0.03 mg/kg/day. At low dose (0.005 mg/kg every 4 hours) a slower onset of foot discomfort may be tolerated with mild complaints of tight-fitting shoes and a sensation of bruised soles of the feet (Berger et al 1993). In a recent study of 47 patients receiving ddC in the currently recommended dosing range of 1.0–2.25 mg/day, 34% developed a toxic neuropathy with median onset after drug initiation of 24 weeks

(range 3–51 weeks) (Blum et al 1993). In over two-thirds of patients, symptoms extended beyond the feet to involve legs or hands. Ankle areflexia was found in 55%, diminished vibration thresholds in 85% and hyperpathia in 58%. About two-thirds of patients had a subjective improvement with dose reduction, but none showed any objective improvement in neuropathic signs. The most important risk factor associated with development of ddC-induced toxic neuropathy was pre-existing diabetes mellitus, and neither weight loss nor CD4 counts were predictive.

Current doses of both drugs (ddI 200–250 mg b.d. and ddC 0.375–0.75 mg t.d.s.) are much lower than used in the initial dose ranging studies which reported very frequent neuropathy, and the incidence of toxic neuropathy is correspondingly lower. Nonetheless, because so many patients are now switched to either drug when zidovudine fails, the frequency of toxic neuropathy poses a serious problem. The development of toxic neuropathy may be more common in patients with pre-existing neuropathies and when ddI is administered more frequently than once daily. After stopping the antivirals, neuropathic symptoms may continue to escalate ('coasting') for 3–6 weeks (Dubinsky et al 1989). In one phase I/II study, 43 children with symptomatic HIV infection received oral ddI in doses from 60 to 540 mg/m^2. Peripheral neuropathy was not encountered.

Malnutrition, weight loss and diarrhoea are common in AIDS and may lead to deficiencies of vitamins B_{12} or E. Excessive doses of pyridoxine (B_6), however, can produce a sensory neuropathy, so daily doses should be limited to less than 200 mg.

Some of the neuropathic symptoms seen in AIDS may result from antimicrobial use. Neuropathies have been linked to a number of these, including isoniazid, dapsone, metronidazole (Coxon & Pallis 1976), nitrofurantoin (Lhermitte et al 1963), and possible sulphonamides (Goldstick et al 1985). Table 6.8 lists the major neurotoxic drugs.

INFLAMMATORY DEMYELINATING POLYNEUROPATHIES

Besides the relatively well-characterized oppor-

Table 6.8   Major neurotoxic drugs

- Dideoxyinosine (ddI)
- Dideoxycytidine (ddC)
- Stavudine (D4T)
- Isoniazid
- Metronidazole
- Vincristine
- Dapsone
- Excessive B_6

tunistic infections and neoplastic involvement of the nervous system, a number of possible immune-mediated phenomena have been described in association with HIV infection, including inflammatory demyelinating polyneuropathies (IDP) (Cornblath et al 1987, Miller et al 1989) and thrombocytopenia. Both disorders often occur at a relatively early stage of HIV infection before profound immunoincompetence, and probably result from immune dysregulation. Clinically recognized IDP is uncommon and the majority of reported cases have presented in the early stages of HIV infection without constitutional symptoms. However, there does not seem to have been a major shift of the incidence of Guillain-Barré syndrome in areas of high prevalence of HIV infection, so its true incidence must be low in HIV infection. Sometimes the neuropathy is a manifestation of the acute seroconversion illness (Cornblath et al 1987) and usually develops in the otherwise asymptomatic patient with normal CD4 counts. Patients may be unaware of their HIV infection when they develop progressive limb and/or facial weakness, generalized areflexia and mild distal sensory changes.

The presentations of IDP take two forms, either an acute demyelinating neuropathy (AIDP or the Guillain-Barré syndrome) or a more chronic, sometimes relapsing course with predominantly motor weakness (CIDP). The AIDP patients develop progressive limb and/or facial weakness, with generalized areflexia and mild distal sensory changes. CIDP is encountered more frequently and occurs typically when there has been some decline in CD4 counts. CIDP usually remits as immunodeficiency progresses. The clinical picture is a much slower evolution of motor deficits, which may be diffuse or patchy. The presentation is identical to CIDP in HIV-seroneg-

ative patients with symmetrical leg weakness, which may be proximal or distal, and reduced or absent reflexes. Sensory symptoms are minor but there may be vibration loss distally. Nerve conduction studies reveal patchy slowing of conduction velocities and F waves, with diagnostic conduction block. At an early stage, if all the pathological process is concentrated in the roots, there may be little or no abnormality detected in the periphery. The diagnosis should not be rejected; rather the studies should be repeated as should the lumbar puncture if the protein is not raised in the first week. HIV is not generally detected by culture or more sensitive techniques like PCR. Among the CSF changes that distinguish patients with HIV-1-related IDP from IDP unrelated to HIV infection is the CSF pleocytosis (mean, 23 white blood cells (WBC)/mm^3 in one series) (Cornblath et al 1987), which contrasts with the normocellular CSF found in HIV-seronegative patients (Cornblath et al 1987). There is probably nothing mysterious about this as it may merely reflect the chances of finding a cellular CSF in HIV-infected patients in the first years of their illness. The CSF total protein is usually markedly elevated (mean, 178 mg/dl) similar to IDPs occurring in uninfected individuals.

Nerve biopsies typically show active demyelination with demyelinated internodes and paranodes with variable degrees of axonal loss and inflammatory change (Figs 6.8 and 6.9). A comparison of morphometry from sural nerve biopsies (Fig. 6.10A) highlights the reduction in large fibre density in HIV-seropositive CIDP. (By contrast unmyelinated nerve fibre density is significantly reduced in HIV predominantly sensory neuropathy (Fig. 6.10B).) Electron microscopy shows vesicular myelin degeneration, usually with macrophages containing myelin debris. Examples of myelin 'stripping' with macrophage processes intercalated between the intraperiod lines of internodal myelin may be identified (Griffin et al 1994c). Wallerian-like degeneration is also present, varying in degree from case to case. The immunopathology of IDPs and the pathological features distinguish Guillain-Barré syndrome (GBS) from CIDP. The GBS cases have extensive T lymphocyte infiltrations, which are predominantly CD8+ lymphocytes as well as

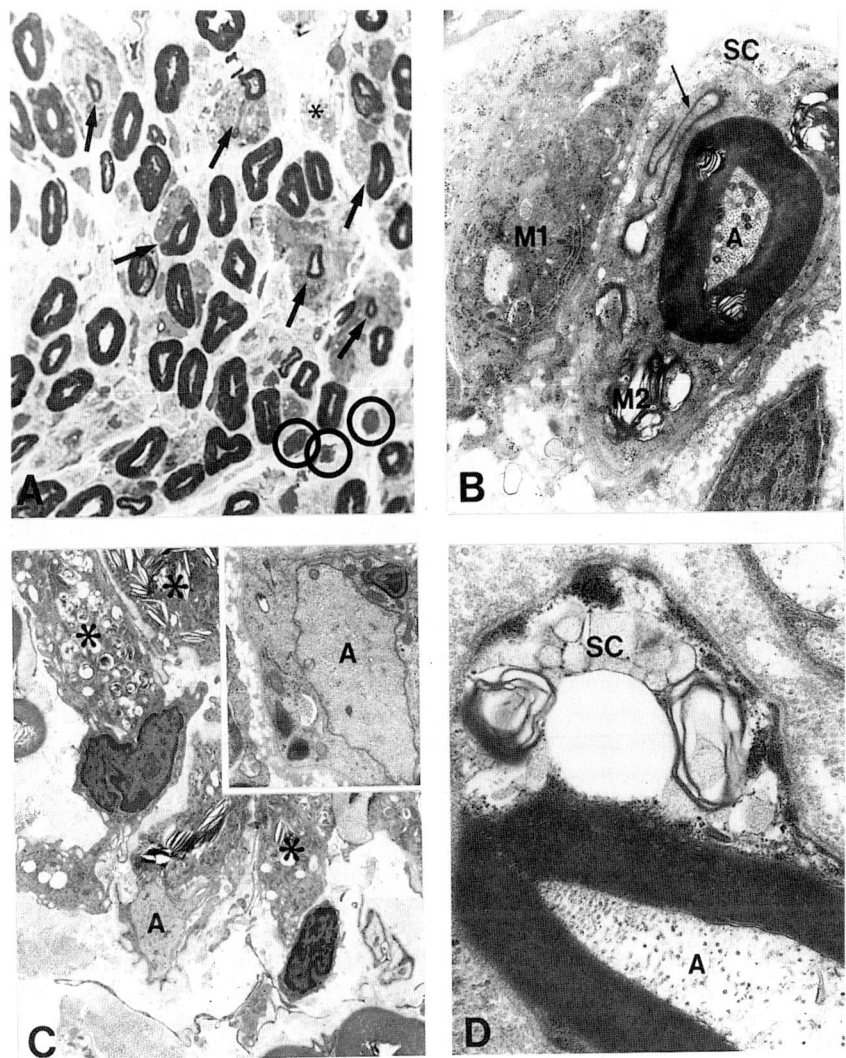

Fig. 6.8 Pathological changes within sural nerve biopsies in inflammatory demyelinating polyneuropathies. (Reproduced from Cornblath et al 1987 with permission of Little, Brown & Co.)
A Light micrograph illustrating macrophage infiltration (*), demyelination (arrows) and lymphocytes in the endoneurial space (circles) (×470). **B** Electron micrograph showing macrophage-mediated demyelination. M1/M2, macrophages; SC, Schwann cell (×10070). **C** Electron micrograph demonstrating complete demyelination. A, axon;*, macrophage (×8280). **D** Electron micrograph of a dead or dying Schwann cell (SC) and a nerve fibre whose axon (A) and myelin sheath are intact (×18566).

activated macrophages. The CIDP cases had less florid lymphocytic infiltration (Cornblath et al 1990). In a unique study of nerve obtained at autopsy from patients presenting 4–5 years earlier with CIDP (Griffin et al 1994a), the evolution of the neuropathological changes can be traced. By the time of death several years after neurological presentation, active demyelination had stopped and the proportion of remyelinated internodes had markedly increased, with 'onion bulbs' composed of Schwann cells.

The features of sensory and demyelinating neuropathies are compared in Table 6.9 and a diagnostic work-up is outlined in Table 6.10.

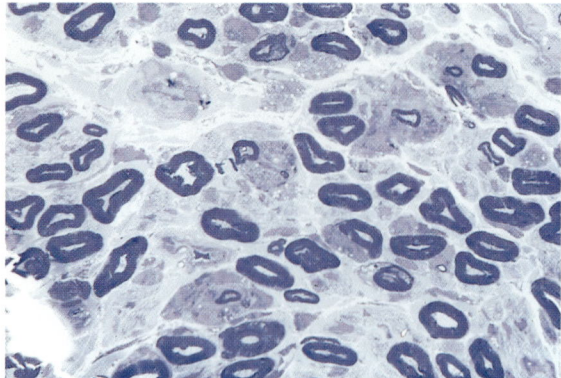

Fig. 6.9 Sural nerve biopsy showing variable thickness of myelin sheaths in a case of demyelinating neuropathy associated with HIV infection.

The pathogenesis of the demyelinating process is unclear even though circulating anti-peripheral nerve antibodies have been identified in some patients (Table 6.5) (Kiprov et al 1986, Miller et al 1989). These probably represent an epiphenomenon rather than being the primary cause of the neuropathy. Griffin and colleagues (1994b) used reverse transcriptase PCR to demonstrate increases in macrophage-derived cytokines, TNF-α and IL-1β transcripts within the nerves. This corresponds with the infiltration of the activated macrophages that appear to be responsible for myelin stripping and removal. Both GBS and

CIDP in HIV infection are distinguishable from the widespread peripheral neuropathy that has been associated with CMV infection (Cornford et al 1992a). This frequently has demyelinating features reflecting the ability of CMV to infect Schwann cells (Dalakas & Pezeshkpour 1988, Said et al 1991).

The recognition of this association between HIV-1 and IDPs means that a careful search for risk factors for HIV-1 infection and serological testing should be made in any patient presenting with IDP, especially if there is an unexpected CSF pleocytosis. At present, plasmapheresis is the treatment of choice because it is less likely than corticosteroids to aggravate existing immunological dysfunction. In GBS, a course of five plasma exchanges are given (Cornblath et al 1987). With CIDP, an induction course is followed by maintenance exchanges as needed. Where plasmapheresis is impractical or unavailable, short courses of corticosteroids or intravenous gammaglobulin are generally tolerated well in patients without advanced immunodeficiency without triggering opportunistic infections. Treatment with human immunoglobulin as used in non-HIV-related cases of relapsing or chronic inflammatory demyelinating neuropathy can be strikingly successful (Faed et al 1989), although the relapse rate may be higher than after plasmapheresis (Irani et al 1993). I.V. immunoglobulin

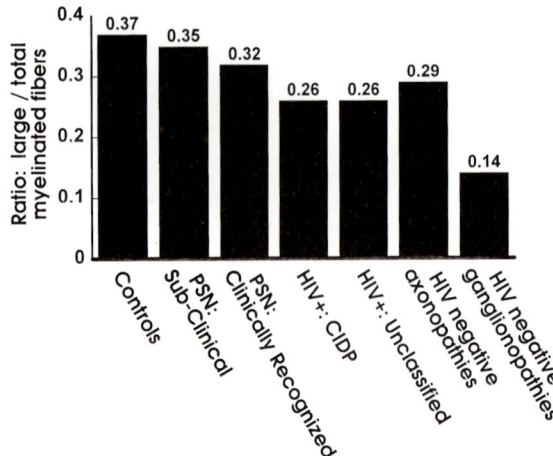

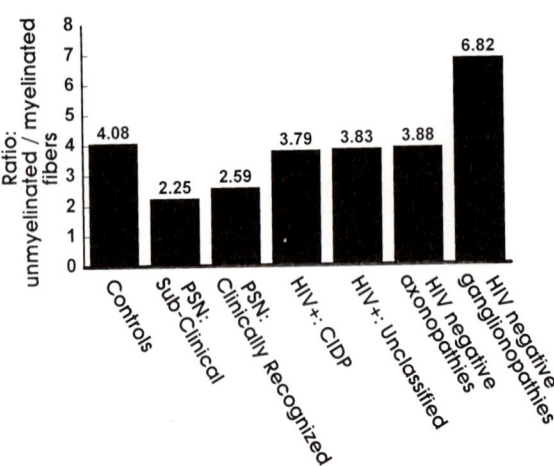

A   B

Fig. 6.10 Morphometric analysis of changes in large (**A**) and unmyelinated (**B**) nerve fibres from sural nerve biopsies. Note the reduction in large fibre density in HIV-positive CIDP and ganglionopathies. Unmyelinated nerve fibre density is significantly reduced in HIV predominantly sensory neuropathy. (Reproduced from Griffin et al 1994a with permission of Oxford University Press.)

Table 6.9   Clinical and pathological features of AIDS-related neuropathies

	Sensory neuropathy	Inflammatory demyelinating neuropathy
Prevalence	30%	<1%
Onset	Late HIV infection/AIDS	Early: asymptomatic seropositive
Symptoms	Pedal paraesthesias, dysaesthesias, 'burning feet'	Weakness, sometimes acute GBS or CIDP
Signs	Abnormal distal vibratory sensation, hyperalgesia, hyperpathia, absent or reduced ankle reflexes	Weakness, areflexia, later wasting
NCV/EMG	Axonal degeneration, secondary demyelination	Marked slowing compatible with primary demyelination
CSF	Protein: 40–60 mg/dl Cells: 0–10 WBC/mm^3	Protein: 50–200 mg/dl Cells: 10–40 WBC/mm^3
Pathology	Dying-back axonopathy (gracile tract degeneration), macrophage infiltration	Internodal demyelination, intense macrophage infiltration
Pathogenesis	Probably immunopathogenic (?): macrophage hyperresponsiveness leading to local cytokine release	Immunopathogenic: macrophage-mediated demyelination
Treatment	Symptomatic	Plasmapheresis

GBS, Guillain-Barré syndrome; CIDP, chronic inflammatory demyelinating polyneuropathy; WBC, white blood cells; NCV, nerve conduction velocity; EMG, electromyography.

Table 6.10   Diagnostic approach to patients with suspected neuropathy

Work-up	Diagnostic study	Implication
Blood studies	Vitamin B$_{12}$, E	Replacement therapy
	VDRL	Appropriate antibiotics
	Thyroid studies	Replacement therapy
	CD4+ count	Degree of immunosuppression
	Serology HIV, HTLV-I	Serostatus
CSF studies	Cells	10–50 WBC/mm^3 with IDP
	Total protein	50–200 mg/dl with IDP
	VDRL	+ with neurosyphilis
	CMV cultures	+ with CMV radiculitis
Electrodiagnostics	NCV	Marked slowing and conduction block with IDP
	EMG	Axonal degeneration and denervation with PSN
	SSEPs	Posterior column dysfunction
Nerve biopsy	Microscopy	Internodal demyelination, and macrophage infiltration with IDP; less intense macrophage infiltration and dying-back axonopathy with PSN

NCV, nerve conduction velocity; EMG, electromyography; SSEPs, somatosensory evoked potentials; WBC, white blood cells; IDP, inflammatory demyelinating polyneuropathy; PSN, peripheral sensory neuropathy.

is extremely expensive, and has been associated with renal failure in patients with pre-existing renal disease. Our recommendation would be to use plasmapheresis where available and reserve intravenous immunoglobulin only for patients in whom plasmapheresis cannot be performed safely or is not tolerated. In those with a sudden and severe illness, recovery is less likely and residual disability the usual outcome.

MONONEUROPATHIES

Mononeuritis multiplex is another rare type of peripheral neuropathy that has been recognized in HIV-1 infection. It typically affects patients with symptomatic HIV-1 disease who have not yet developed frank AIDS (Table 6.1) (Cornblath et al 1987). The patients develop individual nerve lesions, which may coalesce to mimic a diffuse neuropathy. The history usually makes the diagnosis clear if a symmetrical glove or stocking sensory loss begins as patchy asymmetrical deficits in the territory of a single nerve. Typically, motor and sensory deficits develop in an asymmetrical pattern over a few weeks; for example, a foot drop is followed by an ulnar nerve lesion or cranial nerves may be involved, as may the recurrent laryngeal nerve (this may also be due to CMV). The differential diagnosis when limb nerves are affected includes multiple pressure palsies in a bed-ridden or very cachectic patient, or the combination of an IDP with superadded pressure palsies due to the vulnerability of such neuropathic nerve trunks to the additional trauma of entrapment or external pressure. Electrophysiological studies show local lesions in nerves often at common entrapment sites, but also affecting nerves that are not mechanically vulnerable. Nerves that are not clinically affected may prove to show clear-cut conduction disturbances. Nerve biopsies show necrotizing arteritis like that seen in polyarteritis nodosa with what is essentially infarction of the nerve.

Lipkin et al (1985) described 11 AIDS-related complex patients with mononeuritis multiplex who had occasional CNS findings, mixed axonal-demyelinating conduction studies, and nerve biopsies showing a spectrum of pathological changes ranging from axonal degeneration to mixed axonal degeneration and demyelination. One-third of these patients later progressed to AIDS and several appeared to develop a more widespread peripheral neuropathy with features of CIDP. It seems likely that some cases of mononeuritis multiplex in HIV infection represent a variant of HIV-related CIDP while others are a true 'mononeuritis multiplex'. These latter cases have marked vasculitic changes (Fig. 6.11), and centrofascicular degeneration and circulating immune complexes may play a causative role. HIV (Gherardi et al 1989) and CMV (Said et al 1991) have both been incriminated, but many of these vasculitic cases are probably due to hepatitis B immune complex deposition (Gocke et al 1970). Faced with progressive weakness a nerve biopsy should be performed and steroids or intravenous immunoglobulin considered. Lymphomatous infiltration of peripheral nerve(s) is excessively rare, but should be considered in a

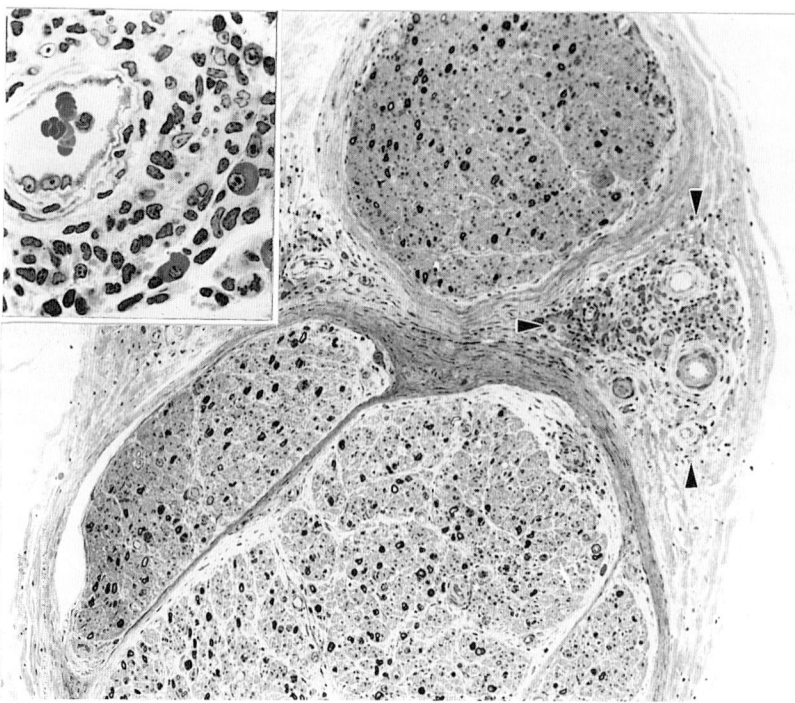

Fig. 6.11 Vasculitis in an HIV-positive female IVDU who was hepatitis B antigen positive. This sural nerve biopsy shows severe reduction in fibre density with inflammation around blood vessels (arrowheads) and destruction of blood vessel walls (insert). (Courtesy of Dr John Griffin.)

patient with systemic lymphoma. KS can also involve nerves locally.

Herpes group radiculitis

Five to ten per cent of patients with HIV-1 infection will develop herpes zoster radiculitis representing reactivation of latent h. zoster infection. While a single attack of shingles can occur in a patient with normal immunity, recurrent shingles should point to an underlying immune destruction and should trigger HIV testing. Uncomplicated dermatomal zoster can be treated with acyclovir 800 mg five times daily. This has been shown to speed lesion healing and reduce acute pain (Shepp et al 1986). Intravenous acyclovir is not necessary unless there is severe involvement of cervical or lumbar dermatomes. In this setting, a severe myeloradiculitis can develop, leading to permanent motor deficits, and intravenous acyclovir (30 mg/kg/day) should be used. The development of post-herpetic neuralgia may require the use of pain-modifying agents such as amitriptyline or carbamazepine. After the vesicles have completely healed, topical capsaicin can reduce the neuralgic pains. Ophthalmic involvement is common with the development of herpetic keratitis or retinitis and severe facial/ocular pain. It should be treated aggressively with topical antivirals and systemic acyclovir.

CMV causes a progressive radiculopathy involving lumbar and sacral roots (Miller et al 1990, Eidelberg 1986). Typically occurring in patients with advanced immune deficiency and CD4 counts < 100, a flaccid paralysis of the lower extremities develops over days or weeks with sacral or sciatic pain, paraesthesias and sphincter dysfunction. A herniated disc syndrome should not be confused as the clinical signs point to involvement of multiple roots. Sphincter impairment, sacral sensory loss and loss of the anal reflex accompany the progressive lower motor neurone weakness of the legs, which is quite unlike the sudden effect of central disc prolapse. The differential diagnosis includes involvement of the cauda equina by lymphoma and other infectious radiculopathies due to herpes zoster or syphilis. Investigations should include imaging of the cauda equina by myelography or contrast MRI,

which in CMV radiculitis may show nodular thickenings on multiple roots (Fig. 6.12) with enhancement of the pia on MRI (Fig. 6.13) (Talpos et al 1991). Early in the syndrome, imaging studies may be normal. The CSF typically contains greatly elevated protein, low glucose and a polymorphonuclear pleocytosis. CMV can be cultured in up to 50% of cases (Miller et al 1990, Cohen et al 1993). Cytopathology should be performed to check for lymphoma cells and may occasionally demonstrate cytomegalic cells (Glass & Erozan 1993). It may be fruitful to repeat the lumbar puncture in difficult cases, even if the initial CSF analysis is relatively normal. In some cases the CSF changes evolve over 1–2 weeks from normal to abnormal after neurological signs (Cohen et al 1993). The CSF formula consisting of a mixed pleocytosis with prominent polymorphonuclear leucocytes,

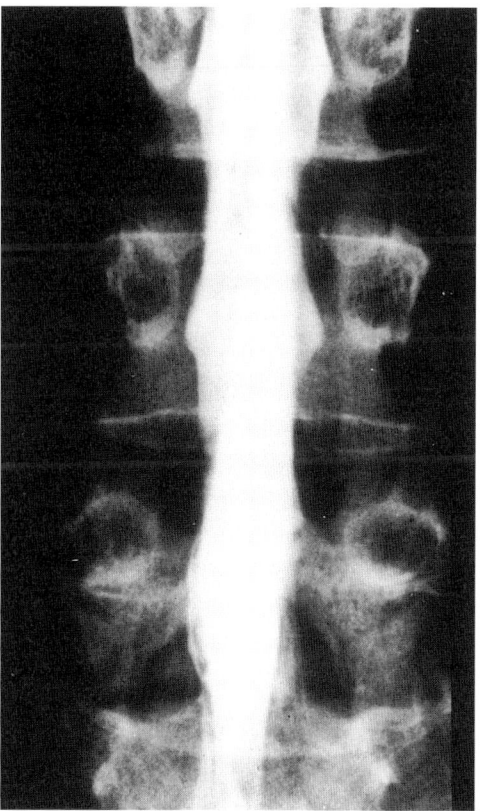

Fig. 6.12 Visible abnormality of lumbar roots on Iohexol myelography in a case of CMV radiculopathy. (Reproduced from Kendall 1993 with permission of Springer Verlag.)

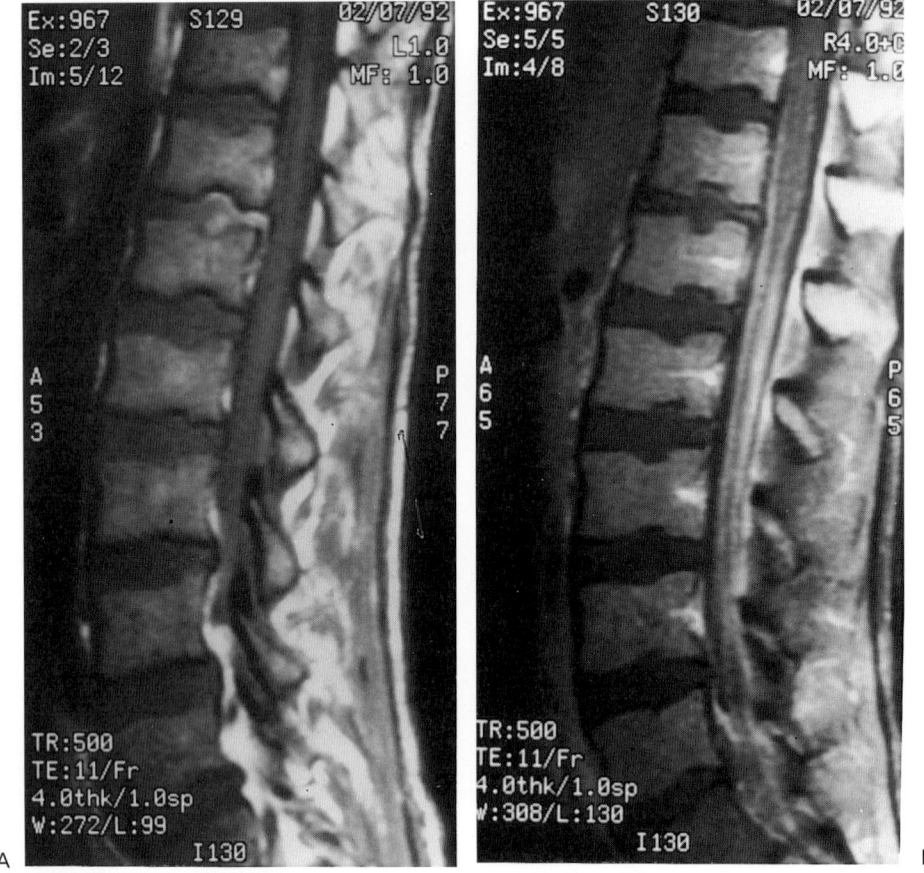

Fig. 6.13 **A** Pre- and **B** post-gadolinium T1-weighted MR images from a patient with CMV polyradiculitis with positive CMV cultures in blood and CSF showing enhancement in the cauda equina. (Courtesy of Dr Roland Lee, Johns Hopkins Hospital.)

elevated protein and hypoglycorrhachia is characteristic (Eidelberg et al 1986, Singh et al 1986, Behar et al 1987, Miller et al 1990). EMG studies typically demonstrate features of an axonal neuropathy with denervation changes and diminished compound muscle action potentials. F waves may be delayed or absent, with reduced evoked sensory nerve action potentials. Cohen and colleagues (1993) described three patients and reviewed the existing literature. Sixteen of 31 patients with CMV polyradiculitis were treated with ganciclovir. Clinical improvement occurred in six patients and stabilization in three. In patients successfully treated with ganciclovir, polymorphonuclear pleocytosis declined after induction therapy. Successfully treated patients had received ganciclovir within 2 weeks of onset of neurological symptoms. Four ganciclovir-treated patients who failed to respond showed persistent polymorphonuclear pleocytosis, hypoglycorrhachia and persistently positive CMV cultures. Foscarnet is an alternative anti-CMV drug, if a patient has already been receiving ganciclovir for CMV retinitis or is severely neutropenic.

Neuropathological features (Fig. 6.14) include acute and chronic inflammation in the ventral and dorsal nerve roots with CMV inclusions in Schwann cells and endothelia with foci of microvascular thrombosis and inflammation (Miller et al 1990). Necrotizing radiculomyelitis occurs and focal myelitis with anterior horn cell loss can be seen.

Patients with histologically proven CMV infec-

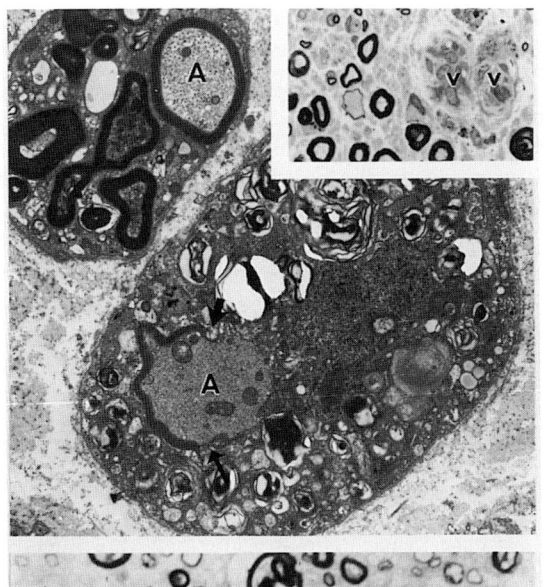

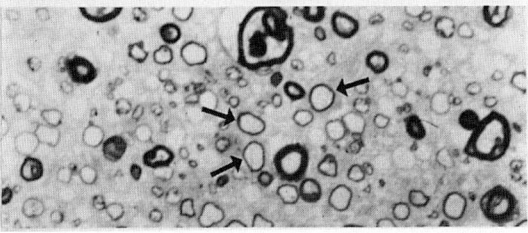

Fig. 6.14 Neuropathological features of CMV infection of nerve (upper panel) and lumbar roots (lower panel). The sural nerve biopsy from a case of multifocal demyelinating CMV neuropathy shows occluded vessels (v), demyelination and enlarged thinly myelinated fibres (inset), and extensive myelin debris (EM). The lumbar spinal root is from an autopsy 6 months after partially successful treatment of CMV polyradiculopathy with ganciclovir. Arrowed are thinly remyelinated fibres. (Reproduced from Griffin 1994 with permission of Raven Press.)

tion of lumbosacral roots (Fig. 6.14) usually have CMV retinitis, CMV viraemia and CD4 counts <100/mm³. The absence of such signs of systemic CMV infection is thus a pointer against the diagnosis. The physician should have a low threshold for entertaining this diagnosis, however, because of the therapeutic possibilities.

Cranial neuropathies

Cranial neuropathies are uncommon, affecting only 2–3% of patients with AIDS. Occasionally, cranial neuropathies will occur with HIV seroconversion and HIV-related meningitis (Ho et al 1985, Levy et al 1985). Bell's palsy is a relatively

common presentation, and in a person with risk factors for HIV infection should trigger HIV serological testing. Multiple cranial neuropathies may be a manifestation of chronic inflammatory polyneuropathy or of mononeuritis multiplex, and can develop rapidly with fulminant cryptococcal meningitis. In cryptococcal meningitis, cranial neuropathies herald elevated intracranial pressure and cranial nerve infiltration with fungi. Rarely will lymphomatous meningitis present with cranial neuropathies. In the absence of cryptococcal meningitis or lymphoma cells in repeated CSF samples, a vasculitic cause may be entertained and steroids prescribed.

Entrapment neuropathies

The patient with AIDS and wasting syndrome who is bed-bound is susceptible to nerve compression. There is added vulnerability in the presence of any generalized neuropathy or neurotoxic medication. The most common symptom complexes are (1) cubital tunnel syndrome with ulnar nerve compression at the elbow producing pain and paraesthesias in the forearm and 4th and 5th digits, sometimes with weakness in the intrinsic hand muscles; (2) common peroneal nerve compression at the fibula head resulting in a foot drop with numbness over the lateral lower extremity and dorsum of the foot; (3) meralgia paraesthetica with entrapment of the lateral cutaneous nerve of the thigh at the inguinal ligament and paraesthesiae over the lateral thigh; and (4) tarsal tunnel syndrome with entrapment of the posterior tibial nerve at the ankle and pain or paraesthesiae in the sole of the foot. The latter is very common in cachectic patients and is frequently mistaken for more generalized sensory neuropathies. Ankle reflexes are preserved and the sensory deficit is confined to the sole of the foot.

These entrapment syndromes are recognizable clinically by the distribution of symptoms and Tinel's signs and can be confirmed with electrophysiological testing. Treatment consists of appropriate padding and limb positioning to avoid further trauma. Local nerve blocks with bupivicaine may provide lasting relief, particularly in the tarsal tunnel. Cortisone injections are also useful.

Autonomic neuropathies

An early study of five patients with AIDS proposed that abnormal cardiac reflexes and autonomic neuropathies could occur in HIV disease. In patients with advanced HIV infection, severe cachexia and systemic infections, it is extremely difficult to discern whether there is concurrent autonomic dysfunction. Several studies have suggested, however, that autonomic dysfunction can be identified with a variety of autonomic function tests even in asymptomatic HIV carriers (Cohen & Laudenslagen 1989, Freeman et al 1990), and abnormality can be detected in sympathetic ganglia at autopsy (Chimelli & Scaravilli 1991). Postural hypotension, syncope, incontinence and impotence may all occur as a result of a small fibre neuropathy, but the differential diagnosis of such symptoms includes the effects of medication, prolonged immobility (postural hypotension) and depression. The differential diagnosis of bladder disturbance or impotence includes lumbar radiculopathy due to CMV, but this will be accompanied by root pain, flaccid weakness and loss of lower limb reflexes. Cerebral causes of incontinence and impotence will usually be identifiable as the patients will also have dementia or alterations of mental state, extensor plantars, and may have other 'frontal lobe signs' such as grasp reflexes.

Tests of cardiovascular reflexes are the easiest way to assess autonomic fibres (Cohen & Laudenslagen 1989, Villa et al 1992), with pulse and blood pressure responses to standing up, deep breathing, hand-grip and the Valsalva manoeuvre. In the presence of autonomic neuropathy, care must be taken with medication that may aggravate hypotension or sphincter disturbance. Further study is needed to identify the frequency of clinically significant autonomic abnormalities and whether they are caused directly by HIV-1 or by the numerous medications used in patients with AIDS.

GANGLIONEURITIS

Rare cases have been described of a progressive sensory ataxia clinically resembling the condition sometimes seen as a non-metastatic complication of malignancies (Elder et al 1986). The patients' progressive ataxia resembles a cerebellar syndrome until the severity of joint position sense loss is appreciated on full examination. Tendon jerks are usually lost, but nerve conduction studies may reveal little change. Examination of the dorsal root ganglia at autopsy in unselected cases reveals that inflammation is rarely severe, but cell loss not uncommon, so it is perhaps surprising that this condition is not seen more often (Scaravilli et al 1992).

REFERENCES

Apfel S C, Lipton R B, Arezzo J C, Kessler J A. Nerve growth factor prevents toxic neuropathy in mice. Ann Neurol 1991; 29: 87–90

Asbury A K, Fields H L. Pain due to peripheral nerve damage. An hypothesis. Neurology 1984; 34: 1587–1590

Asbury A K, Porte D. Proceedings of a consensus development conference on standardized measures in diabetic neuropathy. Neurology 1992; 42: 1823–1839

Barohn R J, Gronseth G S, LeForce B R, et al. Peripheral nervous system involvement in a large cohort of human immunodeficiency virus-infected individuals. Arch Neurol 1993; 50: 167–171

Behar R, Wiley C, McCutchan J A. Cytomegalovirus polyradiculoneuropahy in acquired immune deficiency syndrome. Neurology 1987; 37: 557–561

Belec L, Gherardi R, Georges A J, et al. Peripheral facial paralysis and HIV infection: report of four African cases and review of the literature. J Neurol 1989; 236: 411–414

Berger A R, Arezzo J C, Schaumburg H H, et al. 2',3'-Dideoxycytidine (ddC) toxic neuropathy: a study of 52 patients. Neurology 1993; 43: 358–362

Blum A, Dal Pan G, Raines C, et al. DdC-related toxic neuropathy: risk factors and natural history. Neurology 1993; suppl 2: A190–191 (abstr 149s)

Casey K L. Toward a rationale for the treatment of painful neuropathies. In: Dubner R, Gebhart G F, Bond M R, editors. Proceedings of the Vth World Congress on Pain. Amsterdam: Elsevier, 1988.

Chaunu M P, Ratinahirana H, Raphael M, et al. The spectrum of changes on 20 nerve biopsies in patients with HIV infection. Muscle Nerve 1989; 15: 452–459

Chavanet P Y, Giroud M, Lancon J P, et al. Altered peripheral nerve conduction in HIV-patients. Cancer Detect Prev 1988; 12: 249–255

Chimelli L, Scaravilli F. Morphological changes in the autonomic nervous system of patients with AIDS. Proc XIth Int Conf Neuroscience in AIDS, Padova, 1991: 89

Cohen B A, McArthur J C, Grohman S, et al. Neurologic

prognosis in CMV polyradiculomyelopathy in AIDS. Neurology 1993; 43: 493–499

Cohen J A, Laudenslagen M. Autonomic nervous system involvement in patients with human immunodeficiency virus infection. Neurology 1989; 39: 1111–1112

Cornblath D R, Griffin D E, Welch D, et al. Quantitative analysis of endoneurial T-cells in human sural nerve biopsies. J Neuroimmunol 1990; 26: 113–118

Cornblath D R, McArthur J C. Predominantly sensory neuropathy in patients with AIDS and AIDS-related complex. Neurology 1988; 38: 794–796

Cornblath D R, McArthur J C, Kennedy P G, et al. Inflammatory demyelinating peripheral neuropathies associated with human T-cell lymphotropic virus type III infection. Ann Neurol 1987; 21: 32–40

Cornford M E, Ho H W, Vinters H V. Correlation of neuromuscular pathology in acquired immune deficiency syndrome patients with cytomegalovirus infection and zidovudine treatment. Acta Neuropathologica 1992a; 84: 516–529

Cornford M E, Holden J K, Boyd M C, et al. Neuropathology of the acquired immune deficiency syndrome (AIDS) – report of 39 autopsies from Vancouver, British Columbia. Can J Neurol Sci 1992b; 19: 442–452

Cotton P. Compliance problems, placebo effect cloud trials of topical analgesic. JAMA 1990; 264: 13–14

Coxon A, Pallis C A. Metronidazole neuropathy. J Neurol Neurosurg Psychiatr 1976; 39: 403–405

Dalakas M C, Pezeshkpour G H. Neuromuscular diseases associated with human immunodeficiency virus infection. Ann Neurol 1988; 23: S38–S48

Dubinsky R M, Yarchoan R, Dalakas M, Broder S. Reversible axonal neuropathy from the treatment of AIDS and related disorders with 2',3'-dideoxycytidine (ddC). Muscle Nerve 1989; 12: 856–860

Eidelberg D, Sortel A, Vogel H, et al. Progressive polyradiculopathy in acquired immune deficiency syndrome. Neurology 1986; 36: 912–916

Elder G, Dalakas M, Pezeshkpour G, Sever J. Ataxic neuropathy due to ganglioneuronitis after probable acute human immunodeficiency virus infection (letter). Lancet 1986; 2: 1275–1276

Faed J M, Day B, Pollock M, et al. High dose intravenous human immunoglobulin in chronic inflammatory demyelinating polyneuropathy. Neurology 1989; 39: 422–425

Freeman R, Roberts M S, Friedman L S, Broadbridge C. Autonomic function and human immunodeficiency virus infection. Neurology 1990; 40: 575–580

Fuller G N, Jacobs J M, Guiloff R J. Association of painful peripheral neuropathy in AIDS with cytomegalovirus infection. Lancet 1989; 2: 937–941

Fuller G N, Jacobs J M, Guiloff R J. Subclinical peripheral nerve involvement in AIDS – an electrophysiological and pathological study. J Neurol Neurosurg Psychiatr 1991; 54: 318–324

Fuller G N, Jacobs J M, Guiloff R J. Nature and incidence of peripheral nerve syndromes in HIV infection. J Neurol Neurosurg Psychiatr 1993; 56: 372–381

Gastaut J L, Gastaut J A, Pellissier J F, et al. Neuropathies with HIV infection. Prospective study of 56 cases. Revue Neurol 1989; 145: 451–459

Gherardi R, Lebargy F, Gaulard P, et al. Necrotizing vasculitis and HIV replication in peripheral nerves (letter). N Engl J Med 1989; 321: 685–686

Glass J D, Erozan Y S. Rapid diagnosis of cytomegalovirus polyradiculitis in a patient with acquired immunodeficiency syndrome. Ann Neurol 1993; 34: 239

Gocke D J, Hsu K, Morgan C et al. Association between polyarteritis and Australia antigen. Lancet 1970; 2: 1149–1153

Goldstick L, Mandybur T I, Bode R. Spinal cord degeneration in AIDS. Neurology 1985; 35: 103–106

Griffin J W. In: Price R W, Perry S W, editors. HIV, AIDS and the brain. New York: Raven Press, 1994, 159–182

Griffin J W, Cornblath D R, Wesselingh S L, et al. Pathology of HIV-associated Guillain-Barré syndrome and chronic inflammatory demyelinating polyneuropathy. Ann Neurol 1994c; in press

Griffin J W, Crawford T O, Glass J D, et al. Sensory neuropathy in AIDS: I. Neuropathology. Brain 1994a; in press

Griffin J W, Crawford T O, Tyor W R, et al. Sensory neuropathy in AIDS: II. Immunopathology. Brain 1994b; in press

Grossman S A, Sheidler B R. An aid to prescribing narcotics for the relief of cancer pain. World Health Forum 1987; 8 (4): 525–529 Figs 1 and 2

Hall C D, Synder C R, Messenheimer J A, et al. Peripheral neuropathy in a cohort of human immunodeficiency virus-infected patients: incidence and relationship to other nervous system dysfunction. Arch Neurol 1991; 48: 1273–1274

Ho D D, Sarngadharan M G, Resnick L, et al. Primary human T-lymphotropic virus type III infection. Ann Intern Med 1985; 103: 880–883

Irani D N, Cornblath D R, Chaudhry V, et al. Relapse in Guillain-Barré syndrome after treatment with human immune globulin. Neurology 1993; 43: 872–875

Jaffe J H. Drug addiction and drug abuse. In: Gilman A G, Rall T W, Nies A S, editors. The pharmacological basis of therapeutics. New York: Pergamon Press, 1990

Jakobsen J, Smith T, Gaub J, et al. Progressive neurological dysfunction during latent HIV infection. Br Med J 1989; 299: 225–228

Janssen R S, Cornblath D R, Epstein L G, et al. Nomenclature and research case definitions for neurological manifestations of human immunodeficiency virus type-1 (HIV-1) infection. Report of a Working Group of the American Academy of Neurology AIDS Task Force. Neurology 1991; 41: 778–785

Kendall B E. Acquired immune deficiency: neuroradiological imaging. In: Scaravilli F, editor. The neuropathology of HIV infection. London: Springer-Verlag, 1993: 35–52

Kiprov D D, Abrams D, Pfaeffl W, et al. ARC/AIDS-related autoimmune syndromes and their treatment. II International Conference on AIDS 1986; Paris (abstract)

Lambert J S, Seidlin M, Reichman R C, et al. 2',3'-Dideoxyinosine (ddI) in patients with the acquired immunodeficiency syndrome or AIDS-related complex. A phase I trial. N Engl J Med 1990; 322: 1333–1340

Levy R M, Bredesen D E, Rosenblum M L. Neurological manifestations of the acquired immunodeficiency syndrome (AIDS): experience at UCSF and review of the literature. J Neurosurg 1985; 62: 475–495

Lhermitte F, Fritel D, Cambier J. Polyneurites au cours de traitements par la nitrofurantoine. Presse Med 1963; 71: 767

Lipkin W I, Parry G, Kiprov D, Abrams D. Inflammatory neuropathy in homosexual men with lymphadenopathy. Neurology 1985; 35: 1479–1483

Marks R M, Sachar E J. Undertreatment of medical inpatients with narcotic analgesics. Ann Intern Med 1973; 78: 173–181

Max M B, Lynch S A, Muir J, et al. Effects of desipramine, amitriptyline, and fluoxetine in pain in diabetic neuropathy. New Engl J Med 1992; 326: 1250–1256

McAllister R H, Herns M V, Harrison M J G, et al. Neurological and neuropsychological performance in HIV seropositive men without symptoms. J Neurol Neurosurg Psychiatr 1992; 55: 143–148

Miller R G, Storey J, Greco C. Successful treatment of progressive polyradiculopathy in AIDS patients. Neurology 1989; 39 (suppl): 271

Miller R G, Storey J R, Greco C M. Ganciclovir in the treatment of progressive AIDS-related polyradiculopathy. Neurology 1990; 40: 569–574

Parry G J. Peripheral neuropathies associated with human immunodeficiency virus infection. Ann Neurol 1988; 23: S49–S53

Portenoy R K. Issues in the management of neuropathic pain. In: Basbaum A I, Besson J-M, editors. Towards a new pharmacotherapy of pain. New York: John Wiley, 1991: 393–416

Portenoy R K. Drug therapy for neuropathic pain. Drug Therapy 1993; 23: 41–53

Portenoy R K. Iatrogenic addiction. In: Jaffe J H, editor. The encyclopaedia of drugs and alcohol. New York: MacMillan Publishing Company, 1994

Portenoy R K, Foley K M. Chronic use of opioid analgesics in non-malignant pain: report of 38 cases. Pain 1986; 25: 171–186

Rance N E, McArthur J C, Cornblath D R, et al. Gracile tract degeneration in patients with sensory neuropathy and AIDS. Neuroloy 1988; 38: 265–271

Raphael S A, Price M L, Lischner H W, et al. Inflammatory demyelinating polyneuropathy in a child with symptomatic human immunodeficiency virus infection. J Pediat 1991; 118: 242–245

Said G, Lacroix C, Chemouilli P, et al. Cytomegalovirus neuropathy in acquired immunodeficiency syndrome – a clinical and pathological study. Ann Neurol 1991; 29: 139–146

Scaravilli F, Sinclair E, Arango J-C, et al. The pathology of the posterior root ganglia in AIDS and its relationship to the pallor of the gracile tract. Acta Neuropathol (Berl) 1992; 84: 163–170

Schaumburg H H, Arezzo J, Berger A, et al. Dideoxycytidine (ddC) neuropathy in human immunodeficiency virus infection: a report of 52 patients (abstract). Neurology 1990; 40(suppl): 248

Selwyn P A, O'Connor P G. Diagnosis and treatment of substance users with HIV infection. Primary Care 1992; 19: 119–156

Shepp D H, Danliker P S, Meyers J D. Treatment of varicella-zoster virus infection in severely immunocompromised patients. N Engl J Med 1986; 314: 209–212

Simpson D M, Wolfe D E. Neuromuscular complications of HIV infection and its treatment. AIDS 1991; 5: 917–926

Singh B M, Levine S, Yarrish R L, et al. Spinal cord syndromes in the acquired immune deficiency syndrome. Acta Neurol Scand 1986; 73: 590–598

Snider W D, Simpson D M, Nielsen S, et al. Neurological complications of acquired immune deficiency syndrome: analysis of 50 patients. Ann Neurol 1983; 14: 403–418

So Y T, Holtzman D M, Abrams D I, Olney R K. Peripheral neuropathy associated with acquired immunodeficiency syndrome. Prevalence and clinical features from a population-based survey. Arch Neurol 1988; 45: 945–948

Talpos D, Tien R D, Hesselink J R. Magnetic resonance imaging of AIDS-related polyradiculopathy. Neurology 1991; 41: 1996–1997

Vendrell J, Heredia C, Pujol M, et al. Guillain-Barré syndrome associated with seroconversion for anti-HTLV-III (letter). Neurology 1987; 37: 544

Villa A, Foresti V, Confalonieri F. Autonomic nervous system dysfunction associated with HIV infection in intravenous heroin users. AIDS 1992; 6: 85–89

Wechsler A F, Ho D D. Bilateral Bell's palsy at the time of HIV seroconversion. Neurology 1989; 39: 747–748

Winer J B, Bang B, Clarke J R, et al. A study of neuropathy in HIV infection. Q J Med 1992; 83: 473–488

7. Muscle disease

Although the principal neurological complications of HIV infection have been fairly well characterized, controversy surrounds the cause and nature of muscle-related symptoms associated with HIV infection and antiretroviral therapy. Two major forms of myopathy are seen: HIV-associated polymyositis and toxic myopathy secondary to zidovudine. Other forms of myopathy are less common and are usually easily distinguished (Table 7.1). A survey of skeletal muscle pathology at autopsy (Wrzolek et al 1990) reveals a high prevalence of disuse atrophy and examples of denervation associated with peripheral neuropathy. Of 92 autopsied cases, 51 showed a distribution of muscle fibre atrophy within fascicles typical of the results of disuse, and eight had angular fibres indicative of denervation. Three had evidence of infection (cryptococcal, *Mycobacterium avium intracellulare*) and eight had a necrotizing myopathy. In addition, eight had evidence of an inflammatory process. Muscle biopsy series reveal a similar spectrum, though with more florid changes in keeping with their symptomatic state. For example, Gabbai et al (1990) biopsied 50 patients with some degree of muscle wasting. Signs of denervation were prominent (angular fibres in 38, fibre type grouping in 31). Eighteen patients had inflammatory changes accompanied in most cases by fibre necrosis. The spectrum of light and electron microscopic abnormalities is wide (Table 7.2).

Table 7.1 Muscle disorders in AIDS

HIV-associated polymyositis
Zidovudine toxic myopathy
Pyomyositis
Cardiomyopathy
Wasting in advanced AIDS

Table 7.2 Spectrum of biopsy findings

LM	Type 2 fibre loss
	Mild inflammation (macrophages/lymphocytes)
	Necrotic fibres
	Nemaline rods
	Microvacuolar degeneration
	Ragged red-type fibres
EM	Paracrystalline inclusions
	Vesicular changes
	Dilated sarcoplasmic reticulum
	Swollen mitochondria
	Tubuloreticular inclusions in capillary endothelium

LM, light microscopy; EM, electron microscopy.

What remains controversial is the clinical relevance of the structural changes described, and the aetiological role of zidovudine. Clinically recognized cases of HIV-related myopathy or polymyositis (Dalakas et al 1986) were originally considered rare, but in recent years muscle pain, weakness and wasting, particularly of the glutei, have appeared to be more common. Some have related this to a toxic effect of zidovudine, introduced in 1986 (Richman et al 1987). An alternative explanation is that the muscle changes are an effect of the virus (Simpson & Bender 1988) and that the increased incidence results from the extended survival on antiviral treatment. Some of the confusion relates to variable definitional criteria for myopathy, and to difficulties in assessing muscle strength in the presence of systemic disease and pain. Some reports have equated an elevated serum creatine phosphokinase (CPK) level alone with 'myopathy' in asymptomatic subjects. Moderate creatine kinase (CK) elevations are relatively frequent and non-specific, sometimes reflecting heavy exercise or muscle trauma from injury or injections. For example, in one serosurvey of 112 seropositive individuals performed in the Multicenter AIDS Cohort Study (MACS), CK elevations >200 IU/l were found in five of 51 zidovudine recipients and seven of 55 antiretroviral-free men. After neurological examination, only one individual with a CK of 2361 IU/l had true myopathy. Furthermore, many patients had coincidental myelopathy or peripheral neuropathy making neurological and neurophysiological assessment difficult.

HIV-ASSOCIATED POLYMYOSITIS

In 1986, Dalakas et al described an inflammatory polymyositis akin to that seen in simian AIDS which might occur in the asymptomatic phase of the disease when the patients may show a polyclonal hypergammaglobulinopathy. It was concluded that this was an immunologically related disorder, thus representing an example of immune dysregulation analogous to immune thrombocytopenic purpura (ITP) or inflammatory demyelinating polyradiculoneuropathy (IDP). Rare cases showing rhabdomyolysis at the time of seroconversion (Mahe et al 1989) or repeated episodes of myoglobinuria whilst asymptomatic (Younger et al 1989) support this interpretation. The clinical picture (Table 7.3) in these cases of polymyositis included acute proximal weakness accompanied by elevated CK levels, usually in the range of 2–10 times normal values. Simpson claims there is no concordance between the CK levels and the degree of weakness (Simpson & Wolfe 1991). Myalgias are present in many patients but are somewhat less intense than those in zidovudine toxic myopathy. Myopathic EMG changes are seen in most patients with short motor unit potentials, fibrillations and sharp

waves. Biopsy shows numerous inflammatory cells and muscle fibre necrosis (Fig. 7.1). The spectrum of pathological findings includes non-inflammatory myofibre degeneration and the accumulation of nemaline rod bodies and mitochondrial abnormalities (Simpson & Wolfe 1991). The impression gained from many of our biopsies is that the predominant muscle change is of fibre atrophy (sometimes most obvious in type 2 fibres), together with occasional inflammatory reactions. The fibre atrophy is similar to that seen in a wide range of conditions including cachexia and malnutrition. It may often simply reflect the general catabolic state of these patients, as seen in autopsy series (Wrzolek et al 1990). There is probably a spectrum from mild atrophic change through a 'bland' myopathy to an inflammatory polymyositis. The specificity of these findings and their occurrence with zidovudine myopathy is discussed later. Subsequent to Dalakas' 1986 report, others demonstrated that clinical signs of a myopathy with muscle weakness could occur with little or no inflammatory reaction in the biopsy (Simpson & Bender 1988).

Despite one report of gp41 immunostaining in muscle macrophages (Chad et al 1990), there is no clear evidence of viral infection of muscle fibres. This differs from the polymyositis associated with HTLV-I, where in situ hybridization has clearly demonstrated viral sequences within the muscle fibres (Wiley et al 1989). The

Table 7.3   HIV-associated polymyositis

- Any stage of HIV infection
- Progressive proximal weakness, myalgias, thighs
- CK: 2–6 × normal
- EMG: myopathic; brief MUPs with fibrillations and sharp waves
- Biopsy: myofibre necrosis with inflammatory infiltrates, myofibre degeneration, nemaline rod bodies, and possibly ragged red-type fibres

MUPs, motor unit potentials.

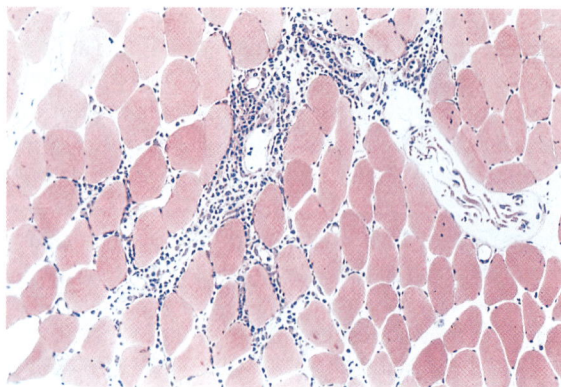

Fig. 7.1   Striking infiltration of muscle biopsy specimen by inflammatory cells in a case of inflammatory myopathy associated with HIV infection. (Courtesy of Dr Ralph Kinch, Johns Hopkins University.)

inflammatory response consists of CD8 cells (Dalakas et al 1986) and macrophages. It has recently been proposed that the latter are dysfunctional because iron accumulates, which is not seen in non-AIDS cases of polymyositis (Lacroix & Said 1992). It has been suggested that HIV-infected CD8 cells produce cytokines that expose muscle fibre antigens against which there is no self-tolerance. It is also possible that there is some homology between the viral gag protein and muscle ribonucleoproteins, which could trigger an autoimmune process. The resulting immunological reaction leads to a self-sustaining cellular infiltration and myofibre damage and necrosis (Illa et al 1991).

Simpson et al (1993b) have studied the effect of steroids in patients with HIV polymyositis and found that prednisone-treated patients had significant relief of myalgias and decreases in CK compared with placebo-treated patients. Dalakas also reported a response in five patients treated with prednisone with no precipitation of opportunistic infections. Pulse intravenous steroids (methylprednisolone 15 mg/kg) have been used, but not in a controlled fashion. Our own experience in four patients was that it was not particularly effective and in one precipitated *Listeria* meningitis. Plasmapheresis and intravenous immunoglobulin have also been suggested as immunomodulatory therapy (Viard et al 1992) and both would probably be better tolerated than high-dose corticosteroids. At this point, we would treat a patient with functionally limiting polymyositis with oral corticosteroids. If there was no response, intravenous immunoglobulin would be tried, or plasmapheresis considered.

ZIDOVUDINE TOXIC MYOPATHY

Since the introduction of zidovudine, muscle problems have appeared to be much more prevalent. There is clearly some toxic effect from zidovudine, which manifests as a painful proximal myopathy, usually after several months (at least) of zidovudine therapy. As with toxic neuropathies, there appears to be a dose–duration effect, and the impression is that zidovudine myopathy was more common in the period 1987–1989 when 'standard' doses of zidovudine were 1000–1500 mg/day, rather than today's 600 mg/day. Muscle pain in thighs and calves was recorded in the first clinical trial (Richman et al 1987), and anecdotal accounts of patients with muscle necrosis whilst on treatment began to appear (Bessen et al 1988, Gertner et al 1989). These reports were more frequent when doses of zidovudine were higher. The incidence may have decreased now that the recommended dose has been reduced to 600 mg daily, as one would expect with a dose-dependent phenomenon. Fischl et al (1989) reported that 30% of patients on long-term zidovudine developed a myopathy, although most patients were not examined in detail to confirm the diagnosis. In some series an elevated CK level appeared to precede clinical signs (Peters et al 1989). In other patients, weight loss and an elevated serum lactate has appeared before weakness (Jay et al 1992). Additional evidence for zidovudine's role comes from the effect of a drug holiday, and rechallenge.

Withdrawal of zidovudine is usually followed by prompt reduction in both myalgic symptoms and CK elevations. Peters et al (1993) reported a prospective study of 118 patients, 88 of whom were receiving zidovudine. Seven of the 41 patients who had taken zidovudine for at least 270 days, but no other individuals, developed clinical and biochemical evidence of myopathy. Stopping treatment often led to a reduction in muscle pain within a week, normalization of serum CPK in 4 weeks, and improved power in 8–10 weeks. Muscle wasting rarely reversed. Histology of biopsies showed mitochondrial abnormalities that were partially reversible. Chalmers et al (1991) stopped zidovudine in 15 myopathic patients on treatment. Muscle pain resolved in all 10 in whom it had been a presenting feature within 1–2 weeks, but strength recovered more slowly (6–20 weeks), and not universally, with three patients showing persistent weakness. Recovery has not been the universal experience (Simpson et al 1993a) and it has often been impossible from the clinical presentation or CK level to predict the biopsy appearance, or from any of the parameters to predict the effect of zidovudine withdrawal or steroid treatment.

'Characteristic' changes of zidovudine myotoxicity on muscle biopsy have been reported by some (Dalakas et al 1990) but not by others. Dalakas found ragged red-type fibres on trichrome-stained sections, which reflect the accumulation of abnormal mitochondria in the sub-sarcolemmal space. His group did not find such changes in biopsies from myopathic patients who had not received zidovudine. Both groups of patients showed mild inflammatory changes (Fig. 7.2) and some had nemaline rods. The number of ragged red-type fibres seemed to correlate with the clinical severity, and in two patients who improved on cessation of the drug, biopsies also improved. Simpson and Bender (1988) found few ragged red-type fibres and were unable to tell whether biopsies came from zidovudine-treated or untreated cases. Panegyres et al (1990) found vesicular changes in both treated and untreated patients but suggested they could be distinguished under electron microscopy. The vesicles in four zidovudine-treated patients were due to swollen mitochondria, with proliferation and disorganization of their cristae, whilst the superficially similar vesicular appearance in two untreated cases was due to dilatations of the sarcoplasmic reticulum with normal-looking mitochondria. Pezeshkpour et al (1991) compared the biopsy appearances in 13 myopathic patients on zidovudine with those of five patients on no anti-viral treatment. Both groups showed disorganization of myofibrillar structures with nemaline rods, vacuolation and inflammation. Blind reading of the biopsies confirmed that the treated cases had sub-sarcolemmal proliferation of abnormal mitochondria with proliferation and disorganization of their cristae.

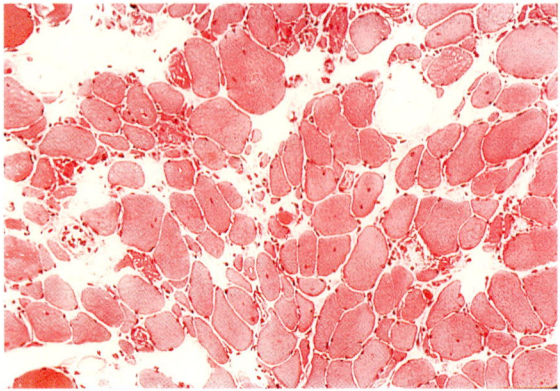

Fig. 7.2 Fibre necrosis with mild cellular infiltration in a biopsy from a case of zidovudine-related myopathy. (Courtesy of Dr Ralph Kinch, Johns Hopkins University.)

Cytoplasmic bodies occurred in all zidovudine-treated patients, but only one other patient. Dalakas has also shown a decrease in mitochondrial DNA in muscle biopsies from patients on zidovudine compared with myopathic patients off treatment and controls (Arnaudo et al 1991). The ratio of mDNA to total rDNA was 1.1 ± 0.5 for zidovudine-related biopsies compared with 2.3 ± 0.2 for controls. Patients with ragged red-type fibres on biopsy had an 80% reduction in their mitochondrial DNA expressed as a fraction of DNA, reflecting total cellular DNA. This fits with zidovudine's mode of action as a DNA polymerase and protein synthesis inhibitor. In addition, there is now evidence from muscle cells in tissue culture (Miranda et al 1990) and from an animal model that zidovudine causes mitochondrial damage (Lamperth et al 1991). Proliferation of mitochondria was caused by exposing cultured myocytes to zidovudine (mean 27.5 ± 8 mitochondria/ 16 μm^2 surface area, compared with 12.8 ± 4; $p<0.001$). Animals given zidovudine developed elevated CPK levels, and high levels of the drug were found in skeletal and cardiac muscle, again with enlarged mitochondria with damaged cristae. Biochemical studies pointed to uncoupling of oxidative metabolism. There is further evidence that cardiac muscle is also affected (Lewis et al 1991). Thus rats given zidovudine after 35 days had cardiac mitochondrial swelling with disorganized cristae, and depressed levels of cytochrome-b mRNA expression. Interestingly the effect was time and dose dependent, and showed no recovery over a 14-day period after withdrawal of the drug.

Patients exposed to zidovudine also show metabolic changes on ^{31}P spectroscopy suggesting impairment of mitochondrial function (Weismann et al 1991). Phosphate spectra were obtained from the calf muscles of eight patients treated with zidovudine, only one of whom had any clinical suspicions of myopathy, and seven age-matched controls. They exercised a foot on a modified ergometer at half maximum effort with ischaemia induced by a thigh cuff for 2 minutes or to the point of subjective fatigue. The spectra showed a fall of PCr of about 50% in both groups. After release of the cuff, PCr levels recovered exponentially. The calculated time constant revealed significantly slower regeneration of PCr in the group of zidovudine-treated patients (time constant 43.3 ± 12.5 s compared with 24.4 ± 3.9 s; $p < 0.001$). Delayed recovery after exercise is characteristic of a number of mitochondrial myopathies (Nishikawa et al 1989). Such a metabolic problem during recovery after exercise may underlie some of the complaints of fatiguability and exercise-related muscle pain. The evidence strongly suggests therefore that zidovudine does affect muscle mitochondrial structure and function (Mhiri et al 1991), but the precise clinico-pathological correlation of the ultrastructural and biochemical changes remains unclear.

The clinical data are somewhat confused. Myalgia is commonly reported and equated with myopathy even when there is no weakness or pathology on biopsy (Miller et al 1991). Some studies equate an elevated CK level with myopathy despite the tendency for levels to fluctuate widely. The best clinical evidence for a pathological effect of zidovudine on muscle would clearly be if symptoms were unique, followed shortly after initiation of treatment, resolved in parallel with laboratory markers on cessation, and recurred with rechallenge. These criteria have been met by some patients (Fig. 7.3) (Till & MacDonell 1990), but not by others whose presentation seemed identical (Helbert et al 1988). Zidovudine does not appear to cause major myotoxic effects in uninfected individuals, so the myopathic effect may be peculiar to HIV-infected muscle (Gertner et al 1989), and such a double insult hypothesis would go some way towards explaining the conflicting evidence. In the clinic, myopathy is uncommon unless the patient has been taking zidovudine in doses of 600 mg/day or more for at least 9 months. The comparison between HIV myopathy and zidovudine-related myopathy is shown in Table 7.4.

The lack of consistent muscle change in relationship to muscle pain is not surprising as there is often little relationship between extent of visible muscle fibre pathology and pain in other muscle diseases. Most patients with mitochondrial myopathies and those with defects of glycolysis complain of acute pain related to exercise rather than of chronic muscle ache as reported by the HIV patients. Muscular dystrophy is usually painless despite extensive fibre damage, whilst the pain of polymyositis is very variable. On the other hand,

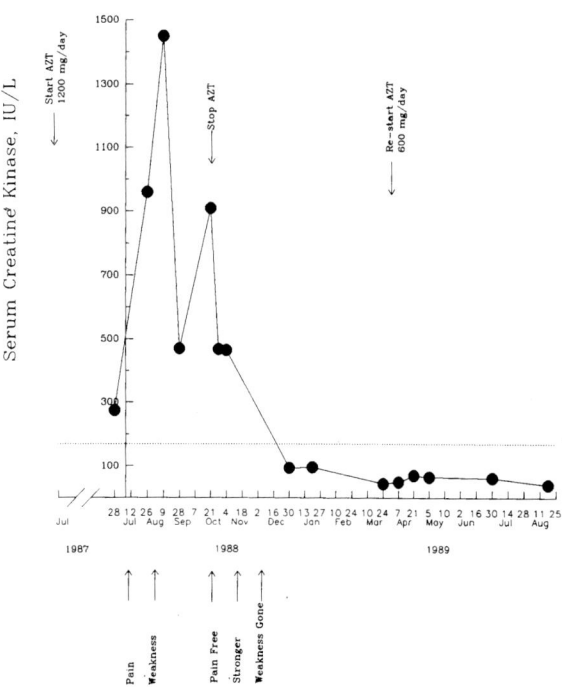

Fig. 7.3 CPK profile in zidovudine toxic myopathy. A patient receiving zidovudine 1200 mg/day for months developed myalgias, followed by weakness and CPK elevation to >1400 IU/l. A zidovudine drug holiday was initiated with prompt resolution in myalgias, followed by improvement in strength. CPK normalized within 4 weeks. (Courtesy of Dr Ralph Kinch, Johns Hopkins University.)

connective tissue disorders such as systemic lupus erythematosus (SLE), with which AIDS has so many parallels (Kaye 1989), can give rise to severe muscle pain with remarkably little muscle fibre pathology on biopsy, or on EMG. This raises the possibility that the pain in the HIV patient group may represent more of a connective tissue disorder.

Simpson et al (1993a) have recently described the clinical, laboratory, electrophysiological and pathological features and the effects of zidovudine in 50 patients with HIV-associated myopathy. At the time of diagnosis of myopathy, 21 patients had AIDS, 12 symptomatic HIV infection (ARC) and 17 asymptomatic HIV infection. Thirty-eight of the 50 patients were gay men, and another nine had used injection drugs. Thirty-one subjects with myopathy had received zidovudine, while 19 had never received the antiretroviral. Among the 31 zidovudine users, the mean daily dose was 1.1 g, with a mean duration of 15.5

Table 7.4   Findings in 50 patients with HIV-associated myopathy with or without zidovudine

	Zidovudine (n = 31)	No zidovudine (n = 19)
Clinical stage		
Asymptomatic	26%	47%
Symptomatic/AIDS	74%	53%
Clinical features		
Proximal weakness	97%	95%
>10% weight loss	42%	37%
Myalgias	61%	26%
Associated neurological disorders		
Sensory neuropathy	48%	53%
Myelopathy	13%	16%
Laboratory features		
CK median (interquartile range)	485 (689)	471 (1736)
EMG:		
myopathic	93%	94%
irritative	90%	61%
Muscle biopsy:		
myofibre degeneration	93%	100%
marked inflammation	27%	45%
ragged red-type fibres	rare	rare
Response		
Drug holiday	NA	7/15
Prednisone	7/7	1/2

(After Simpson et al 1993a)

months, and a mean cumulative close of 515 g. The severity of muscle weakness did not distinguish zidovudine-users from zidovudine-free individuals. Two other HIV-associated neurological disorders occurred concurrently: sensory neuropathy in 25 patients and myelopathy in seven. The pattern of weakness was that of a symmetrical, mainly proximal muscle weakness involving neck flexors and lower extremities more than upper extremities. Myalgias (mainly in the thighs) were present in 24 patients. Generally, symptoms developed over several months. Twenty patients had sufficient weight loss to fulfil criteria for wasting syndrome with greater than 10% body weight loss. CPK levels did not correlate with the severity of weakness and did not differentiate zidovudine users from non-users. EMG showed myopathic motor unit potentials with early recruitment and full interference patterns. In two-thirds of patients, fibrillation potentials, positive sharp waves and complex repetitive discharges suggested an irritative myopathy and was slightly more common among zidovudine users. Quadri-

ceps muscle biopsies were performed in 26 patients and myopathic features were present in 25. Interstitial inflammatory infiltrates were present in 58% and marked inflammation was significantly more common in the zidovudine-negative biopsies. HIV was not demonstrated in muscle fibres by electron microscopy, immunohistochemistry or in situ hybridization. Myofibre degeneration was present in 25 out of 26 of the biopsies. The degenerating myofibres were not necrotic, often contained fibrillar sarcoplasmic inclusions, and were seldom associated directly with inflammation. Fibrillar inclusions, either nemaline rod bodies or commonly cytoplasmic bodies, were seen and probably reflect disorganization of contractile and cytoskeletal filaments. In contrast to Dalakas et al, ragged red-type fibres (with modified Gomori's trichrome stain) were not frequent, and similar mitochondrial abnormalities were present in both zidovudine-users and zidovudine-free biopsies (Fig. 7.4).

In seven zidovudine-free patients, severe progressive weakness developed and prednisone therapy (60 mg/day) was used. Marked improvement in strength and reduction in CPK levels was seen in all. Treatment was complicated by cryptococcal meningitis in one patient, developing after 2 months of prednisone. Eight additional patients did not receive corticosteroids. One remitted spontaneously; the other seven had progressive weakness. In 15 zidovudine users with myopathies, a drug holiday of 4–12 weeks was used. Eight had no significant clinical improvement; seven patients had either improvement in strength, reduction in CPK levels or lessening of myalgias. Among 16 zidovudine-users who did not discontinue the antiretroviral, two remitted spontaneously.

In summary, Simpson's series suggests that the clinical, laboratory and pathological features of myopathy in HIV infection do not reliably distinguish HIV-associated myopathy from zidovudine toxicity. The mitochondrial abnormalities previously noted by Dalakas et al were seen infrequently and may be non-specific markers of myofibre degeneration. From a therapeutic standpoint, the benefits of the zidovudine drug holiday are not clear cut and unless a dramatic response to zidovudine withdrawal is seen within 2–4

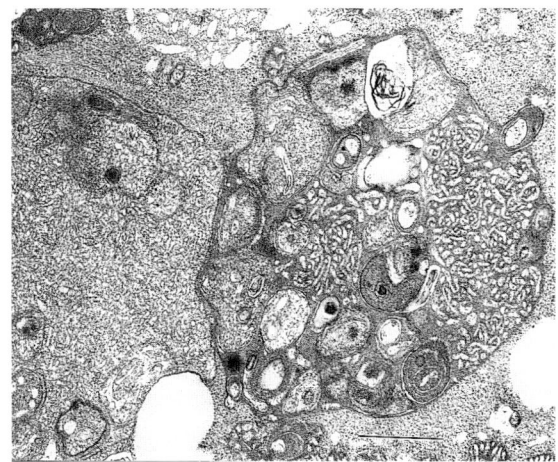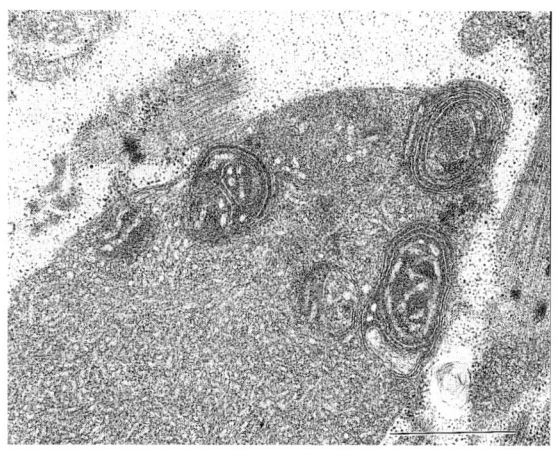

A

B

Fig. 7.4 Mitochondrial abnormalities seen in non-necrotic degenerating myofibres in HIV-associated myopathy, independent of zidovudine use. These include double-membrane bounded profiles containing tubular, circinate and otherwise convoluted cristae and amorphous dense inclusions in quadriceps muscle. **A** Zidovudine user; **B** no zidovudine use. (Bar = 1 μm.) (Reproduced from Simpson et al 1993a with permission of *Neurology*.)

weeks, we would recommend reinstituting anti-retroviral therapy.

Simpson et al (1993b) have also reported the preliminary findings of a controlled interventional study. Ten patients with myopathy unassociated with zidovudine use were randomized to prednisone or placebo. The five patients given steroids lost their pain, regained strength and their CPK levels fell. Of the first six patients with myopathy on zidovudine, five were randomized to withdrawal of therapy, but there was no resultant response of strength, pain or CPK level. This pattern of response suggests a polymyositis type of illness predominated in this group of patients. It is hoped that this ongoing trial will help define the relative roles of zidovudine and HIV in muscle disease and reveal the best therapeutic strategy for the different types of pathology encountered.

WASTING IN AIDS

Simpson has suggested that some cases of terminal 'wasting' attributed to cachexia are in fact examples of myopathy (Simpson et al 1990, Simpson & Wolfe 1991), though few such patients are investigated with this in mind. Certainly, diffuse muscle weakness is seen in cachectic patients with wasting syndrome, but generally the muscle strength is proportionate to bulk and CK

levels are normal. High circulatory cytokine levels, particularly of tumour necrosis factor, may play a role in the muscle wasting. Metabolic (Grunfeld & Feingold 1992) and endocrine (Grinspoon & Bilezikian 1992) factors also play a role in weight loss analogous to the cachexia of other infections and malignancies. An anabolic steroid, dianazole, is currently under trial for weakness in the wasting syndrome.

INFECTIONS IN MUSCLE

Pyomyositis can develop in AIDS as a result of Gram-negative bacteria or staphylococci that develop in some injection drug users who have dysfunctional neutrophils. This diagnosis is suggested by very intense localized muscle pain and swelling in a patient with a low fever. The investigation of choice is an ultrasound scan, which also shows normal subcutaneous tissues ruling out cellulitis, with which it can be confused. Magnetic resonance imaging (MRI) of pyomyositis can show enhancing abscesses typically in quadriceps muscle. Denervation also causes MRI changes. Toxoplasmosis affecting skeletal muscles has been reported (Gherardi et al 1992) and should be considered when there is fever, encephalopathy, multi-organ failure, and elevated serum CK and *Toxoplasma* serology.

CARDIOMYOPATHY

AIDS patients may develop congestive cardio-myopathy and cardiac failure. Whilst some have evidence of a myocarditis related to HIV infection (Grody et al 1990), a toxic cardiomyopathy should obviously be considered in those on long-term high-dose zidovudine treatment in view of the animal data (Lamperth et al 1991, Lewis et al 1991). In children, selenium deficiency can cause or contribute to cardiomyopathy.

MANAGEMENT PLAN (Fig. 7.5)

1. Patients with isolated elevation of CK discovered on screening can simply be followed. A steadily rising level would raise the question of a trial of withdrawal of zidovudine or a biopsy if the patient was not on treatment or failed to respond to withdrawal of therapy.

2. If muscle pain with or without associated CK rise does not respond to simple anti-inflammatory drugs, a similar strategy may be followed. Muscle pain in patients on zidovudine sometimes stops after withdrawal. It may be possible to restart it at lower dose, or switch to an alternate anti-viral drug.

3. If muscle weakness is found, it is appropriate to stop zidovudine for at least a month. If there is no sign of recovery a biopsy should be considered. Any sign of inflammatory change will strengthen the argument in favour of a trial of steroids. If a biopsy is not possible for any reason

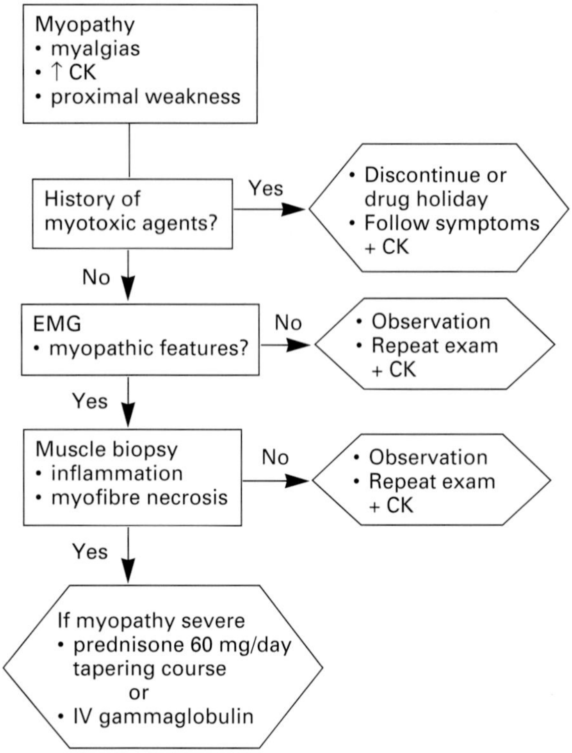

Fig. 7.5 Scheme for management of muscle disorders.

(thrombocytopenia, patient refusal, etc.), these sequential therapeutic steps should be followed 'blind'. It is hoped that an ongoing formal study of these options will reveal which, if any, of the interventional steps are beneficial (Simpson et al 1993b).

REFERENCES

Arnaudo E, Dalakas M, Shanske S, et al. Depletion of muscle mitochondrial DNA in AIDS patients with zidovudine-induced myopathy. Lancet 1991; 337: 508–510

Bessen L J, Greene J B, Louie E, et al. Severe polymyositis-like syndrome associated with zidovudine therapy of AIDS and ARC. New Engl J Med 1988; 318: 708

Chad D A, Smith T W, Blumenfeld A, et al. Human immunodeficiency virus (HIV)-associated myopathy: immunocytochemical identification of an HIV antigen (gp41) in muscle macrophages. Ann Neurol 1990; 28: 579–582

Chalmers A C, Greco C M, Miller R G. Prognosis in AZT myopathy. Neurology 1991; 41: 1181–1184

Dalakas M C, Isabel I, Pezeshkpour G H, et al. Mitochondrial myopathy caused by long term zidovudine therapy. N Engl J Med 1990; 322: 1098–1105

Dalakas M C, Pezeshkpour G H, Gravekk M, et al. Polymyositis associated with AIDS virus. JAMA 1986; 256: 2381–2383

Fischl M, Gagnon S, Uttamchandani R, et al. Myopathy associated with long-term zidovudine therapy. Proceedings of Vth International Conference on AIDS, Montreal, 1989: 276

Gabbai A, Schmidt B, Castelo A, et al. Muscle biopsy in AIDS and ARC analysis of 50 patients. Muscle and Nerve 1990; 13: 541–544

Gertner E, Thurn J R, Williams D N, et al. Zidovudine-associated myopathy. Am J Med 1989; 86: 814–818

Gherardi R, Baudrimont M, Lionnet F, et al. Skeletal muscle toxoplasmosis in patients with acquired immunodeficiency syndrome: a clinical and pathological study. Ann Neurol 1992; 32: 535–542

Grinspoon S K, Bilezikian J P. HIV disease and the endocrine system. New Engl J Med 1992; 327: 1360–1365

Grody W W, Cheng L, Lewis W. Infection of the heart by the human immunodeficiency virus. Am J Cardiol 1990; 66: 203–206

Grunfeld C, Feingold K R. Metabolic disturbances and wasting in the acquired immunodeficiency syndrome. New Engl J Med 1992; 327: 329–337

Helbert M, Fletcher T, Pedle B, et al. Zidovudine-associated myopathy. Lancet 1988; i: 689–690

Illa I, Nath A, Dalakas M. Immunocytochemical and virological characteristics of HIV-associated inflammatory myopathies – similarities with seronegative polymyositis. Ann Neurol, 1991; 29: 474–481

Jay C, Ropka M, Hench K. Prospective study of myopathy during prolonged low dose AZT. Neurology 1992; 42 (suppl): 146

Kaye B R. Rheumatologic manifestations of infection with human immunodeficiency virus (HIV). Ann Intern Med 1989; 111: 158–167

Lacroix C, Said G. Muscle siderosis in AIDS: a marker for macrophage dysfunction. J Neurol 1992; 239: 46–48

Lamperth L, Dalakas M C, Dagani F, et al. Abnormal skeletal and cardiac muscle mitochondria induced by zidovudine (AZT) in human muscle in vitro and in an animal model. Lab Invest 1991; 65: 742–751

Lewis W, Papoian T, Gonzalez B, et al. Mitochondrial ultrastructural and molecular changes induced by zidovudine in rat hearts. Lab Invest 1991; 65: 228–236

Mahe A, Bruet A, Chabin E, Fendler J-P. Acute rhabdomyolysis coincident with primary HIV-1 infection. Lancet 1989; 2: 1454–1455

Mhiri C, Baudrimont M, Bonne G, et al. Zidovudine myopathy: a distinctive disorder associated with mitochondrial dysfunction. Ann Neurol 1991; 29: 606–614

Miller R G, Carson P J, Moussavi R S, et al. Fatigue and myalgia in AIDS patients. Neurology 1991; 41: 1603–1607

Miranda A F, Sancho S, Tanji K, et al. Mitochondrial studies in tissue culture: effects of 3′-azido-3′-deoxythymidine (AZT). J Neurol Sci 1990; 98 (suppl): 110

Nishikawa Y, Takahashi M, Yorifuji S, et al. Long term coenzyme Q10 therapy for a mitochondrial encephalomyopathy with cytochrome C deficiency: a ^{31}P NMR study. Neurology 1989; 39: 399–403

Panagyres P K, Papadimitrou J M, Hollingsworth P N, et al. Vesicular changes in the myopathies of AIDS. Ultrastructural observations and their relationship to zidovudine treatment. J Neurol Neurosurg Psychiatr 1990; 53: 649–655

Peters B, Wilson G, Pinching A. Zidovudine myopathy. A prospective study. Proceedings of Vth International Conference on AIDS, Montreal, 1989: 266

Peters B S, Winer J, Landon D N, et al. Mitochondrial myopathy associated with chronic zidovudine therapy in AIDS. Q J Med 1993; 86: 5–15

Pezeshkpour G, Illa I, Dalakas M C. Ultrastructural characteristics and DNA immunocytochemistry in human immunodeficiency virus and zidovudine-associated myopathies. Hum Pathol 1991; 22: 1281–1288

Richman D D, Fischl M A, Grieco M H, et al. The toxicity of azidothymidine (AZT) in the treatment of patients with AIDS and AIDS-related complex: a double-blind placebo controlled trial. New Engl J Med 1987; 317: 192–197

Simpson D M, Bender A N. Human immunodeficiency virus-associated myopathy: analysis of 11 cases. Ann Neurol 1988; 24: 79–84

Simpson D M, Wolfe D E. Neuromuscular complications of HIV infection and its treatment. AIDS 1991; 5: 917–926

Simpson D M, Bender A N, Farraye J, et al. Human immunodeficiency virus wasting syndrome may represent a treatable myopathy. Neurology 1990; 40: 535–538

Simpson D M, Citak K A, Godfrey E, et al. Myopathies associated with human immunodeficiency virus and zidovudine: can their effects be distinguished? Neurology 1993a; 43: 971–976

Simpson D, Godbold J, Hassett S, et al. HIV associated myopathy and the effects of zidovudine and prednisone: preliminary results of placebo-controlled trials. Clin Neuropathol 1993b; 12 (suppl 1): S20

Till M, MacDonell K B. Myopathy with human immunodeficiency virus type 1 (HIV-1) infection: HIV-1 or zidovudine? Ann Intern Med 1990; 113: 492–494

Viard J-P, Vittecoq D, Lacroix C, Bach J-F. Response of HIV-1 associated polymyositis to intravenous immunoglobulin (letter). Am J Med 1992; 92: 580–581

Weismann J D, Constantinitis I, Hudgins P, Wallace D C. [31]P magnetic resonance spectroscopy suggests impaired mitochondrial function in AZT-treated HIV-infected patients. Neurology 1992; 42: 619–623

Wiley C A, Nerenberg M, Cros D, Soto-Aguilar M C. HTLV-I polymyositis in a patient also infected with human immunodeficiency virus. New Engl J Med 1989; 320: 992–995

Wrzolek M A, Sher J H, Kozlowski P B, Roa C. Skeletal muscle pathology in AIDS: an autopsy study. Muscle and Nerve 1990; 13: 508–515

Younger D S, Hays A P, Uncini A, et al. Recurrent myoglobinuria and HIV seropositivity: incidental or pathogenic association. Muscle and Nerve 1989; 12: 842–844

8. Opportunistic infections – fungi

CRYPTOCOCCAL MENINGITIS

Epidemiology

About 10% of AIDS patients develop crypto-coccal meningitis with an early mortality that approaches 15% even with treatment. Survival data compiled by the Centers for Disease Control (CDC) for 3022 patients with extrapulmonary cryptococcosis (81% with meningitis) showed a median survival of 8.4 months (Horsburgh & Selik personal communication). It is the most common fungal infection of the central nervous system (CNS) seen in AIDS, and in the USA it is the presenting AIDS-defining illness in about 5%. In Africa, it is one of the most common oppor-tunistic infections (Desmet et al 1989). The organism *Cryptococcus neoformans* (Treseler & Sugar 1990) is a ubiquitous budding encapsulated solid yeast present in soil, and especially prevalent in pigeon excreta. It is 4–7 μm in diameter surrounded by a 3–5 μm capsule. Virtually all cryptococcal disease in AIDS patients is caused by serotypes A and D, rather than B and C, which occur in normal hosts and are more common in tropical and subtropical areas related to the preva-lence of eucalyptus trees. It gains access to the body through the respiratory tract, though the pulmonary infection is usually asymptomatic. Blood-borne spread can then affect any organ but the CNS is preferentially targeted. It causes a sporadic granulomatous meningitis sometimes associated with small cerebral cysts in Virchow-Robin spaces or granulomatous cryptococcomas, and, in non-immunosuppressed hosts, produces an indolent dementing syndrome. In the USA some 50% of meningitis cases are immunosup-pressed, compared with 15% in the UK.

Clinical features

Cryptococcal meningitis is the third most com-mon neurological presentation of AIDS (Larsen 1990), and in 45% of patients is the first AIDS-defining illness (Chuck & Sande 1989). It rarely develops with a CD4 count above 200. It may only be manifest as a pyrexia of uncertain origin (PUO), but the usual presentation (Table 8.1) is of an ill, febrile patient with the recent onset of bad headache who may be photophobic and confused. Systemic manifestations of cryptococ-cosis include pneumonitis and occasionally disseminated cutaneous infection. The cutaneous lesions may present as relatively bland papulo-

Table 8.1 Features of meningeal cryptococcosis in 89 patients

Feature	Number	%
Concurrent PCP	12	(13)
First AIDS manifestation	40	(45)
Symptoms		
Fever	58	(65)
Malaise	68	(76)
Headache	65	(73)
Stiff neck	20	(22)
Nausea or vomiting	37	(42)
Photophobia	16	(18)
Altered mentation	25	(28)
Focal deficits	5	(6)
Seizures	4	(4)
Cough or dyspnoea	28	(31)
Diarrhoea	19	(21)
Signs		
Temperature > 38.4°C	50	(56)
Meningeal signs	24	(27)
Altered mentation	15	(17)
Focal deficits	13	(15)

PCP, *Pneumocystis carinii* pneumonia.
(Reproduced from Chuck & Sande 1989)

nodular lesions. The length of the history is from a few days to about 3 weeks, in most cases. Frank meningism occurs in 27% of patients, but neck stiffness can be mild or absent. Altered mentation is common, ranging from disorientation to coma. Ten to 20% of patients have signs of raised intracranial pressure with papilloedema, but focal signs are unusual, occurring in only 15% in one series (Chuck & Sande 1989). Cranial nerve involvement can occur very rapidly in fulminant cryptococcal meningitis with onset of blindness and deafness from involvement of cranial nerves II and VIII. This is a poor prognostic sign and reflects massive infiltration of parenchyma and cranial nerves with the yeast. Another possibility for hyperacute visual loss or deafness in cryptococcal meningitis is vascular compromise associated with a constrictive arachnoiditis (Lipson et al 1989). Papilloedema rarely causes abrupt visual loss, but may cause a gradual enlargement of the blind spot. One autopsy study of a patient who developed sudden hearing loss with cryptococcal meningitis showed marked infiltration with cryptococcal organisms of the internal auditory canal with necrosis of the cochlear and vestibular nerves (Kwartler et al 1991). Optic neuropathy in

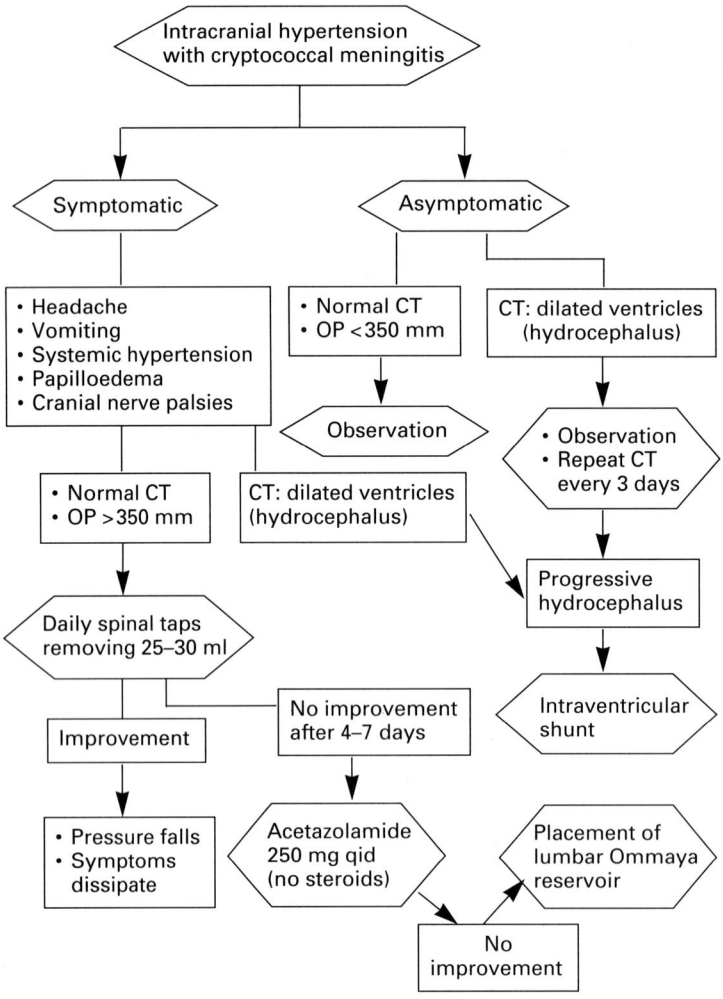

Fig. 8.1   Treatment of elevated intracranial pressure in cryptococcal meningitis. OP, opening pressure. (Modified from Dr Charles van der Horst (personal communication) and from Denning et al 1991.)

cryptococcal meningitis may be reversible with prompt treatment. Golnik et al (1991) described three patients with acute or subacute loss of central vision presumed to result from crypto-coccal invasion of the visual pathways and not from elevated intracranial pressure who res-ponded to amphotericin B therapy.

Fulminant cryptococcal meningitis, which carries a much higher mortality rate approaching 50%, typically develops when symptoms have been unrecognized and diagnosis and prompt treatment are delayed. In the USA, this frequently occurs among individuals who have limited access to medical care who may delay reporting symp-toms of meningitis until late in the infection. In addition to severe refractory headache and altered mentation, elevated intracranial pressures in fulminant cryptococcal meningitis leads to papill-oedema with enlargement of the blind spot, visual blurring and occasionally blindness. The elevated intracranial pressure develops from a combination of brain swelling, the mass effect of collections of active *C. neoformans*, and from obstruction to cerebrospinal fluid (CSF) absorption. Non-communicating hydrocephalus is relatively un-common. The fungal burden within the brain and meninges probably alters brain compliance and is itself enough to make it possible for small changes in volume to make large changes in pressure. The presence of unrelieved headache, cranial nerve signs, papilloedema and high opening pressures should alert one to the possibility that raised intracranial pressure will need direct therapy (Denning et al 1991; Fig. 8.1). If there is no evidence of hydrocephalus or focal abscesses, lumbar puncture with removal of large volumes of CSF is therapeutic, rapidly reducing intracranial pressure in most patients. Placement of an Ommaya reservoir in the lumbar area may facili-tate regular removal of CSF to reduce pressure. In one surgical series of placement of a ventricular peritoneal shunt in non-AIDS cryptococcal meningitis with hydrocephalus, 10 of 14 patients had bilateral papilloedema and five showed gradual resolution of papilloedema after shunting. Ventri-cular peritoneal shunting did not restore vision in one patient and two other patients developed optic atrophy and blindness. This suggests that direct invasion of the optic pathways by

C. neoformans or opto-chiasmatic arachnoiditis, rather than the pressure itself, may cause the visual failure (Tang 1990). Some 10–20% of HIV-infected patients with cryptococcal menin-gitis will need treatment for raised pressure with lumbar punctures, acetazolamide or shunting.

Because headache and fever are common symptoms in advanced HIV infection, the key pointers to development of cryptococcal menin-gitis are: (1) new onset of headache which is unusually severe or of a different pattern and is associated with nausea or vomiting; (2) daily fevers; and (3) development of stiff neck, blurred vision or confusion. Relapse of meningitis after successful treatment tends to have a lower inci-dence of headache and neck stiffness, so must be considered if there is a recrudescence of fever alone without clearer pointers to a meningitic illness (Sugar et al 1990).

There is extensive meningeal invasion with huge numbers of budding yeast forms (Fig. 8.2). Because *C. neoformans* produces a thick polysac-charide capsule (seen as a 'halo' on India ink preparations of the CSF, Fig. 8.3), there is frequently minimal tissue reaction to the presence of the yeast forms. Thus, microscopically, foci of cryptococcal meningitis (Fig. 8.4) are usually not surrounded by an inflammatory response (Fig. 8.5). In advanced or fulminant cases of cryptococcal meningitis, the yeast invades the brain parenchyma along the Virchow-Robin spaces (Fig. 8.5). Clusters of budding yeasts

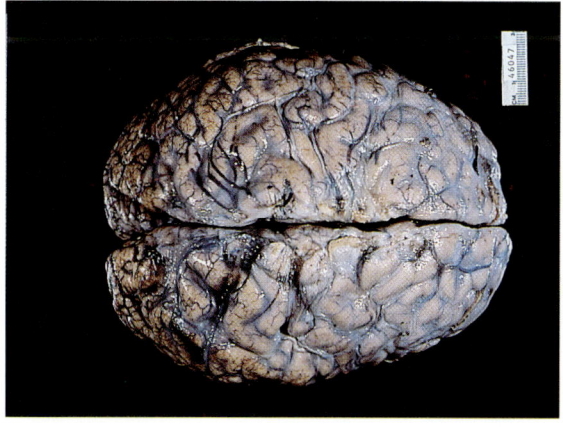

Fig. 8.2 Post-mortem appearance of brain in a case of cryptococcal meningitis.

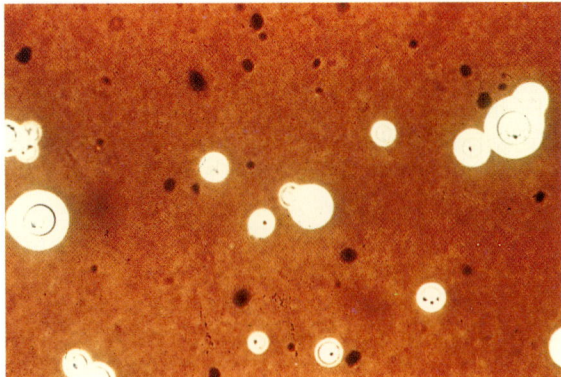

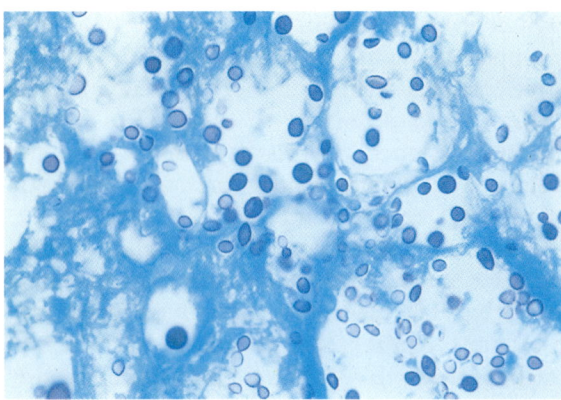

Fig. 8.3   India ink preparation of CSF showing encapsulated cryptococci. The budding forms indicate viable yeast. (Courtesy of Dr W. Merz, Johns Hopkins Hospital.)

Fig. 8.4   Cryptococci in the leptomeninges in a case of cryptococcal meningitis.

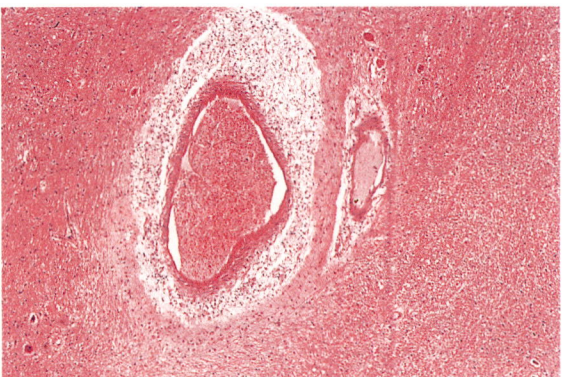

Fig. 8.5   Cryptococci in a dilated perivascular space.

develop within the basal ganglia and may coalesce to form cryptococcomas (Fig. 8.6). When large, these may act as mass lesions or 'gelatinous pseudocysts' producing hemiparesis or seizures. In fulminant cases, diffuse cerebral swelling with elevated intracranial pressure and a risk of herniation occurs. Tien et al (1991) and Mathews et al (1992) have reviewed the radiological findings. Tien et al (1991) found magnetic resonance imaging (MRI) (10/10) to be more sensitive than computed tomography (CT). Nine of 29 CT scans were normal and 13 only showed atrophy. Mathews et al (1992) (Table 8.2) reported on the radiological/pathological correlations in 13 cases. Punctate hyperintensities were seen in all patients, with MRI corresponding to autopsy findings of dilated perivascular spaces and cryptococcomas.

Cryptococcomas were irregularly marginated lesions that contained mucinous material, inflammatory cells and organisms, and replaced brain parenchyma. They were frequently confluent. A dilated perivascular space was a well-marginated circular space within the brain tissue with a vessel located in this space. Contrast enhancement was uncommon, but sometimes seen in the meninges rather than around cryptococcomas. Both CT and MRI tend to underestimate the extent of disease, probably due to the small size of lesions and the lack of inflammatory response.

Cerebrospinal fluid

The principal diagnostic measure in cryptococcal meningitis is CSF analysis demonstrating the

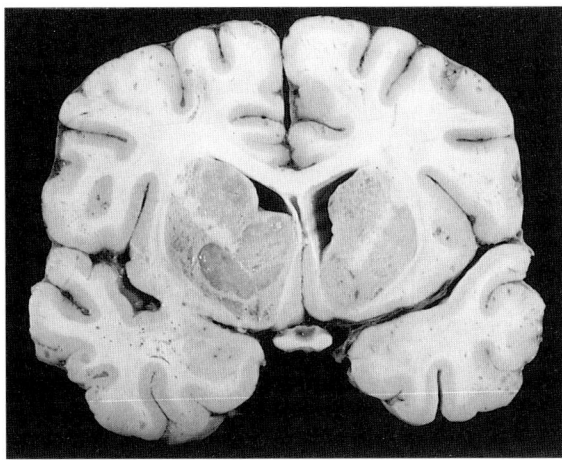

Fig. 8.6 Post-mortem appearance of cryptococcal infection of the brain showing dilated Virchow-Robin spaces and cryptococcomas, particularly in the basal ganglia.

organism or its capsular polysaccharide. Lumbar puncture should be performed promptly in patients suspected of cryptococcal meningitis because response to treatment depends on how early it is started. The fungus is difficult and slow to culture, so early diagnosis depends on other measures. In non-AIDS-related cryptococcal meningitis, the CSF classically shows an elevated protein level and a pleocytosis with low sugar (Table 8.3), but in AIDS it is often normal (Shaunak et al 1989); opening pressures are elevated in two-thirds of patients. In one series (Kovacs et al 1985), two-thirds of patients had no

Table 8.3 Laboratory findings in cryptococcal meningitis

Feature	%
Hyponatraemia	22*
Extrameningeal Cryptococcosis	68*
Antigen >1:1024	39
Opening pressure ⩾ 200	66
Glucose < 40	24
Protein > 45	55
WBC ⩾20	21

* Associated with poor prognosis.
(Reproduced from Chuck & Sande 1989 with permission of The New England Journal of Medicine)

pleocytosis and one-third had normal protein levels. Assay of cryptococcal antigen is highly specific and sensitive and should be performed on all samples from HIV-seropositive individuals with suspected meningitis, irrespective of normalcy of other CSF constituents. In patients with fulminant cryptococcal meningitis, the titre can be >1:1 000 000. Fungal cultures are positive in over 85% of patients and India ink staining of the CSF reveals the fungi in about 75%, but the detection of cryptococcal antigen in the spinal fluid is far more reliable, being positive in some 95% of patients (Nelson et al 1990). Persistently positive cultures are indicative of treatment failure. The latex agglutination test is highly specific and suitable for rapid diagnosis, but may remain persistently positive at a lower titre despite effective induction therapy.

Serum cryptococcal antigen

Serum detection of cryptococcal antigen can be used as a screening tool in febrile patients or those with new-onset headache in whom there is a relative contraindication to lumbar puncture such as thrombocytopenia. In one study, screening for serum cryptococcal antigen in febrile patients was an accurate and sensitive index of cryptococcal meningitis, but no more helpful than recognition of meningism (headaches, neck stiffness, pyrexia) (Nelson et al 1990) (Table 8.1). In this study, serum cryptococcal antigen titres were measured in 828 HIV-positive patients with fever, 69 of whom had meningism. The serum cryptococcal antigen was positive in 17 patients, 16 of whom had meningism and a clinical diagnosis of menin-

Table 8.2 Findings on final imaging study before autopsy in 13 patients with CNS cryptococcosis

Finding	CT	MRI
Normal	1	0
Atrophy	3	2
Punctate lesions (<3 mm)	0	5
Masses (> 1 cm)		
Enhancing	1[a]	0
Non-enhancing	1	1
No contrast	1	0
Abnormal meningeal enhancement	0	1[b]

[a] Pathologically found to be primary CNS lymphoma.
[b] This patient had focal cerebritis and adjacent vascular congestion.
(Reproduced from Mathews et al 1992 with permission of American Journal of Neuroradiology, © American Society of Neuroradiology.)

gitis. All 16 patients had CSF analysis and proven cryptococcal meningitis. The only false positive patient did not develop cryptococcal meningitis. In a separate study from Denmark (Hoffmann et al 1991), 530 routine serum specimens from 334 patients with symptomatic HIV infection were assayed. None had symptoms or signs of cryptococcosis; all were negative. This suggests that routine serum cryptococcal antigen assay in patients without meningism from areas of relatively low prevalence is not useful. In contrast, in a study from Zaire (Desmet et al 1989), routine serum cryptococcal antigen screening was positive in 12.2% of 450 HIV-positive/AIDS patients and cryptococcal meningitis was confirmed in 66%. The positive predictive value increased with increasing serum antigen titres and was 92% for titres greater than 1:128. In summary, routine serum cryptococcal antigen testing does not appear to be useful or cost effective in patients with AIDS without any symptoms of cryptococcosis, except perhaps in very high-risk populations in Africa where there

may be a higher environmental exposure to *C. neoformans*. In a symptomatic immunosuppressed (CD4 <200) patient with frank meningism, headache, fever and stiffness, lumbar puncture should be performed. Serum cryptococcal antigen assay may be helpful in prioritizing the 'urgency' of lumbar puncture in a patient with milder symptoms, for example only fever and headache. If the serum cryptococcal antigen titre is greater than 1:128, urgent lumbar puncture should be performed. If serum cryptococcal antigen is negative or of low titre, the patient can be managed conservatively.

Radiology

Contrast-enhanced MRI and CT may demonstrate meningeal enhancement or small hyperintensities (on T2-weighted MRI) that are believed to correspond to Virchow-Robin spaces dilated by organisms (Fig. 8.7). Rarely, larger non-enhancing masses are seen, which are cryptococcomas

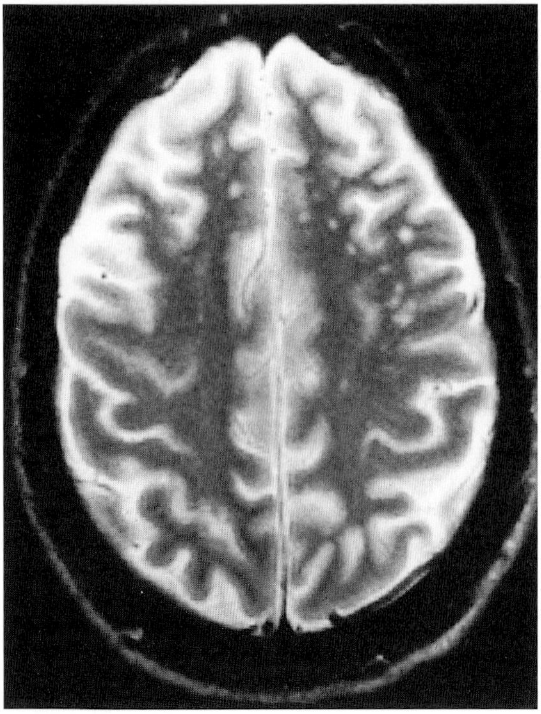

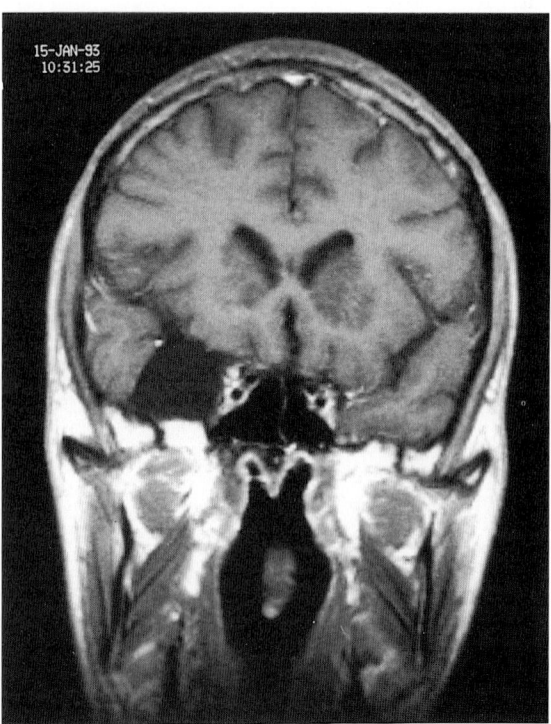

Fig. 8.7   T2-weighted MRI showing small high-intensity lesions thought to be due to cryptococcal infection.

Fig. 8.8   T1-weighted MRI showing the dilated Virchow-Robin spaces in the basal ganglia of cryptococcal infection. Note coincidental arachnoid cyst.

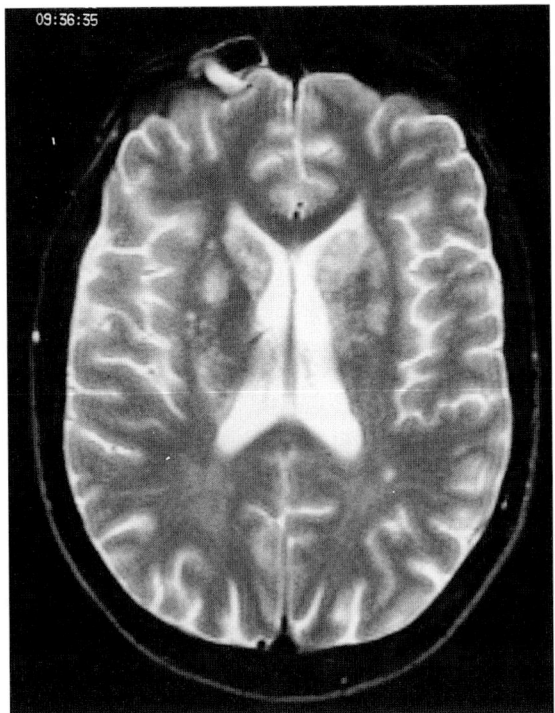

Fig. 8.9   T2-weighted MRI showing effect of cryptococcal infection in the basal ganglia. Note similarity to pathological appearance in Figure 8.6.

(Figs 8.8 and 8.9). These are typically in the basal ganglia. Hydrocephalus may follow obstruction of CSF spaces by large numbers of organisms.

Antifungals

Amphotericin B is a parenteral polyene antibiotic with a high degree of binding to ergosterol. This is the mechanism by which it achieves its antifungal effect. In addition to intravenous administration, the intrathecal route has been used for treatment of cryptococcal meningitis. The most important adverse effect of amphotericin B is its effect on the glomerular filtration rate, which decreases in about 80% of patients, sometimes sufficiently to cause renal failure. The glomerular filtration rate decreases by about 40% soon after initiation of therapy, stabilizing at 20–60% after multiple doses. The effect on renal function is usually reversible after amphotericin B has been discontinued, although most patients are left with mild persistent reduction in glomerular filtration rate,

have a tendency to waste potassium and magnesium, and may develop renal tubular acidosis (Sugar et al 1990). Amphotericin B is often poorly tolerated because of chills, rigors and fever, and other side-effects include pulmonary oedema, phlebitis, seizures and vomiting. Liposomal amphotericin has been used to attenuate some of its nephrotoxicity, but its efficacy is probably unchanged (Saag M, personal observation).

5-Flucytosine causes diarrhoea and marrow toxicity, a problem that is aggravated by the renal impairment from the amphotericin B causing higher than intended serum drug levels. Drug-induced hepatitis and, rarely, severe enterocolitis have been reported. Regular monitoring of renal function and levels of 5-flucytosine is desirable. Most of the adverse effects associated with 5-flucytosine occur with serum levels above 100 μg/ml, particularly when 5-flucytosine is given with amphotericin B. Serum peak levels should be kept below 100 μg/ml (Sugar et al 1990) and serum levels should be checked regularly. Resistance develops to 5-flucytosine in up to 30% of patients with cryptococcosis, limiting its use to combination therapy (Block et al 1973). As many of the patients already have marrow suppression, 5-flucytosine often has to be omitted when the absolute neutrophil count is 500/m^3 or less. The benefits of combining flucytosine with amphotericin over the use of amphotericin alone are under trial at the present time (ACTG 159).

The development of modern antifungal azoles has produced effective triazoles (Larsen 1990). Fluconazole was originally tested in patients unable to tolerate amphotericin and proved effective clinically and in sterilizing the CSF. Fluconazole is a water-soluble triazole whose mode of action is inhibition of the demethylase enzyme involved in the synthesis of ergosterol, a critical component of the fungal cell wall. Because of its relatively low molecular weight and high degree of water solubility, it penetrates easily into the CSF and other body compartments. The CSF concentrations of fluconazole are 60–80% of serum concentration, independent of meningeal inflammation. In addition, its long half-life permits once-daily administration (Arndt et al 1988). Fluconazole is excreted primarily in the urine as unchanged active drug. It has a half-life of 26 hours. The drug is extremely well tolerated with only minor side-effects reported in some patients. An important drug interaction is an increase in dilantin (phenytoin) levels and additional monitoring is required to avoid dilantin toxicity.

Other agents

Itraconazole and ketoconazole both have identical modes of action to fluconazole, but both have poor CSF penetration with a serum: CSF concentration of 0.1 or less. Itraconazole is highly active against *C. neoformans*, although fungicidal activity is quite variable (Denning et al 1989). Itraconazole is lipophilic, and despite its limited CSF penetration, tissue concentrations may be the critical factor in its action because of tissue accumulation. One potential advantage of itraconazole over fluconazole is that it has a much lower minimal inhibitory concentration for *C. neoformans* than fluconazole in vitro (de Gans et al 1988). In one study, 26 patients with AIDS and cryptococcosis were treated with 200 mg b.i.d. Ten of 14 patients with cryptococcal meningitis had complete responses, three partial responses, and therapy failed in one. In all of these patients, conventional therapy had failed or was avoided because of potential toxicity. Ketoconazole was the first broad-spectrum antifungal that could be administered orally. Absorption is unpredictable, particularly if gastric pH is not normal and ketoconazole does not readily enter the CSF except in very high doses (800–2000 mg daily), which are poorly tolerated. Ketoconazole requires gastric acid for absorption. It should not be taken at the same time as didanosine (which contains an acid buffer) or with antacids or H_2 blockers. Ketoconazole's absorption can be enhanced by administration with orange juice or other low pH juices. Despite its lack of efficacy for treatment of cryptococcal meningitis, because ketoconazole is widely used for treatment of oral candidiasis, it may have some protective effect against the development of cryptococcal meningitis (Chuck & Sande 1989).

Liposomal amphotericin B has been developed to allow a higher dose to be administered without increased toxicity. In a study of fungal infections in 144 immune compromised patients (12 with AIDS), liposomal amphotericin was sometimes successful after failure of standard treatment (Ringden et al 1992, Vincent et al 1992).

Treatment (Table 8.4)

No vaccine is available for *C. neoformans*; however, the more widespread use of azole antifungals for treatment of oropharyngeal candidiasis may reduce the incidence of cryptococcal meningitis. Antifungal therapy is less effective in AIDS-related cryptococcal meningitis than in non-AIDS cryptococcal meningitis. In the Chuck and Sande study (1989) of 108 patients with AIDS and cryptococcosis, the presence of abnormal mental status, extraneural sites of infection and hyponatraemia were most predictive of a poor response to therapy. Regimes consisting of either ampho-

Table 8.4 Treatment regimes for cryptococcal meningitis

Induction treatment for severe cryptococcal meningitis	
Medication	Amphotericin B 0.5–0.7 mg/kg/day (usually administered into a central vein in 5% dextrose–premedication with phenergan + demerol may be needed). With or without 5-flucytosine 100–150 mg/kg/day in four divided doses
Course	2–4 weeks until symptoms resolve and CSF cultures negative
Monitoring side-effects	Electrolytes, renal function, blood count, hepatic enzymes, peak serum levels of 5-flucytosine
Side-effects	Amphotericin B: fever, rigors, seizures, hypokalaemia, hypomagnesaemia, reduced glomeruli filtration rate, renal failure, anaemia 5-Flucytosine: nausea, vomiting, diarrhoea, hepatitis, renal failure, marrow suppression
Alternative induction treatment (mild cryptococcal meningitis)	
Medication	Fluconazole 400 mg i.v. daily
Course	2–4 weeks until symptoms resolve and CSF cultures are negative
Monitoring side-effects	Liver function tests, potential interactions with dilantin, phenytoin and warfarin
Maintenance regime	
Medication	Fluconazole 200–400 mg p.o. daily

tericin B alone (0.6 mg/kg/day) or, in fulminant cases, a combination of amphotericin B (0.7 mg/kg/day) and flucytosine (150 mg/kg/day) have been used for 6 weeks with response rates of about 60% (Kovacs et al 1985, Zuger et al 1986) (Table 8.4). In an early comparison in non-AIDS cryptococcal meningitis, amphotericin B alone was compared with amphotericin B plus flucytosine in 78 patients. The combination of amphotericin B (0.3 mg/kg/day) and flucytosine (150 mg/kg/day) was more effective than amphotericin B alone at 0.4 mg/kg/day. There was significantly more rapid sterilization of the CSF in the combination group, fewer deaths and the incidence of nephrotoxicity was lower; however, nearly one-third of patients failed to respond to this combination. A subsequent study in 91 patients with cryptococcal meningitis compared 4 vs. 6 weeks of combination therapy with failure rates of 27% and 16% respectively (Dismukes et al 1987). In this study, in the pre-AIDS era, a favourable outcome was linked to certain features: headache at presentation, normal mental status and CSF white blood cells (WBC) >20.

Recent trials of AIDS-related cryptococcal meningitis have directly compared fluconazole with amphotericin for initial induction therapy. In an early study (Larsen et al 1990) comparing fluconazole (400 mg/day) or amphotericin (0.7 mg/kg/day) plus flucytosine (150 mg/day), eight of 14 patients assigned to fluconazole failed compared with none of six treated with amphotericin plus flucytosine. Mortality was higher in the fluconazole-treated group and the mean duration of positive CSF cultures was 41 days compared with 16 days in those receiving the amphotericin regime. In this study, the amphotericin regime appeared to have superior mycological and clinical efficacy. In a larger study (Saag et al 1992), 131 patients received fluconazole (200 mg/day) and 63 amphotericin B (0.4 mg/kg/day). Treatment success (defined by resolution of symptoms with two consecutive negative CSF cultures) occurred in only 34% of the fluconazole recipients compared with 40% of those assigned to amphotericin B. Early mortality in the first 2 weeks was higher in the fluconazole group, 15% compared with 8% in the amphotericin group. A major difficulty in interpreting

the results of this trial is that both fluconazole and amphotericin treatment groups received relatively low dosages of antifungals. Thus, the mortality is unusually and unacceptably high and treatment was unsuccessful in most patients. The most important predictive factors for high risk of death were abnormal mental status, obtundation, CSF cryptococcal antigen titre >1:1024 and CSF WBC < 20 cells/mm^3. In an open label study (Sugar et al 1990), 35 patients with cryptococcal meningitis received 150–200 mg/day or 400 mg/day of fluconazole. Resolution of symptoms often began quickly and was complete by the third week of treatment; however, two of 13 patients receiving the high-dose regime continued to have positive cultures after 45 days of treatment.

Based on the inconclusive results from these studies and clinical experience, current policy is to continue to use amphotericin B with 5-flucytosine for induction therapy in most cases of cryptococcal meningitis. The combination should certainly be used in cases of fulminant cryptococcal meningitis with elevated intracranial pressure or cranial neuropathies. For severely ill patients, rapid increments in the dose of amphotericin B are suggested: initial test dose is 1 mg in 20 ml of 5% dextrose given over 10–20 minutes with careful monitoring of vital signs for 4 hours. At 4 hours, the next dose of 0.3 mg/kg may be given over 2–6 hours and subsequent doses are 0.7 mg/kg/day. For patients with milder cryptococcal meningitis who are clinically more stable, the dose is generally increased by 5–10 mg/day up to 0.5–0.7 mg/kg/day. Rigors can generally be prevented by meperidine (15–20 mg i.v.) plus phenergan (25 mg i.v.) given before the amphotericin infusion. One thousand units of heparin are usually added to the infusion to reduce phlebitis. Monitoring should include measurements of serum creatinine, potassium, electrolytes and a complete blood count two to three times each week. The daily dose of amphotericin B should be reduced or suspended if serum creatinine rises above 3 mg/dl. 5-Flucytosine is used in the dosage 25 mg/kg orally every 6 hours in patients with an absolute neutrophil count >1000/mm^3. It should be discontinued when the absolute count is 500/mm^3 or less. Regular serum levels should be checked to keep peak levels below

100 µg/ml. CSF sterilization usually requires 0.75–1.0 g over 2–3 weeks. The aim of treatment is resolution of symptoms and reversion of CSF cultures to negative. In particular, when CSF cryptococcal antigen is very high (>1:2056) it may not become negative.

Milder forms of cryptococcal meningitis in patients with normal intracranial pressure and low CSF cryptococcal antigen can be treated initially with fluconazole in doses of 400 mg/day intravenously for the first several weeks, followed by 200mg/day.

Fulminant cryptococcal meningitis with elevated intracranial pressure, cranial neuropathies and formation of cryptococcomas may require surgical intervention with ventricular shunting. The use of corticosteroids has not been tested and may accelerate the meningitis; however, in patients with marked cerebral oedema and imminent herniation, they may have some role. Dexamethasone 0.6 mg/kg/day in four divided doses is used. Patients with persistent intracranial pressure elevations may require daily lumbar punctures with removal of large volumes of CSF to control symptoms of headache from elevated intracranial pressure. If daily lumbar punctures are required for longer than 2–3 weeks, placement of an Ommaya reservoir in the lumbar canal is a more convenient method of drainage.

Maintenance therapy of cryptococcal meningitis

Maintenance therapy is always essential; otherwise, relapse will occur within a few weeks after successful induction therapy. Suppressive treatment must be continued for life with fluconazole. Initially, amphotericin given via Hickman catheter twice weekly was the only available maintenance therapy. As with induction therapy, this was poorly tolerated because of nephrotoxicity and the side-effects associated with amphotericin administration. In addition, the indwelling catheter was frequently a source for line-associated sepsis. Fluconazole has now been proven to be more effective and better tolerated than amphotericin for maintenance therapy in cryptococcal meningitis. In one of the initial studies (Sugar & Saunders 1988) using 200 mg fluconazole daily,

only two of 106 patients relapsed compared with 13 of 77 receiving amphotericin maintenance treatment.

COCCIDIOIDOMYCOSIS

Coccidioidal meningitis

Coccidioides immitis is a dimorphic fungus that is endemic in low altitude, warm, arid areas, which, in the USA, includes the Southwest, California, New Mexico and Texas. Infection is acquired through the respiratory route and meningitis occurs early, with particular risk among non-Caucasians (Bouza et al 1981). Ampel et al (1993) followed-up 170 patients in an endemic area (Tucson, Arizona). Thirteen developed active coccidiomycosis with an estimated incidence after 41 months of 25%. A CD4 count below 250 and a diagnosis of AIDS proved predictive of active infection. Prior infection, a positive skin test and long-term residence in the area did not appear to be risk factors. This suggests that AIDS patients are at risk of primary infection, not just reactivation. Coccidioidal meningitis can present as either an acute or chronic meningitis with fever, headache, weight loss and, in about 50%, encephalopathy. Meningismus is less common than with cryptococcal meningitis and is seen in one-third of patients. Papilloedema, cranial nerve signs and other focal findings are seen in approximately 10% of cases. Skin and lung lesions are fairly frequent, and the CSF shows a lymphocytic pleocytosis with elevated protein and hypoglycorrhachia, and culture is positive in one-half of patients. The CSF pleocytosis is variable from 50 to 200 cells/mm^3 and occasionally several thousand cells/mm^3 are seen in the late stages. Polymorphonuclear reaction predominates early, but later response is mononuclear. The diagnosis is established by serologies: any positive CSF titre, complement fixation (CF) titre or a serum titre of 1:16 is suggestive. Approximately 75% of patients with coccidioidal meningitis have detectable antibody in CSF; sensitivity can be increased to 95% with an overnight binding CF assay and to 100% with radioimmunoassay (RIA) (Gade et al 1992). Rising CF titres in serum or CSF are associated with disease progression, while falling titres parallel clinical improvement. Enzyme immunoassay (EIA) using a combination of coccidioidal antigens is the method of choice for diagnosis of infection and in CSF yields a sensitivity of 100% and specificity of 96%, as well as providing information about disease stage (Gade et al 1992). False negative serological reactions appear to be uncommon. The recommended treatment is amphotericin B 1.5 mg/kg/day i.v. and amphotericin B 0.5 mg intrathecally, two doses per week, or intraventricular amphotericin B. *C. immitis* is not sensitive to flucytosine. Treatment is continued for several months until the CSF has normalized (Zealear & Winn 1967, Post et al 1985). Therapeutic response should be monitored by lumbar puncture and not by analysis of CSF obtained from the ventricular reservoir, because ventricular fluid may be relatively normal while lumbar fluid is markedly abnormal (Goldstein et al 1972). In coccidioidomycosis, fluconazole had been tried; however, a collaborative trial by the NIAID Mycosis Study Group was closed after 20 patients treated with 50–100 mg/day of fluconazole did not improve. A higher dose, 200–400 mg/day, is under trial. Coccidioidal meningitis has previously been treated with intrathecal amphotericin B (Labadie & Hamilton 1986). Fluconazole and itraconazole are currently under trial for coccidioidal meningitis (Tucker et al 1990a, b).

HISTOPLASMOSIS

Histoplasmosis occurs in 2–5% of AIDS patients from endemic areas of central USA, Latin America and the Caribbean. Cases may occur outside endemic areas. Outdoor workers, e.g. construction, farming, where there is contact with the soil-containing spore, are at particularly high risk. Most AIDS-related histoplasmosis occurs with a CD4 count less than 100. *Histoplasma capsulatum* is a typical dimorphic yeast present in soil, bird and bat faeces in endemic areas, which are usually river valleys, including Ohio, Mississippi and St Lawrence. Infection develops after inhalation of air-borne spores. Although histoplasmosis remains a common cause of deep-seated fungal infections in North America, CNS abscesses or histoplasmoma are unusual (Goodwin

et al 1980, Walpole & Gregory 1987). A more common neurological manifestation is meningitis, which is seen in up to 8% of all cases and one-quarter of those with disseminated disease. In 1987, extrapulmonary histoplasmosis was added to the CDC list of AIDS-defining illnesses (CDC 1987). Histoplasmosis in AIDS is usually a severe disseminated infection (Table 8.5), often resembling septicaemia. In the largest review (Wheat et al 1990), 72 patients with AIDS and histoplasmosis were reviewed (Table 8.6). Fifty-three per cent had pulmonary involvement, 13% a septicaemia-like syndrome, 26% hepatomegaly and 18% CNS involvement. These included encephalopathy, meningitis and focal abscesses. Eight of 13 patients with CNS histoplasmosis died of the infection. The diagnosis of histoplasmosis was made by positive fungal cultures for *H. capsulatum* in over 90% of the cases and in the remainder, by the detection of histoplasma polysaccharide antigen (HPA) in body fluids (detected in 97%). The regular measurement of HPA in serum and

Table 8.5 Clinical findings of severe histoplasmosis in AIDS

- Hypotension
- Hypoxia
- Altered mentation
- Rhabdomyolysis
- Coagulopathy
- Pancytopenia
- Hepatic enzyme elevation
- Renal failure

Table 8.6 Clinical findings of histoplasmosis

Finding	Wheat series (n = 72)		Literature (n = 51)	
	No.	%	No.	%
Respiratory system	38	52.8	8	15.7
Hepatomegaly	19	26.4	15	29.4
Splenomegaly	9	12.5	18	35.3
Lymphadenopathy	12	16.7	19	37.3
Central nervous system	13	18.0	7	13.7
Skin	1	1.4	9	17.6
Septicaemia-like syndrome	9	12.5	5	9.8
Gastrointestinal tract	2	2.8	6	11.8
Mucosa	1	1.4	0	0

(Reproduced from Wheat et al 1990)

urine is helpful in identifying a relapse of disseminated histoplasmosis in AIDS. An increase in HPA in urine or serum of > 2 units heralded most relapses in this series. HPA was detected in six of nine cases in this series. Eighty per cent of cases improved after induction therapy with amphotericin B, most defervescing within 1 week. Ketoconazole was effective in preventing relapse. The organism can be cultured from bone marrow, nodes or ulcers. However, the most sensitive test is the RIA or EIA to detect HPA in urine. Results are expressed as HPA units and values of > 1 are considered positive. Sensitivity is 90–97% (Wheat et al 1986). Serological diagnosis by antibody detection is not reliable because of high false positive rates in patients from endemic areas and in patients with other fungal or bacterial infections. In patients with AIDS and histoplasmosis, increases in antigenuria or antigenaemia herald relapses (Wheat et al 1991). Treatment of histoplasmoma is a combination of surgical drainage and intravenous amphotericin (0.6–1.0 mg/kg/day) extended until there has been radiological improvement.

BLASTOMYCOSIS

Blastomyces dimethitis is another dimorphic yeast that is endemic in the south and south-central USA and the Great Lakes area. Seeding of the CNS can occur after dissemination from a respiratory focus has developed. Meningitis occurs in about 5% of cases and mass lesions or blastomycomas can develop occasionally. CSF culture is rarely positive. An EIA using purified antigen A has a high sensitivity for blastomycosis and good specificity distinguishing blastomycosis from coccidioidomycosis. False positives, however, occur in some cases of histoplasmosis and sporotrichosis (Green et al 1980).

NOCARDIA ASTEROIDES

Nocardia asteroides is an aerobic saprophytic actinomycete that exhibits fungal characteristics (true aerial hyphae), but is considered a higher bacterium because its cell wall contains peptidoglycans. It appears as a thin (0.5–1.0 µm) branching, often beaded Gram-positive rod. It is found ubiquitously in soil and infection is usually acquired through inhalation with haematogenous dissemination in immunosuppressed HIV-positive patients. This is an uncommon opportunistic infection in AIDS and clues to its occurrence should be the presence of an acute necrotizing pneumonia commonly associated with cavitation. Patients are usually systemically ill with fever, cough and weight loss. The most common presentation of dissemination to the brain is with focal cerebritis and contrast-enhancing mass lesions. Differential diagnosis includes neoplasms, tuberculosis and fungal disease. Serological diagnosis is limited because of cross-reactivity with other related organisms including diactinomyces and mycobacteria. Histological confirmation from tissue and culture are the gold standard. Species identification can be accomplished by a combination of biochemical tests. Culture grows slowly so culture plates should be held for at least 10 days. *Nocardia* is extremely sensitive to sulphonamides and clinical improvement should begin within 7–10 days of treatment. Trimethoprim sulphamethoxazole (1 double strength b.i.d.) is used and should be continued life-long. In patients who are allergic to sulpha drugs or in whom the *Nocardia* is resistant, an alternative is minocycline 200 mg b.i.d. For severely ill patients, the combination of cefotaxime (2 g intravenously every 8 hours) with imipenem–cilastatin (500 mg i.v. every 6 hours) appears to have in vitro synergism. Amikacin, an aminoglycoside, also has very good activity against *Nocardia*.

OTHER FUNGAL INFECTIONS

Despite the frequency of oropharyngeal and oesophageal candidiasis in AIDS, brain abscess is relatively rare and candidal meningitis has not been described. Several patients with AIDS with candidal microabscesses have been reported (Snider et al 1986). Diagnosis should be suspected when multiple microabscesses develop in the setting of *Candida* septicaemia. Diagnosis is confirmed by culture of tissue from biopsy. Despite the relative frequency of *Aspergillus* infections in patients with haematological neoplasms or neutropenia or receiving iatrogenic immunosuppression, CNS infections with *Aspergillus* species are rare in AIDS. Like other moulds, *Aspergillus* has a predilection to invade blood vessel walls (see Fig. 13.5, p. 201) and cause thrombosis, infarction and haemorrhage. Meningitis without cerebritis is uncommon. Because of the vasocentric nature of the infection, the neurological presentation is often with stroke or subarachnoid haemorrhage. Generally, infection is spread haematogenously with multiple small abscesses and microabscesses (Fig. 8.11). The CSF is non-specifically abnormal and CSF culture is usually negative (Boon et al 1991). Current serological tests are insensitive, although immunoassays based on *A. fumigatus* antigens are being developed (Kurup & Kumar 1991). The diagnosis of aspergilloma should be strongly suspected in an immunosuppressed HIV-positive patient who presents with a stroke or an intracranial haemorrhage and has multiple contrast-enhancing lesions. As with *Candida* infection, treatment remains a combination of surgery and amphotericin B. Concomitant therapy with rifampicin or 5-flucytosine has been tried.

MANAGEMENT PLAN

Patients with overt meningitis or with a short history of headaches, confusion or fever may have a fungal infection. After scanning to rule out unexpected mass lesions, a lumbar puncture should note the pressure, and the fluid should be screened with appropriate stains including India

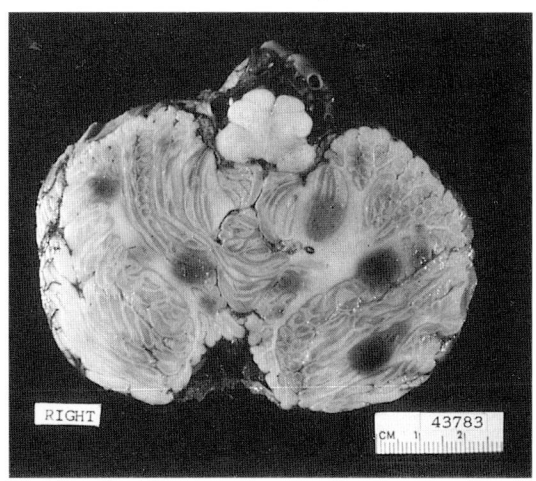

Fig. 8.10 Post-mortem appearance of cerebellum showing multiple *Aspergillus* abscesses.

ink, cultured on appropriate media, and cryptococcal antigen titres measured. MRI may show dilated Virchow-Robin spaces or cryptococcomas. If any of these investigations point to a cryptococcal infection, amphotericin should be prescribed, to which flucytosine may have to be added. After a satisfactory clinical response, prophylaxis against relapse requires continuing treatment with fluconazole. Some patients do badly and need intensified antifungal treatment and management of raised intracranial pressure. In endemic areas, CSF coccidio antibody and blood and urine HPA should be sought. Amphotericin is again the mainstay of treatment.

REFERENCES

Ampel N M, Dols C L, Galgian J N. Coccidioidomycosis during human immunodeficiency virus infection: results of a prospective study in a coccidioidal endemic area. Am J Med 1993; 94: 235–240

Arndt C A S, Walsh T J, McCully C L, et al. Fluconazole penetration into cerebrospinal fluid: implications for treating fungal infections of the central nervous system. J Infect Dis 1988; 157: 178–180

Block E R, Jennings A E, Bennett J E. 5-Fluorocytosine resistance in *Cryptococcus neoformans*. Antimicrob Agents Chemother 1973; 3: 649–656

Boon A P, O'Brien D, Adams D H. Ten year review of invasive aspergillosis detected at necropsy. J Clin Pathol 1991; 44; 452–454

Bouza E, Dreyer J S, Hewitt W L, Meyer R D. Coccidioidal meningitis. An analysis of 31 cases and review of the literature. Medicine 1981; 60: 139–172

Centers of Disease Control. Revision of the CDC surveillance case definition for acquired immunodeficiency syndrome. MMWR 1987; 36 (suppl 1S): 3S–15S

Chuck S L, Sande M A. Infections with *Cryptococcus neoformans* in acquired immunodeficiency syndrome. N Engl J Med 1989; 321: 794–799

de Gans J, Eeftinck Schattenkerk J K, van Ketel R J. Itraconazole as maintenance treatment for cryptococcal meningitis in the acquired immune deficiency syndrome. Br Med J 1988; 296: 339

Denning D W, Armstrong R W, Lewis B H, Stevens D A. Elevated cerebrospinal fluid pressures in patients with cryptococcal meningitis and acquired immunodeficiency syndrome. Am J Med 1991; 91: 267–272

Denning D W, Tucker R M, Hanson L H, et al. Itraconazole therapy for cryptococcal meningitis and cryptococcosis. Arch Intern Med 1989; 149: 2301–2308

Desmet P, Kayembe K D, De Vroey C. The value of cryptococcal serum antigen screening among HIV-positive/AIDS patients in Kinshasa, Zaire. AIDS 1989; 3: 77–78

Dismukes W E, Cloud G, Gallis H A, et al. Treatment of cryptococcal meningitis with combination amphotericin B and flucytosine for four as compared with six weeks. New Engl J Med 1987; 317: 334–341

Gade W, Ledman D W, Wethington R, Yi A. Serological responses to various coccidioides antigen preparations in a new enzyme immunoassay. J Clin Microbiol 1992; 39: 1907–1912

Goldstein E, Winship M S, Pappagianis D. Ventricular fluid and the management of coccidioidal meningitis. Ann Intern Med 1972; 77: 243–246

Golnik K C, Newman S A, Wispelway B. Cryptococcal optic neuropathy in the acquired immune deficiency syndrome. J Clin Neuro Ophthalmol 1991; 11: 96–103

Goodwin R A, Shapiro J L, Thurman G H, et al. Disseminated histoplasmosis: clinical and pathological correlations. Medicine 1980; 59: 1–33

Green J H, Harrell W K, Johnson J E, Benson R. Isolation of an antigen from Blastomyces dermatiditis that is specific for the diagnosis of blastomycosis. Curr Microbiol 1980; 4: 293–296

Hoffmann S, Stenderup J, Mathiesen L R. Low yield of screening for cryptococcal antigen by latex agglutination assay on serum and cerebrospinal fluid from Danish patients with AIDS and ARC. Scand J Infect Dis 1991; 23: 697–702

Kovacs J A, Kovacs A A, Polis M, et al. Cryptococcosis in the acquired immunodeficiency syndrome. Ann Intern Med 1985; 103: 533–538

Kurup V P, Kumar A. Immunodiagnosis of aspergillosis. Clin Microbiol Rev 1991; 4: 439–456

Kwartler J A, Linthicum F H, Jahn A F, Hawke M. Sudden hearing loss due to AIDS-related cryptococcal meningitis – a temporal bone study. Otolaryngol Head Neck Surg 1991; 104: 265–269

Labadie E L, Hamilton R H. Survival improvement in coccidioidal meningitis by high dose intrathecal amphotericin B. Arch Intern Med 1986; 146: 2013–2018

Larsen R A. Azoles and AIDS. J Infect Dis 1990; 162: 727–730

Larsen R A, Leal M A, Chan L S. Fluconazole compared with amphotericin B plus flucytosine for cryptococcal meningitis in AIDS. A randomized trial. Ann Intern Med 1990; 113: 183–197

Lipson B K, Freeman W R, Beniz J, et al. Optic neuropathy associated with cryptococcal arachnoiditis in AIDS patients. Am J Ophthalmol 1989; 107: 523–527

Mathews V P, Alo P L, Glass J D, et al. AIDS-related CNS cryptococcosis: radiologic-pathologic correlation. AJNR 1992; 13: 1477–1486

Nelson M R, Bower M, Smith D, et al. The value of serum cryptococcal antigen in the diagnosis of cryptococcal infection in patients infected with the human immunodeficiency virus. J Infect 1990; 21: 175–181

Post M J, Kursunoglu S J, Hensley G T, et al. Cranial CT in acquired immunodeficiency syndrome: spectrum of disease and optimal contrast enhancement technique. AJR 1985; 145: 929–940

Ringden O, Tollemar J, Tyden G. Liposomal amphotericin B (letter). Lancet 1992; 339: 374

Saag M S, Powderly W G, Cloud G A, et al. Comparison of amphotericin B with fluconazole in the treatment of acute AIDS-associated cryptococcal meningitis. New Engl J Med 1992; 326: 83–89

Shaunak S, Schell W A, Perfect J R. Cryptococcal meningitis with normal cerebrospinal fluid. J Infect Dis 1989; 160: 912

Snider W D, Simpson D M, Neilsen S, et al. Neurological complications of acquired immune deficiency syndrome: analysis of 50 patients. Ann Neurol 1986; 14: 403–418

Sugar A M, Saunders C. Oral fluconazole as suppressive therapy of disseminated cryptococcosis in patients with acquired immunodeficiency syndrome. Am J Med 1988; 85: 481–489

Sugar A M, Stern J J, Dupont B. Overview: Treatment of cryptococcal meningitis. Rev Infect Dis 1990; 12 (suppl 3): S338–S348

Tang L-M. Ventriculo-peritoneal shunt in cryptococcal meningitis with hydrocephalus. Surg Neurol 1990; 33: 314–319

Tien R D, Chu P K, Hesselink J R, et al. Intracranial cryptococcosis in immunocompromised patients: CT and MR findings in 29 cases. AJNR 1991; 12: 283–289

Treseler C B, Sugar A M. Fungal meningitis. Infect Dis Clin North Am 1990; 4: 789–808

Tucker R M, Denning D W, Dupont B, Stevens D A. Itraconazole therapy for chronic coccidioidal meningitis. Ann Intern Med 1990a; 112: 108–112

Tucker R M, Galgiani J N, Denning D W, et al. Treatment of coccidioidal meningitis with fluconazole. Rev Infect Dis 1990b; 12 (suppl): S380–S389

Vincent M, Webster M H, Pether J V. Liposomal amphotericin B (letter). Lancet 1992; 339: 374–375

Walpole H T, Gregory D W. Cerebral histoplasmosis. South Med J 1987; 80: 1575–1577

Wheat L J, Kohler R B, Tewari R P. Diagnosis of disseminated histoplasmosis by detection of Histoplasma capsulatum antigen in serum and urine specimens. N Engl J Med 1986; 314: 83–88

Wheat L J, Connolly-Stringfield P A, Baker R L, et al. Disseminated histoplasmosis in the acquired immune deficiency syndrome: clinical findings, diagnosis and treatment and review of the literature. Medicine 1990; 69: 361–374

Wheat T T, Connolly-Stringfield P A, Blair P, et al. Histoplasmosis relapse in patients with AIDS: detection using Histoplasma capsulatum variety capsulatum antigen levels. Ann Intern Med 1991; 115: 936–941

Zealear D S, Winn W A. The neurosurgical approach in the treatment of coccidioidal meningitis. Report of ten cases. In: Allejo L, editor. Coccidioidomycosis. Tucson: University of Arizona Press, 1967: 43–53

Zuger A, Louie E, Holzman R S, et al. Cryptococcal disease in patients with the acquired immunodeficiency syndrome. Diagnostic features and outcome of treatment. Ann Intern Med 1986; 234–240

9. Opportunistic infections – viruses

HERPES SIMPLEX ENCEPHALITIS

Herpes simplex encephalitis (HSE) is the most common cause of fatal encephalitis in the Western world and many hundreds of cases are seen each year. The acute disease may present with confusion, disorientation and bizarre behaviour suggesting an acute dementing illness, and long-term survivors frequently show evidence of memory impairment, personality change or frank dementia (Oxbury & MacCallum 1973, Hierons et al 1978).

The herpes simplex virus (HSV) is a large enveloped double-stranded DNA virus. The virion has a dense central core surrounded by a trilayered membrane that makes it look like a bull's eye target. HSV1 and HSV2 are closely related, but have subtle immunological and biological differences.

HSE affects all sections of the adult community, and all ages. It is estimated to affect 1 in 250 000 to 1 in 500 000 of the population each year. Most victims have previously been well, and the prevalence of a history of recurrent herpetic skin lesions (herpes labialis) is probably no greater than in the general public. The pathogenesis is somewhat mysterious. Both primary and recurrent infections can give rise to HSE. Primary infection probably accounts for one-third of cases and most of these are under 18 years of age. The route of infection into the central nervous system (CNS) is disputed. Both the olfactory tracts and the trigeminal ganglia are supported by pathological studies.

The clinical presentation in the immunocompetent reflects the focal nature of the parenchymatous infection. Thus the familiar mental state and conscious level changes of encephalitis in general are compounded by the features of frontal, temporal or brainstem infection. Thus hemiparesis, dysphasia, visual field loss or cranial nerve signs were recorded in 96 of 113 biopsy-proven cases in the National Institute of Allergy and Infectious Disease Collaborative Antiviral Study Group (NIAID) study (Whiteley et al 1982). The other 17 cases had behavioural changes and evidence of localized CNS involvement on neuroimaging. The most common clinical findings were headache, fever, personality change, seizures, hemiparesis and ataxia, all of which affected more than 50% of victims.

The cerebrospinal fluid (CSF) virtually always has a pleocytosis and is also often haemorrhagic. Leucocyte counts of $10-1000/mm^3$ are seen. Electroencephalograms (EEGs) may be helpful as the predilection for the temporal lobes seen in HSE can be seen in the occurrence of focal repetitive complexes. The complexes (Figs 9.1 and 9.2) are of simple morphology and can be independent on the two sides. They are not uniformly encountered and are not necessarily detected at presentation. Serial records may be necessary. The complexes may precede flattening of the record due to necrosis. The sensitivity of EEGs in the diagnosis of HSE has been estimated at 84%, but the specificity in the NIAID studies was only 32.5%. Localization to the temporal lobes may be seen on nucleotide and computed tomographic (CT) scans. Magnetic resonance imaging (MRI) is more sensitive, and bilateral high signal in the temporal lobes with some swelling is very suggestive of the diagnosis.

None of these tests is sufficiently diagnostic,

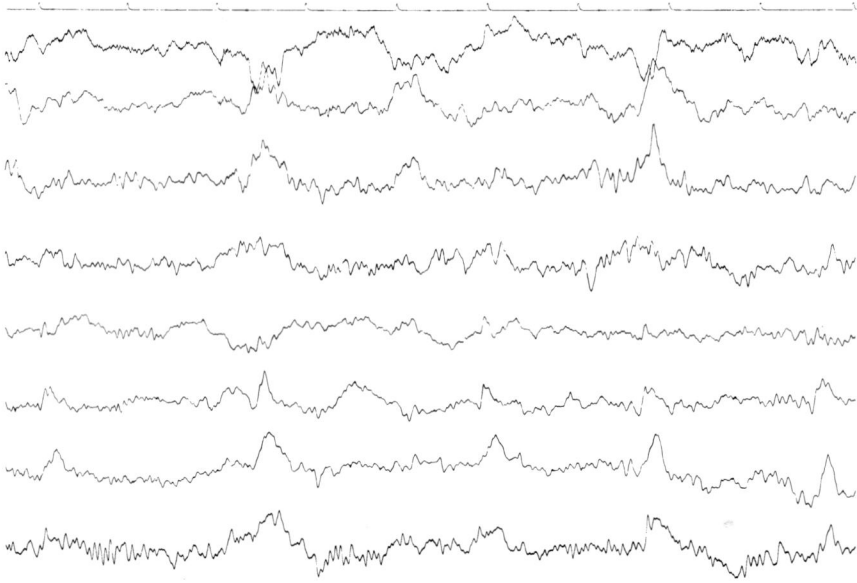

Fig. 9.1 EEG early in the course of HSE (non-AIDS case). Disorganized recording with suggestion of repetitive complexes. (Upper four channels from right temporal lobe, lower four from the left.)

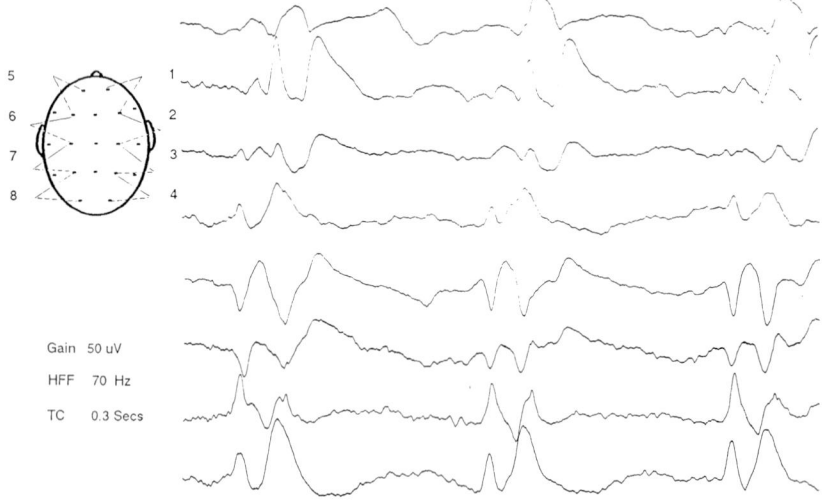

Gain   50 uV

HFF   70 Hz

TC   0.3 Secs

Fig. 9.2 EEG late in the course of HSE (non-AIDS case). Loss of all normal activity and repetitive complexes.

however, and proof of the diagnosis has traditionally depended on brain biopsy (Soong et al 1991). The continued need for histological proof of the diagnosis is challenged by two developments. Firstly, rapid identification of herpes virus in the CSF has become possible by polymerase chain reaction (PCR) (Rowley et al 1990). Secondly, successful antiviral treatment is now available with an agent of low toxicity so that it may be prescribed without prior proof of diagnosis (Sawyer & Ellner 1988).

In the context of AIDS, encephalitis or meningitis may be due to HSV1 or 2. The illness is less acute than in the immunocompetent individual, and often appears to be less severe, raising the possibility that the pathogenesis of cerebral damage in the immunocompetent includes an autoimmune response. The encephalitic illness is less haemorrhagic and less often produces focal deficit. MRI and CT less often reveal oedema or necrosis of the temporal lobe, the EEG less often shows repetitive complexes, and the CSF may show little, if any, abnormality. Detection of the virus in the CSF or biopsy therefore remain the best way of making the diagnosis in this context. PCR techniques have been used for the early detection of HSV in CSF and, in some hands, positive results have been obtained as early as the second day of neurological symptoms (Aurelius et al 1991). The measurement of the intrathecal synthesis of antibodies to HSV by comparing concentrations of immunoglobulins in serum to CSF is not useful in the acute setting because of the delay in production of antibodies and the critical need for early initiation of treatment for success (van Loon et al 1989, Whitley et al 1991). Persistent parenchymatous and periventricular changes (Figs 9.3–9.5) were seen in a personally followed biopsy-proven case.

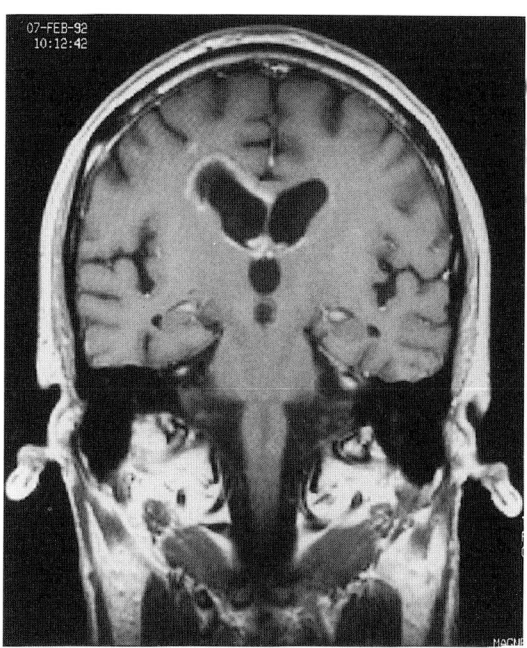

Fig. 9.4 T1-weighted MRI with gadolinium enhancement of ventricular wall in a case of HSE in a patient with AIDS.

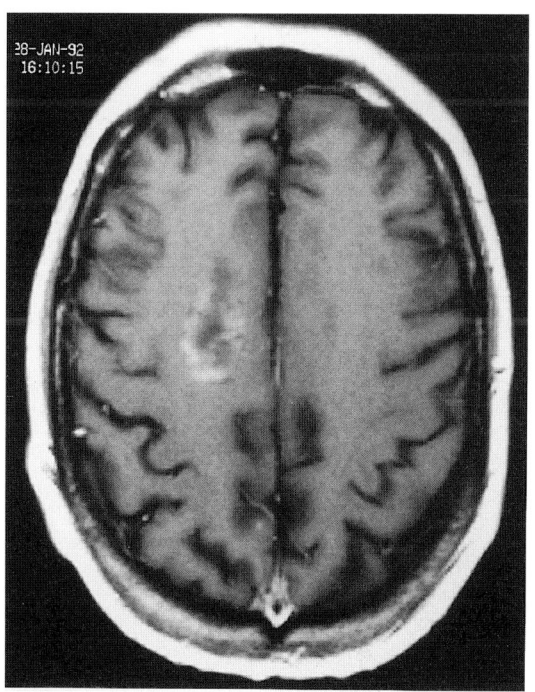

Fig. 9.3 T1-weighted MRI with gadolinium enhancement of abnormal area due to HSE in AIDS.

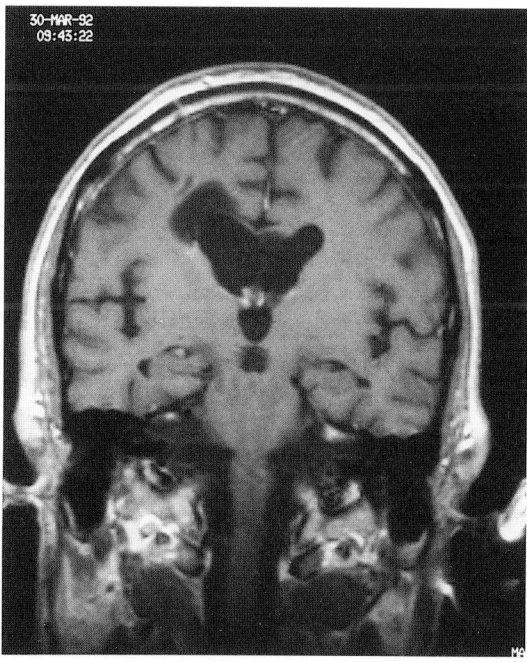

Fig. 9.5 T1-weighted MRI with gadolinium enhancement of the same case as shown in Figs 9.3 and 9.4 after treatment with acyclovir.

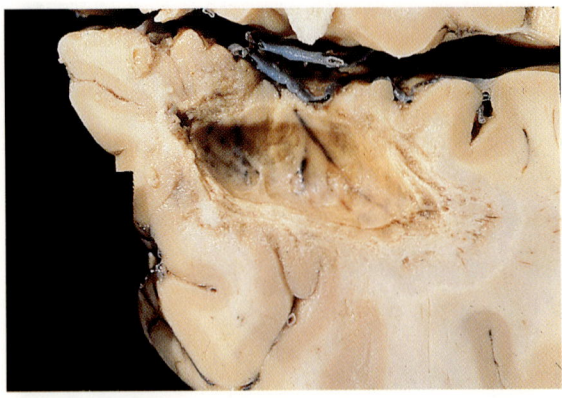
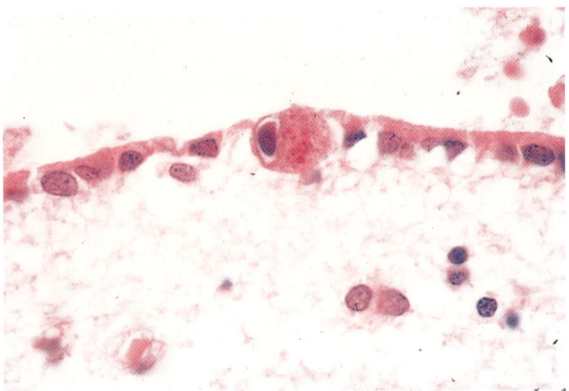

A   B

Fig. 9.6   A Post-mortem appearance of CMV ventriculitis. **B** Cytomegalic cells from the subependymal region in a case of CMV ventriculitis.

Treatment involves the use of acyclovir, which is phosphorylated by virus-encoded thymidine kinase in virus-affected cells to an active anti-DNA metabolite. Relapses have occurred even in the immunocompetent so the treatment period is now considered to be 21 rather than 10 days (Van Landingham et al 1988). In AIDS, treatment needs to be maintained orally after a therapeutic intravenous regimen.

CMV ENCEPHALITIS/RETINITIS/RADICULITIS

Almost all homosexual patients have circulating antibodies to cytomegalovirus (CMV), and signs of CMV infection in the brain (Fig. 9.6) rank amongst the most common autopsy findings (about 30%). Multiple organs can be affected, including the lungs, eyes and adrenals.

CMV causes an encephalitis (Hawley et al 1983, Snider et al 1983, Moskowitz et al 1984, Levy et al 1985, Vinters et al 1989), which is probably under-recognized because of difficulty in pre-mortem diagnosis and because the presentation can be confused with HIV-1 dementia. The course is often rapidly progressive with prominent periventriculitis (Fig. 9.7) and encephalitis in the setting of CMV retinitis or disseminated CMV infection. Kalayjian et al (1993) reviewed six patients with ependymal necrosis attributable to CMV coinfection in AIDS. A clinical picture emerged of a subacute or acute presentation with

lethargy and confusion and signs of brainstem involvement. Cranial nerve palsies and nystagmus were often accompanied by a cellular CSF with low glucose level. Holland et al (1994) found 14 autopsied cases to contrast with 17 with HIV-associated dementia in a 10-year period at Johns Hopkins Hospital. The mean duration of symptoms was 3.5 weeks with apathy, confusion and disorientation, whilst those with HIV dementia had more insidious presentations. Both groups

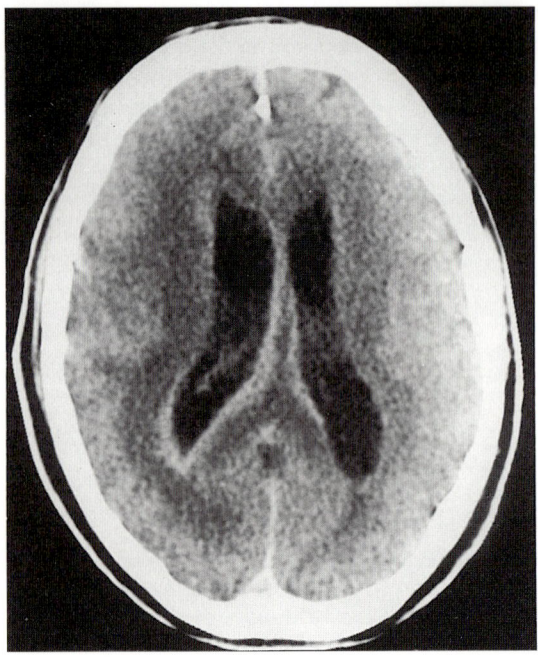

Fig. 9.7   CT scan with contrast showing ventriculitis.

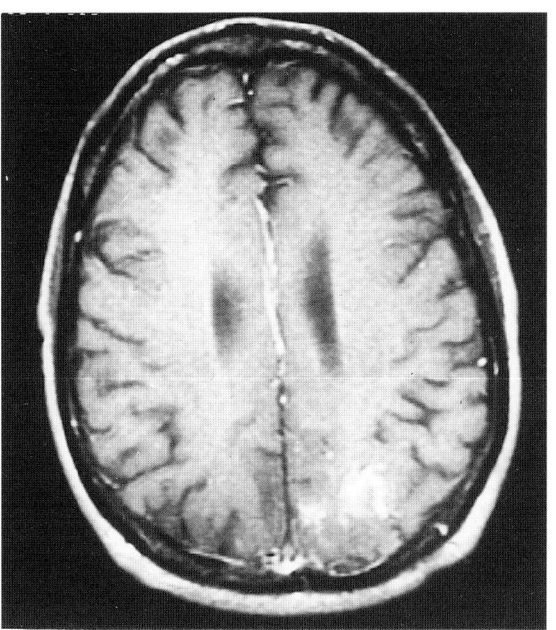
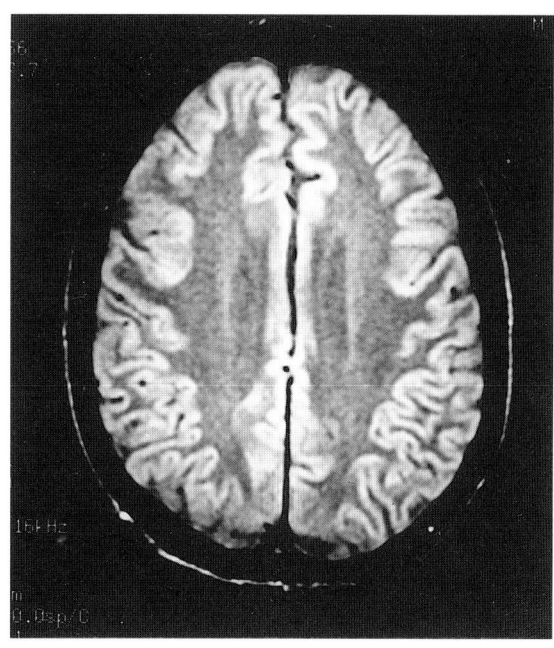

A   B

Fig. 9.8   MRI scan of a case of CMV encephalitis showing gadolinium enhancement (T1) of an abnormal occipital area (**A**) which resolves after treatment with ganciclovir (**B**).

complained of memory problems. As in Kalayjian's cases, cranial nerve lesions were a pointer to CMV infection. Most cases had CMV elsewhere at autopsy. The clinical counterpart to the usual CMV adrenalitis was a tendency to hyponatraemia. Cell counts in the CSF failed to distinguish those with CMV, but 33% had positive PCR for CMV. Radiological studies show periventricular rarefaction (CT) or white matter hyperintensity (T2-weighted MRI), and contrast-enhancing lesions in subependymal and cortical regions (Post et al, 1986) (Fig. 9.8). Serial images showed progressive ventriculomegaly (Kalayjian et al 1993). CSF analysis is not diagnostic because cultures are usually negative (Power et al 1992); however, PCR for CMV has been found to be positive in 30–100% of cases (Cinque et al 1992, Gozlan et al 1992, Wolf et al 1992, Holland et al 1994). Fiala et al (1993) showed high levels of intrathecal synthesis of CMV antibodies in patients with CMV encephalitis. It is possible that this may become a simpler and more useful test for the early diagnosis of CMV encephalitis. At this point, however, neither the sensitivity nor specificity of CSF CMV serology is known (Luer et al 1988). Reverse transcriptase PCR for CMV

RNA is under development and will probably become a much more reliable measure of active CMV infection.

Neuropathological findings are variable, ranging from rare isolated CMV inclusions, which may be found in up to 50% of AIDS brains, to severe necrotizing ependymitis (Figs 9.6 and 9.9) and meningo-encephalitis (Vinters et al 1989). Usually cytomegalic cells within microglial nodules are detectable. In a proportion of cases, however, either in situ hybridization or immuno-cytochemistry may be necessary to demonstrate CMV DNA or antigens. Schmidbauer et al (1989) showed that a third of cases with nodular encephalitis without cytomegalic cells had signifi-cant amounts of CMV DNA detectable by in situ hybridization. Typical lesions of HIV encephalitis do not show local co-infection with CMV. Microglial nodules are found in the grey matter and the subcortical white matter. An acyclovir analogue, ganciclovir, is licenced for treatment of CMV retinitis and, in the setting of suspected CMV encephalitis, could be initiated. Ganciclovir crosses the blood–brain barrier with up to 40% of blood levels detected in the CSF, and at autopsy 38% in the brain (Shepp et al 1985). Controlled

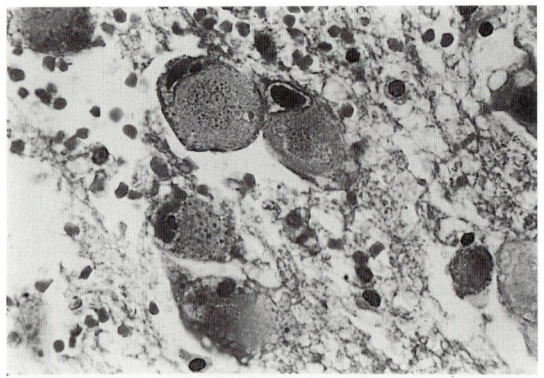

Fig. 9.9 Pathological appearance of CMV encephalitis. Numerous cytomegalic cells in the subependymal region with surrounding inflammation and necrosis. Note the typical owl's eye inclusions in the cytomegalic cells.

clinical trials are lacking, although some open-label use (Fig. 9.8) has suggested some efficacy (Peters et al 1992, Novak et al 1989). The prognosis has been poor, however, which in some cases may be due to a degree of resistance associated with prolonged exposure to the drug used to contain CMV retinitis (Holland et al 1994).

Fiala et al (1993) reported seven patients with progressive encephalopathy considered to be caused by CMV encephalitis. In all cases there was a rapid progression of neurological findings, usually in a patient with CMV retinitis with sensory polyneuropathy and elevated CMV antibodies in the CSF. CMV viraemia was present in five of eight patients with CMV encephalitis. Intrathecal CMV antibodies were found to be elevated in three of the CMV encephalitis cases (although it is not certain how many were actually tested), with markedly elevated ratios of CSF to serum. The successful use of combined ganciclovir and foscarnet was reported in 10 patients with AIDS and progressive CMV retinitis or gastrointestinal disease (Dieterich et al 1993). Nine of 10 patients had received ganciclovir and foscarnet monotherapy before receiving combination therapy. Anaemia was more common with combination therapy, but other toxicities were similar. Treatment with ganciclovir was begun with an induction dose of 5 mg/kg every 12 hours for 2 weeks, then 5 mg/kg each day. Foscarnet was begun with an induction dose of 60 mg/kg every 8 hours for 2 weeks, followed by maintenance therapy of 90–120 mg/kg/day. Foscarnet doses

were given with 1 litre of normal saline and dosing adjusted for predicted creatinine clearance. Combination therapy was begun with ganciclovir 5 mg/kg every 12 hours and foscarnet 60 mg/kg every 8 hours. The rate of neutropenia was somewhat higher in those receiving combination therapy than monotherapy. The one patient who did not respond died after 40 days from manifestations of advanced HIV disease. More information is needed on such a strategy, as it should be noted that this was a retrospective study.

CMV encephalitis has been successfully treated in immunodeficiency states other than HIV infection. Bamborschke et al (1992) reported a 40-year-old HIV-negative renal transplant patient with CMV encephalitis who was treated with ganciclovir, anti-CMV immunoglobulins and intrathecal beta-interferon with complete recovery. Interestingly, no intrathecal production of antibodies was detected and CMV encephalitis was diagnosed by in situ hybridization on CSF cell preparations and PCR. Routine use of CMV blood and urine cultures is not recommended because of poor diagnostic and predictive value for the subsequent development of end-organ disease (Zurlo et al 1993). Only 35% of patients with CMV viraemia develop end-organ disease and some patients with proven end-organ disease were not viraemic (45%) although most were viruric (88%).

CMV retinitis is the most common ocular infection in patients with AIDS and causes a

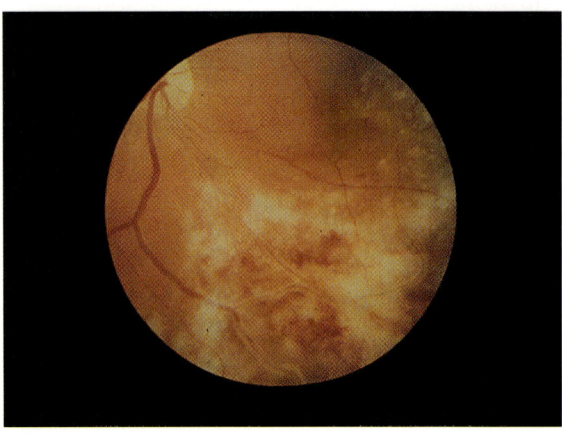

Fig. 9.10 Retinal appearance in CMV retinitis showing haemorrhage and necrosis. (Courtesy of Mr J. Brazier.)

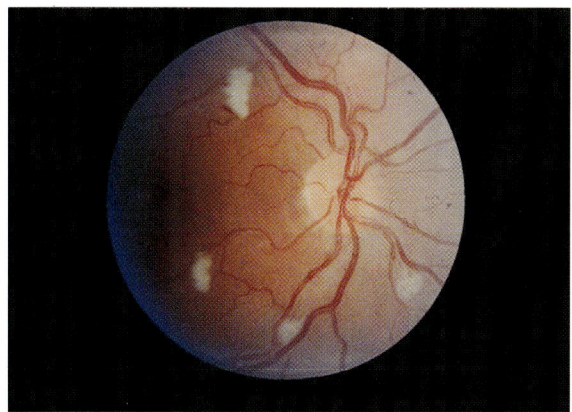

Fig. 9.11   Retinal appearance in HIV infection showing 'cotton wool' spots. No evidence of CMV. (Courtesy of Mr J. Brazier.)

haemorrhagic retinitis in up to 20% (Jabs et al 1989). Kupperman et al (1993) examined 132 patients with AIDS. For those with CD4 counts below 50, 26 out of 87 (30%) had CMV retinitis, while none out of 45 with a count over 50 had retinitis. CMV retinitis is recognized by its characteristic appearance of retinal necrosis admixed with haemorrhage on ophthalmoscopy (Fig. 9.10). In up to 60% it becomes bilateral. Untreated, CMV retinitis is a progressive disease that can lead to blindness. It is important, but sometimes difficult, to distinguish CMV retinitis from cotton-wool spots (Fig. 9.11), which are microinfarcts of the nerve fibre layer of the retina that do not interfere with vision. They occur in 40–92% of patients with AIDS (Newsome et al 1984), are non-infectious in origin, and may be related to immune complex deposition. Kupperman et al (1993) noted that their incidence was also related to CD4 count; 45% had cotton wool spots with a CD4 count of 50 or less, compared with 16% with a count over 50. It is generally possible to culture CMV from either the blood, vitreous or urine of patients with active CMV retinitis.

Treatment of CMV infection

The only currently available form of treatment for CMV retinitis is ganciclovir. Several open-labelled studies have demonstrated the efficacy of ganciclovir in suppressing CMV infection, with a clinical response observed in about 80% (Collaborative DHPG Treatment Study Group 1986). Treatment consists of an initial induction phase for about 2 weeks with the drug being given intravenously twice daily. Subsequently, maintenance therapy, using a once-daily intravenous infusion, must be continued life-long because interruption of ganciclovir almost universally results in the reactivation of active CMV retinitis (Jabs et al 1989). The most significant side-effect of ganciclovir is reversible leucopenia, which occurs to a mild degree in most patients. In an open-label study comparing ganciclovir with foscarnet, a pyrophosphate analogue with in vitro activity against CMV and HIV in CMV retinitis, no difference in the progression of retinitis was found. However, mean survival in the ganciclovir group was significantly shorter than for those receiving foscarnet. The patients in the ganciclovir group received less antiretroviral therapy on average than those in the foscarnet group, although other unidentified factors may be involved in the survival differences (Studies of Ocular Complications of AIDS Research Group 1992).

CMV can also cause a progressive radiculopathy involving lumbar and sacral roots (Miller et al 1990). Typically occurring in patients with advanced immunodeficiency with a CD4 count less than 100, although it may be the first AIDS-defining illness (Mahieux et al 1989), there is usually the subacute onset of flaccid paralysis of the lower extremities with sacral pain, paraesthesias and sphincter dysfunction. MRI or myelography may reveal clumped thickened roots and MR enhancement of roots and the conus may be obvious. Often the imaging is normal. CSF analysis is helpful in diagnosis, frequently but not universally showing a polymorphonuclear pleocytosis (often several hundred), hypoglycorrhachia and elevated protein. Polymorphs were recorded in 24 out of 29 cases reviewed from the literature by Cohen et al (1993). CMV can be isolated by culture in about 40% of cases and cytopathology may demonstrate cytomegalic cells. Necrosis and inflammation with cytomegalic cells and CMV immunoreactivity have been demonstrated in lumbosacral roots (Eidelberg et al 1986, Miller et al 1990) (see Fig. 6.13, p. 104). Disseminated

CMV infection with viraemia and CMV retinitis are frequent concomitants. The differential diagnosis includes HSV2 infection, which may cause urinary retention, a radiculopathy and myelitis. HSV may be cultured from the CSF, but the distinction cannot always be made. Fortunately, treatment with ganciclovir 'covers' both viruses. Toxoplasmosis can occasionally affect the cord or conus, so may produce a similar clinical picture. MRI or myelography may show an abscess, and the CSF may contain antibodies. Lymphomatous meningoradiculitis can be diagnosed by finding lymphoma cells in the spinal fluid, and serology should include the VDRL, as syphilitic radiculitis or cord damage can again mimic the presentation.

If CMV is suspected the acyclovir analogue, ganciclovir, should be prescribed. If initiated early, it can produce stabilization or even improvement, particularly in patients whose course is more indolent. Persistent CSF pleocytosis predicts a poor response to treatment, and may reflect ganciclovir resistance (Cohen et al 1993). Ganciclovir CSF penetration varies from 0 to 41% (Fletcher et al 1986, Laskin et al 1987), which may also affect the response. Foscarnet achieves CSF concentrations adequate for complete inhibition of CMV replication (Hengge et al 1993).

For treatment of CMV infection, HPMPG is a new nucleotide analogue with no requirement for thymidine kinase. It has potent anti-CMV activity and is already phosphorylated so does not require triphosphorylation as do both ganciclovir and acyclovir. The major limiting side-effect is nephrotoxicity; some patients can develop Fanconi syndrome.

Both HSV and varicella zoster virus (VZV) code for thymidine kinase, which phosphorylates acyclovir. CMV does not encode thymidine kinase, but does encode another kinase, the UL-97 gene product, which can phosphorylate ganciclovir and possibly acyclovir. Although acyclovir inhibits the replication of CMV in vitro, much higher concentrations are required than for the suppression of HSV or VZV replication.

BW-256U87 is a pro-drug (the 1-valyl ester of the hydrochloride salt) of acyclovir. It is rapidly converted to acyclovir after oral administration and shows a three- to four-fold increase in acyclovir bioavailability. The absorption of oral acyclovir is slow, variable and incomplete with an estimated total bioavailability of 20% at doses of 200 mg decreasing to 10% at doses of 800 mg. Acyclovir has a terminal plasma half-life of 2–3 hours in patients with normal renal function. In man, the mechanism for conversion of the BW pro-drug to acyclovir has not been determined. The pro-drug is currently under trial (ACTG 204) to evaluate its efficacy in preventing CMV end-organ disease in HIV/CMV co-infected patients with less than 100 CD4 lymphocytes. Other treatments for CMV disease include monoclonal antibodies (murine monoclonal CMV antibodies). These were studied in 1988 in bone marrow transplant recipients with CMV pneumonia. Patients receiving ganciclovir and immune globulin containing CMV antibodies had improved survival (Winston et al 1987, Emanuel et al 1988, Reed et al 1988). One product available in Europe, Cytotect, produced by Biotest Pharma, contains CMV-specific hyperimmune globulin. In the USA, it is categorized as an orphan drug and is manufactured by the Massachusetts Health Biologic Laboratories and distributed by the Red Cross Northeast Region. Triclonal CMV antibodies are being developed and may have broader activity against different strains of CMV. These are currently being developed by Medimorphics. Desiclovir is the acyclovir pro-drug. HOE-602 is a ganciclovir pro-drug produced by Hoescht Roussel. HPMPC is 10-fold more potent than ganciclovir as a selective inhibitor of CMV in vitro (Snoeck et al 1988). This drug is being developed by Bristol Myers. Another agent, FIAC/FIAU, made by O'Classen Pharmaceuticals, has considerable in vitro anti-CMV activity. In previous trials, neurological toxicity and elevated creative phosphokinase (CPK) levels have been found. Another agent, HPMPA, related to HPMPC, is less potent than HPMPC in vitro. Oxetanocin A and G and cyclobut A and G are oxetanocin analogues with broad-spectrum antiviral activity against CMV, other herpes viruses and HIV, which may cross the blood–brain barrier (Hayashi et al 1990). Foscarnet inhibits viral DNA polymerase selectively with lesser effects on cellular DNA polymerase. It does not require phosphorylation by thymidine kinase or other kinases; thus, mutants of HSV and VZV, which are deficient in thymidine kinase (TK-negative) and resistant to acyclovir, remain susceptible to foscarnet. Similarly, CMV mutants resistant to ganciclovir with low levels of phosphorylating enzymes also remain susceptible to foscarnet. Certain acyclovir-resistant HSV strains that are DNA polymerase mutants may also be resistant to foscarnet.

Management plan

A short history compatible with encephalitis or lumbosacral radiculopathy, in the context of CMV retinitis or CMV viraemia, warrants a therapeutic trial of ganciclovir and/or foscarnet. The lumbosacral radiculopathy syndrome is sufficiently specific to warrant treatment even in the absence of evidence of systemic CMV, once syphilis and lymphoma have been excluded. CMV retinitis requires long-term treatment and monitoring by ophthalmologists.

HERPES ZOSTER RADICULITIS

Varicella zoster virus (VZV) is a 100 nM icosahedral nucleocapsid with a host-derived envelope that becomes latent in sensory neurones during primary infection. Five to 10% of patients with HIV-1 infection will develop herpes zoster radiculitis representing reactivation of latent H. zoster infection. Dermatomal H. zoster (Fig. 9.12) does not require antiviral treatment unless cervical or lumbar dermatomes are involved. In this setting, a severe myeloradiculitis can develop leading to permanent motor deficits; therefore, intravenous acyclovir (30 mg/kg/day) should be used. The development of post-herpetic neuralgia may require the use of pain-modifying agents such as amitriptyline or carbamazepine. After the vesicles have completely healed, topical capsaicin can reduce the neuralgic pains. A rare encephalitis has been described with 'plaques' in the white matter and brainstem. After dermatomal zoster, particularly in the trigeminal and cervical areas, a granulomatous angiitis can precipitate thrombotic occlusion, for example of the ipsilateral middle

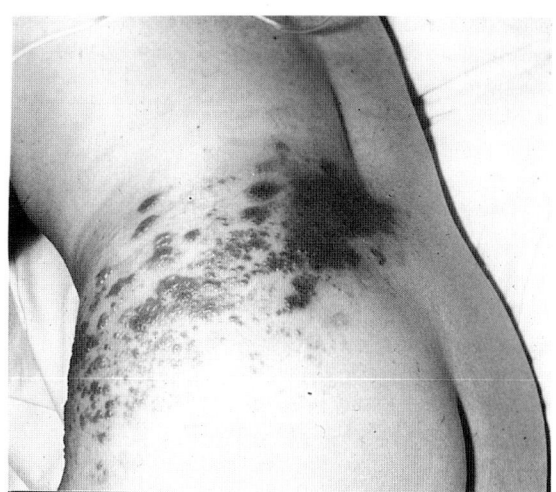

Fig. 9.12   Multidermatomal H. zoster infection.

cerebral artery with subsequent stroke (Chapter 13).

PROGRESSIVE MULTIFOCAL LEUCOENCEPHALOPATHY

In 1958, Astrom, Mancall and Richardson described three cases of an unusual demyelinating disease affecting particularly the posterior parts of the cerebral hemispheres. Two of the patients had leukaemia, the third Hodgkin's disease. The clinical picture was of dementia, with speech and pyramidal tract dysfunction. The CSF remained normal. The course was relentlessly progressive with death in 2–6 months. From the literature they found another five cases including examples in which the underlying disease was sarcoidosis and tuberculosis. In one patient no such systemic disorder was detected (Astrom et al 1958).

Subsequent cases have confirmed the usual association with conditions associated with defects in cell-mediated immunity such as lymphoproliferative disorders (Richardson 1970). Transplant recipients, patients on antineoplastic therapy and those with autoimmune diseases or Whipple's disease have also been described as developing progressive multifocal leucoencephalopathy (PML). The condition is now seen most frequently in the context of AIDS, occurring in 2–3% of such patients (Gillespie et al 1991). Cavanagh et al (1959) suggested that the role of immunosuppression was critical and that a virus was probably responsible. Virions, morphologically identifiable as belonging to a papova virus, were subsequently identified in abnormal oligodendroglial nuclei (Zu Rhein & Chou 1965). The responsible virus was finally grown from a patient whose initials were JC. It was characterized as belonging to the papova group of small non-enveloped double-stranded DNA viruses (Padgett et al 1971). The JC virus, as it was named, is a frequent childhood infection, though usually silent. By the age of 6 years, 50% of children have seroconverted and by middle adulthood 80–90% of the population have been infected. Renal transplant patients frequently have JC virus in their urine. During pregnancy, when many viruses are reactivated, about 1 in 200 women shed JC virus in the urine. It thus seems possible that the kidney is a site of latent infection after the childhood exposure. However, the strain isolated from the kidney is not always the same as that in the affected brain. Entry into the brain, where the virus targets oligo-dendrocytes and astrocytes, appears to be from the bloodstream (the early lesions parallel the distribution of haematogenous abscesses). Houff et al (1988) have shown the presence of JC virus in the B lymphocytes of the marrow and spleen in cases of PML. JC virus and related BK virus (also named after a patient) are not normally patho-genic in the absence of some degree of immuno-suppression. This opportunism as an infective agent in the CNS is particularly well marked in AIDS where PML typically develops when the

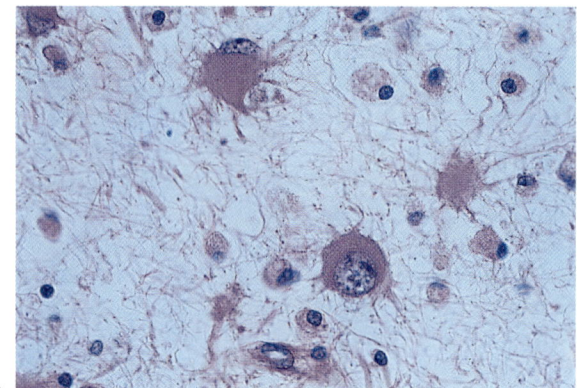

A

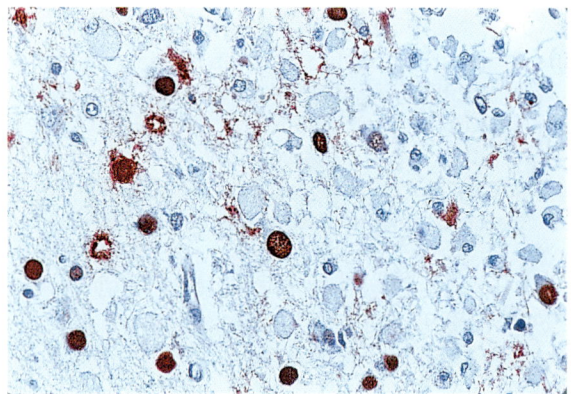

B

Fig. 9.14   **A** Bizarre astrocytes in an area of the brain affected by PML. **B** Infected oligodendrocytes in PML identified by SV40 positivity.

CD4 count is less than 200. In half the cases of HIV-related PML, the latter is the first, and there-fore the AIDS-defining, illness.

The reactivated papovavirus affects the hemispheric white matter and causes patchy foci of demyelination (Fig. 9.13), which may become confluent. The hallmarks of the histological diagnosis are inclusion bodies in deformed oligo-dendroglia, associated demyelination and bizarre giant astrocytes (Fig. 9.14). The lesions are often inflammatory, with many foamy macrophages present and necrosis is common. Immunostaining with SV40 (a cross-reacting antibody) demon-strates the inclusion-bearing oligodendrocytes (Fig. 9.15). Electron microscopy will reveal the collections of virus (Fig. 9.16). The first foci are usually at the junction of grey and white matter. The subcortical areas are usually the first sites of involvement (Fig. 9.17), but the grey matter or

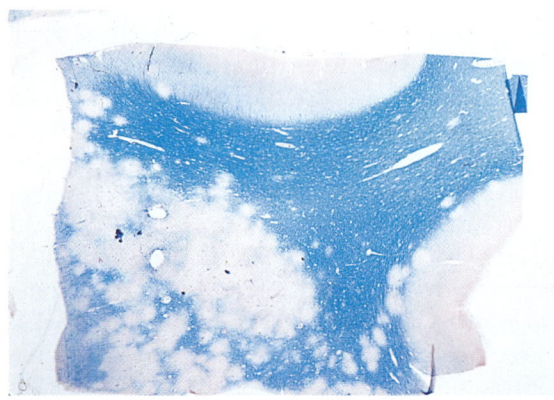

Fig. 9.13   Demyelination in the superior frontal gyrus due to PML (Luxol Fast Blue stain).

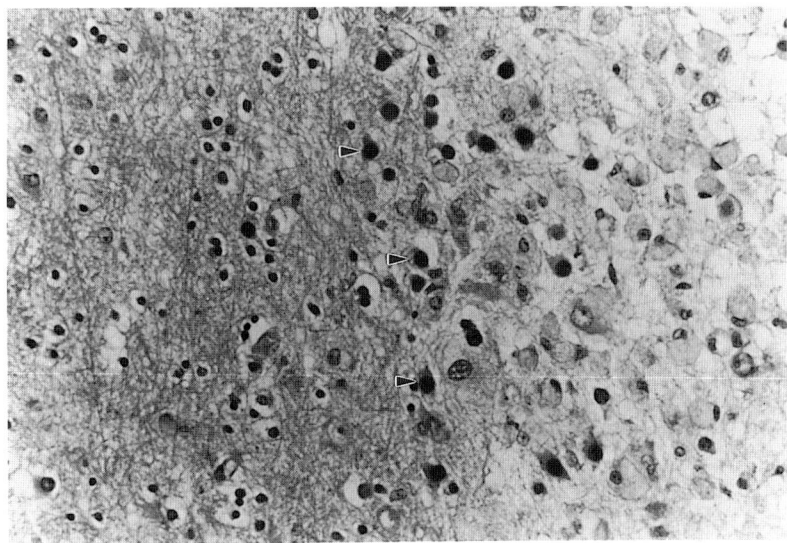

Fig. 9.15   Inclusion bodies in infected oligodendrocytes in a case of PML (arrow heads).

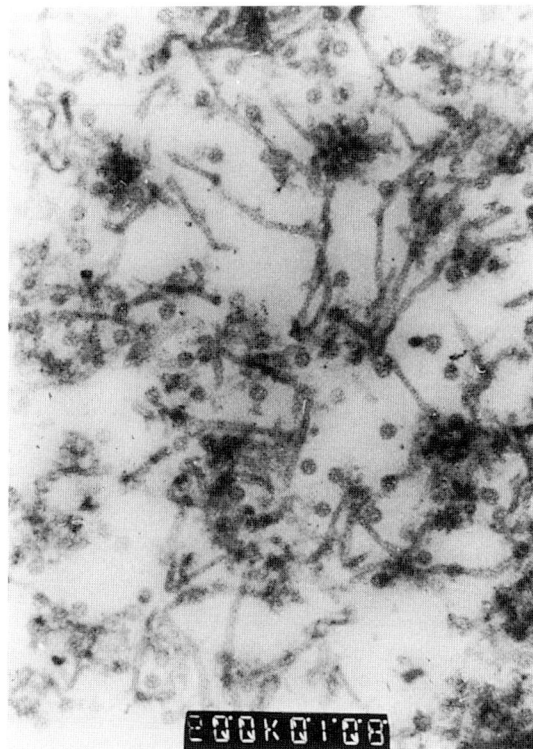

Fig. 9.16   JC virus particles on electron microscopy (× 60 000) in a case of PML. (Courtesy of Dr Susan Silver, Johns Hopkins University.)

periventricular areas may be affected, occasionally even before the typical subcortical lesions are recognized. Infected oligodendroglia are disrupted by viral replication and the shed virions affect neighbouring cells of the same lineage. The area affected grows like a bush fire (Fig. 9.18) creating an ever increasing area of demyelination, which

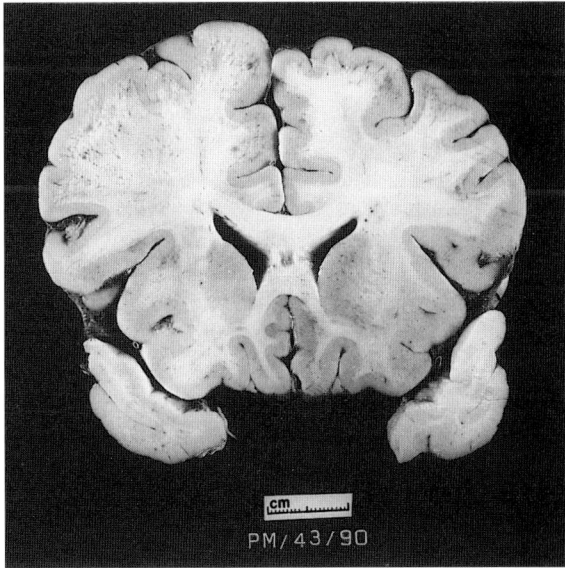

Fig. 9.17   Post-mortem brain showing changes in white matter due to PML.

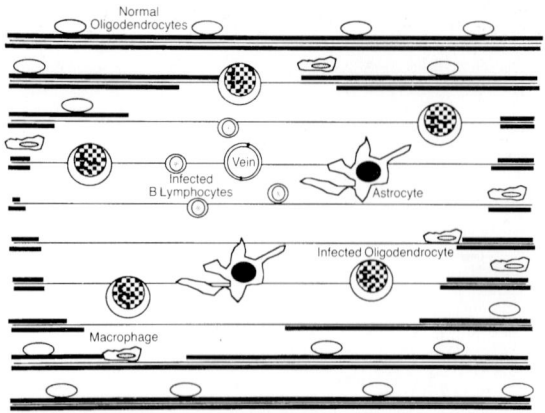

Fig. 9.18 Schematic diagram of pathogenesis of PML in an area of demyelination. Thick lines represent myelin ensheathing nerve fibres. Lymphocytes carrying the virus (asterisks) enter the brain from the blood and infect oligodendroglia and probably astrocytes. Macrophages remove the damaged myelin. The lesion expands out from the perivascular area. (© 1990 American Medical Association Reproduced from Chaisson & Griffin 1990 with permission of the American Medical Association.)

Table 9.1   Presenting symptoms of PML

Symptom	%
Limb weakness	48
Cognitive dysfunction	24
Visual loss	24
Gait disturbance	24
Limb incoordination	16
Headache	16
Speech/language disturbance	16

(Reproduced from Berger et al 1987 with the permission of the American College of Physicians)

also spreads down the tracts of myelinated fibres. The minimal lesion is a small punched-out area of demyelination at the grey/white matter interface with JC virus infected oligodendroglia at its margins. The lesions of PML in AIDS are often more destructive than PML not associated with HIV infection (Rhodes et al 1988). The cerebellum, temporal lobe and spinal cord tend to be spared in non-AIDS cases but not in AIDS. There are more affected oligodendrocytes in the grey matter adjacent to the affected white matter. There appear to be less bizarre astrocytes perhaps suggesting a more acute process. There are also perivascular infiltrates of lymphocytes, but this inflammatory histology is not as predictive of a more benign clinical outlook as it is in non-AIDS material (Aksamit personal communication).

Gillespie et al (1991) provided the first population-based study of PML. Between 1981 and 1989, 94 patients were identified in San Francisco (definite diagnosis in 48, presumptive in 46, 17 diagnosed at autopsy). The most common symptoms at diagnosis were motor abnormalities (67%), mental status changes (66%), hemiparesis (39%) and facial weakness (38%), with median time from first symptom to death of 3.5 months. Nine of 14 patients who later developed PML were JC virus seropositive, an identical seroprevalence to a group of matched controls.

PML typically presents with focal neurological deficits that progress inexorably over weeks or a few months to death (Table 9.1) (Snider et al 1983, Levy et al 1985, Berger et al 1987). PML is rare in children, although there have been scattered reports (Berger et al 1992b). Insidious but progressive limb weakness or visual field defect is common, as is subcortical dysphasia, ataxia and eventually dementia. Features typical of mass lesions such as headache are conspicuously rare, as are those implying grey matter involvement such as seizures. Having said that, it is true that, in the context of AIDS, grey matter involvement is rather more noticeable than is traditionally encountered in the other types of at-risk cases. Thus Gerstmann syndrome, proposagnosia, apraxia, unilateral neglect and spatial disorientation have all been documented in proven HIV-associated cases (Berger et al 1987). Focal presentations are very much the rule, though occasional cases show a rapid dementing illness in which focal problems develop secondarily. Most cases are eventually demented. The distinction in AIDS-related cases from AIDS dementia depends on the focal signs and the results of investigations. The clinical course has usually consisted of relentless progression with death in between 10 days and 18 months with a median survival of 16 weeks (Berger et al 1987), but there have been exceptions (Berger & Mucke 1988). In non-AIDS cases, recovery may attend improvement in the immune status of the patient, e.g. on stopping immunosuppressive treatment or

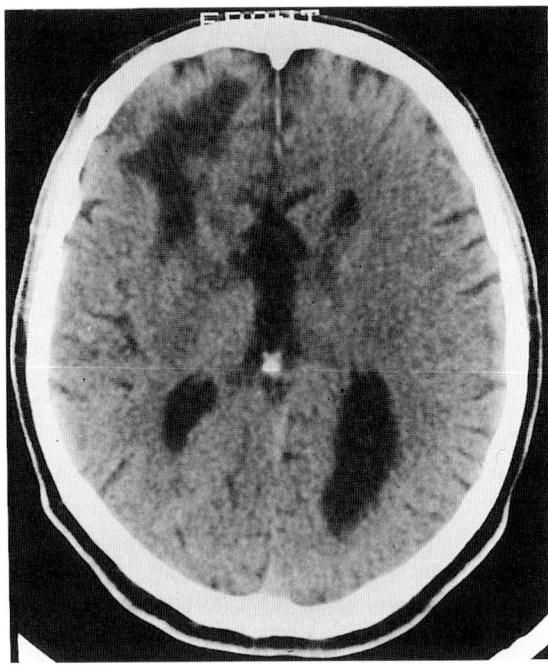

Fig. 9.19   CT scan showing frontal low-density lesion due to PML.

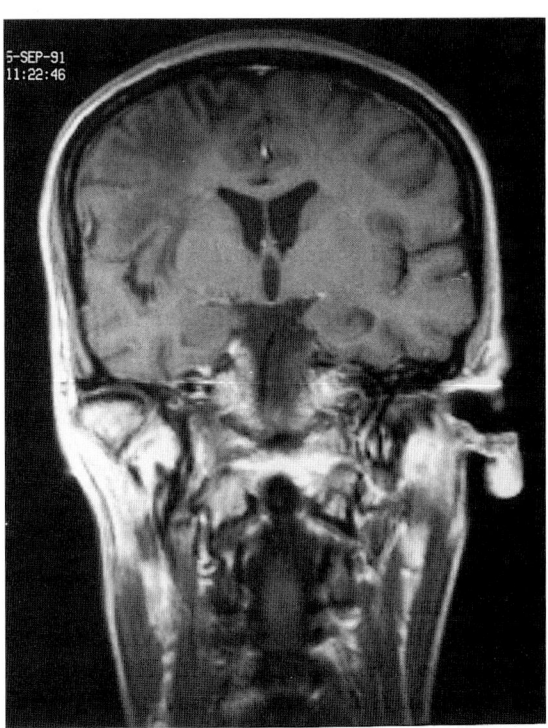

Fig. 9.20   T1-weighted MRI showing lesion due to PML.

in patients whose sarcoidosis, for example, responds to treatment. In some AIDS cases, prolonged survival has been described (Berger & Mucke 1988), e.g. for up to 30 months. Some cases have appeared to fluctuate spontaneously or in response to systemic factors, including response to antiviral therapy aimed at the HIV (Conway et al 1990). It is not known whether there are genetic subtypes of the JC virus that affect outcome. The diagnosis is usually made by recognition of a typical indolent clinical course with imaging studies demonstrating multiple abnormal areas within the subcortical white matter.

EEGs show non-specific slow-wave abnormalities related to the underlying white matter lesion(s). CT scans reveal non-enhancing hypodense white matter lesions (Fig. 9.19) that show no mass effect. Lesions may be single or multiple and may affect cerebral hemispheres or the cerebellum or brainstem. The parieto-occipital area is particularly likely to be affected. MRI is even more sensitive to the demyelination with low signal intensity on T1 (Fig. 9.20) and hyperintensity on T2-weighted images (Fig. 9.21), again lacking mass effect. The abnormal areas are homogenous, but

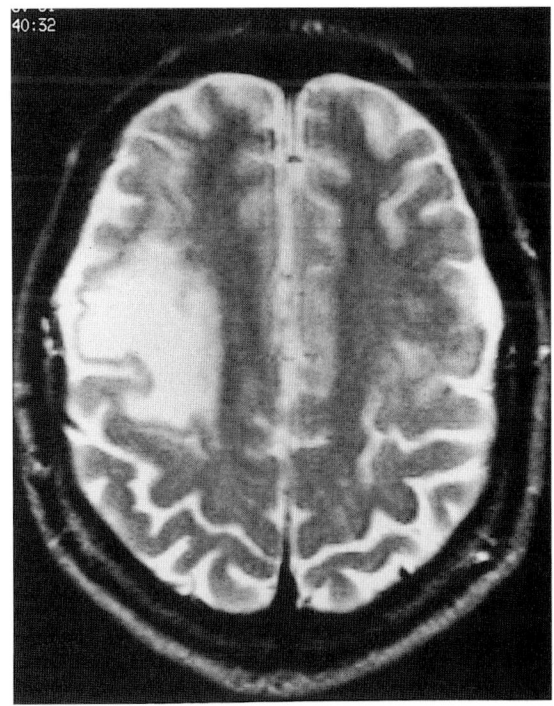

Fig. 9.21   T2-weighted MRI of PML in the hemisphere.

have indistinct margins. The single MR lesion represents a confluence of histological lesions. It has a scalloped appearance in the subcortical region due to involvement of gyral cores. The abnormal signal from the white matter can be seen to follow fibre tracts on review of contiguous slices (Fig. 9.22). In most cases the lesions are bilateral (Fig. 9.23). In 20% or so, there are posterior fossa lesions as well as cerebral ones. Rare cases have disease confined radiologically to the posterior fossa at presentation. Within the cerebral hemisphere the most common sites for imaging lesions are the parieto-occipital and frontal white matter. There is usually associated atrophy. Basal ganglia are visibly affected in about a fifth of cases (Whiteman et al 1993), because of damage to myelin in striopallidal fibres and those interconnecting the globus pallidus and putamen. Enhancement is rare (9% according to White-man), faint and peripheral. Differentiation from white matter disease resulting from HIV leucoen-cephalopathy is usually possible in that PML shows a subcortical scalloped appearance of brighter signal on T2-weighted images, in contrast to the fluffier-looking deeper changes of HIV. PML is also more often of low intensity on

T1, which weighting often 'misses' HIV-related white matter change (Whiteman et al 1993). These features are supported by the association of PML imaging changes with focal deficit, which is usually absent in the case of HIV leucoen-cephalopathy. Routine CSF analysis reveals non-specific changes or may be normal. Biopsy may be necessary to differentiate PML from cerebral toxoplasmosis, other opportunistic infections or CNS lymphoma. Immunostaining with antibody to the related papovavirus SV40 or electron microscopy identification of inclusions is neces-sary for definitive pathological diagnosis. The clinical features and radiological characteristics are so characteristic that biopsy is not necessary in most cases, particularly as there is no effective treatment at this point. The rapid deterioration of most patients with PML ensures that, in any case, most patients would die within a few weeks of the confirmatory biopsy. In one series of 13 patients with PML diagnosed by stereotactic brain biopsy,

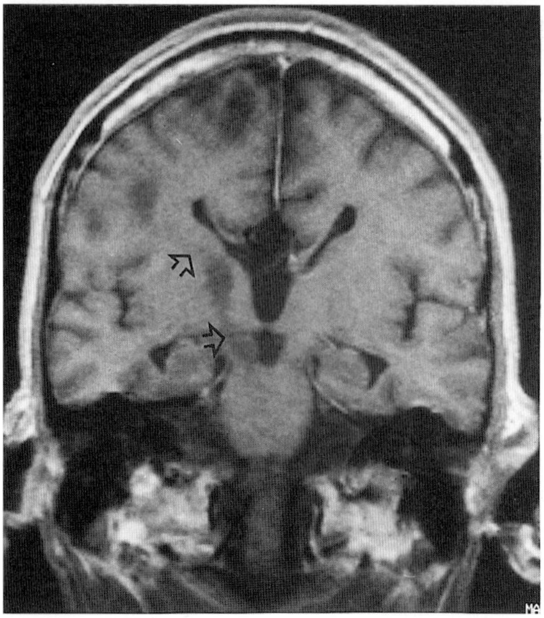

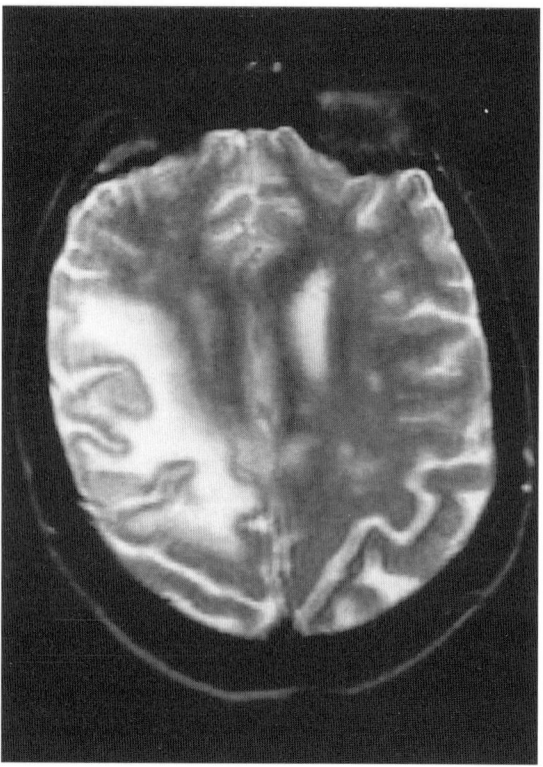

Fig. 9.22 T1-weighted MRI showing how PML outlines white matter tracts (arrowed).

Fig. 9.23 T2-weighted MRI of PML showing bilateral lesions.

death occurred within 3 months for 11 patients, and in only two cases was survival longer than 6 months (Karahalios et al 1992).

Although it was hoped that detection of JC virus in the CSF by PCR (Telenti et al 1992) might prove a valuable diagnostic tool, it has been somewhat disappointing in practice. The PCR primers recognize portions of genome coding for early proteins such as the large T antigen of the JC virus. In one series examining CSF of patients with biopsy or autopsy-proven PML, the sensitivity of CSF PCR was 50% (Aksamit A personal communication). Telenti et al (1990) using primer pairs for the VP1/large T antigen region of JC virus had a much more promising positive sensitivity of 94% in 16 CSF samples and a specificity of 85%. Intrathecal synthesis of JC virus-specific antibody has not proven useful so far for diagnosis. The detection of the virus in peripheral lymphocytes by PCR, however, may become a useful tool. Tornatore et al (1992) using PCR found the JC virus genome in circulating lymphocytes in none of 30 patients with Parkinson's disease, but in 38% of 26 HIV-infected subjects and 89% of 19 patients with biopsy-proven PML. Only three of the

PML patients with JC virus detected in their circulating lymphocytes had it detected in their CSF. These findings suggest that the circulating lymphocytes might be the source of CNS infection, and that patients potentially at risk may be detectable.

There is no effective treatment and the neurological disorder usually progresses inexorably to death over weeks or a few months. Interferons, particularly alpha-interferon, have been used for treatment of PML because papovaviruses appear to be responsive to alpha-interferon. For example, alpha-interferon is used to treat genital warts caused by human papilloma virus. Tashiro et al (1987) reported the apparent stabilization of neurological progression in an HIV-negative woman with PML. Interestingly, the patient did not respond to intravenous adenosine arabinoside (ara-A), cytosine arabinoside (ara-C) or interferon, but stabilized after intrathecal beta-interferon. No controlled trials of interferons have been completed, although several anecdotal reports have suggested that the neurological deterioration may stabilize with alpha-interferon therapy (Fig. 9.24). Confounding the interpretation of these results, of course, is the natural variability of PML and the

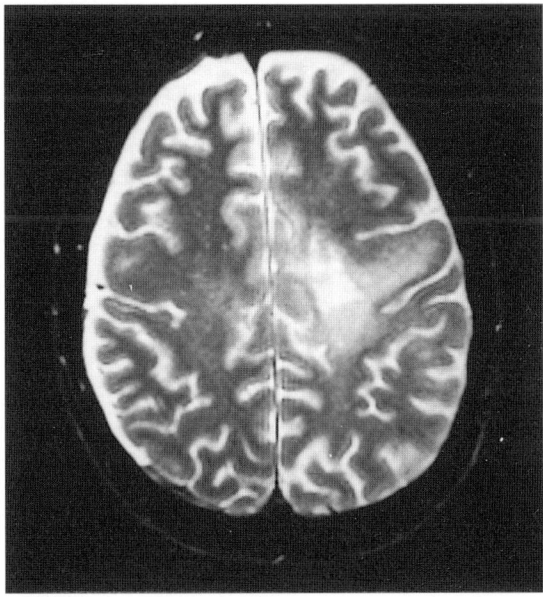 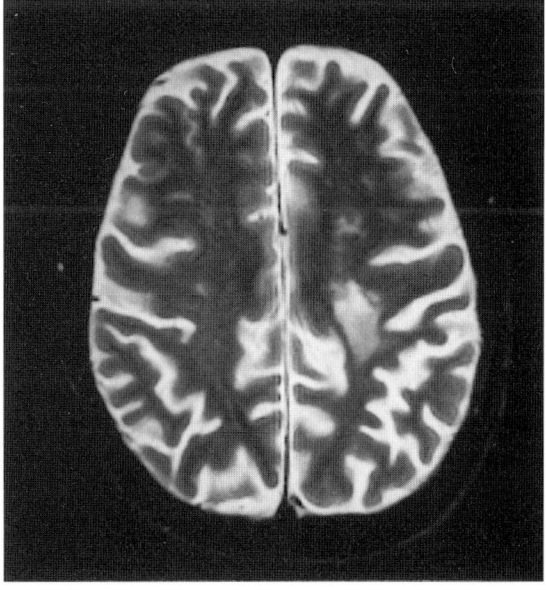

Fig. 9.24   T2-weighted MRI in a case of PML before (left) and after (right) 7 months' treatment with interferon α (3–18 million units daily subcutaneously) showing apparent shrinkage of white matter lesions.

fact that there may be spontaneous remissions (Berger & Mucke 1988, Berger et al 1992a). Recently, attention has swung back to re-examine ara-C, a potent nucleoside analogue principally used for treatment of myeloproliferative disorders. An antiviral effect has been documented in vitro (Major & Tornatelli personal communication). In the pre-AIDS era, case reports linked remission with ara-C, administered either intravenously or via the intrathecal route. In AIDS-related PML, Portegies et al (1991) described clinical improvement with intravenous ara-C (2 mg/kg intravenously for 5 days every 4 weeks). A concern, of course, with intravenous use of ara-C is with its myelosuppressive toxicity. Thus, the intrathecal administration of lower doses has potential advantages. Britton and colleagues (1992) treated 13 patients with biopsy-proven PML with intrathecal ara-C after initially trying to maximize antiretroviral therapy. Eight of the 13 stabilized, four for up to 2 years and four for up to 6 months. The ara-C was administered through an Ommaya reservoir and was well tolerated apart from chemical meningitis in some patients. A randomized open-label study is planned (ACTG 243) in the USA comparing maximal antiretroviral therapy with intravenous ara-C (4 mg/kg daily for 5 days, repeated with intervals of 15 days between each cycle) and intrathecal administration of 50 mg/mm^2 of ara-C through an Ommaya reservoir once weekly for 4 weeks and then every other week for 4 weeks, then monthly.

Amantadine and ara-A have been tried with little success. Other potential treatments that may be developed are various inhibitors of enzymes critical for virion production. Two examples are topotecan and campothecin, which inhibit topoisomerase.

At this point, none of these proposed therapies appear to be particularly useful. Maximizing antiretroviral therapy is probably important and may slow progression by improving immune function somewhat. Interferon α is relatively easy to administer, although patients frequently report 'flu-like' symptoms with subcutaneous administration. Doses between 3 and 18 million units daily subcutaneously have been used in an uncontrolled manner. In a patient with rapidly advancing PML that has been biopsy-confirmed, intravenous or intrathecal ara-C could be considered.

Management plan

The development of focal neurological deficit in an otherwise neurologically well patient should suggest PML. Other patients will be investigated for mental changes, but again without disturbance of the level of consciousness or evidence of raised intracranial pressure. MRI scans can be very suggestive, with hemispheric or posterior fossa areas of high intensity on T2 weighting (low intensity on T1) affecting the white matter without mass effect. JC virus should be sought in blood and CSF. If the patient's prognosis is otherwise reasonable, and the patient is keen for aggressive treatment, a brain biopsy may be needed to confirm the diagnosis, prior to a trial of ara-C or interferon.

REFERENCES

Astrom K-E, Mancall E L, Richardson E P. Progressive multifocal leukoencephalopathy. Brain 1958; 81: 93–111

Aurelius E, Johansson B, Skoldenberg B, et al. Rapid diagnosis of herpes simplex encephalitis by nested polymerase chain reaction assay of cerebrospinal fluid. Lancet 1991; 337: 189–192

Bamborschke S, Wullen T, Huber M, et al. Early diagnosis and successful treatment of acute cytomegalovirus encephalitis in a renal transplant recipient. J Neurol 1992; 239: 205–208

Berger J R, Mucke L. Prolonged survival and partial recovery in AIDS-associated progressive multifocal leukoencephalopathy. Neurology 1988; 38: 1060–1065

Berger J R, Kaszovitz B, Post M J, Dickinson G. Progressive multifocal leukoencephalopathy associated with human immunodeficiency virus infection. A review of the literature with a report of sixteen cases. Ann Intern Med 1987; 107: 78–87

Berger J, Pall L, McArthur J C, et al. Pilot study of recombinant alpha 2a interferon in the treatment of AIDS related progressive multifocal leukoencephalopathy. Neurology 1992a; 42 (suppl 3): 257 (abstr)

Berger J R, Scott G, Albrecht J, et al. Progressive multifocal leukoencephalopathy in HIV-1-infected children. AIDS 1992b; 6: 837–841

Britton C B, Romagnoli M, Sisti M, Powers J M. Analysis of outcome and response to intrathecal ara-C in 26 patients. Neuroscience of HIV infection, Amsterdam 1992

Cavanagh J B, Greenbaum D, Marshall A H E, Rubinstein L J. Cerebral demyelination associated with disorders of the reticuloendothelial system. Lancet 1959; 2: 524–529

Chaisson R E, Griffin D E. Progressive multifocal leukoencephalopathy in AIDS (Technical conference). JAMA 1990; 264: 79–82

Cinque P, Vago L, Brytting M, et al. Cytomegalovirus infection of the central nervous system in patients with AIDS: diagnosis by DNA amplification from cerebrospinal fluid. J Infect Dis 1992; 166: 1408–1411

Cohen B A, McArthur J C, Grohman S, et al. Neurologic prognosis in CMV polyradiculomyelopathy in AIDS. Neurology 1993; 43: 493–499

Collaborative DHPG Treatment Study Group. Treatment of serious cytomegalovirus with 9-(1,2 dihydroxy-2-propoxymethyl) guanine in patients with AIDS and other immunodeficiencies. N Engl J Med 1986; 314: 801–805

Conway B, Halliday W C, Brunham R C. Human immunodeficiency virus-associated progressive multifocal leukoencephalopathy: apparent response to 3-azido-3-deoxythymidine. Rev Infect Dis 1990; 12: 479–482

Dieterich D T, Poles M A, Lew E A, et al. Concurrent use of ganciclovir and foscarnet to treat cytomegalovirus infection in AIDS patients. J Infect Dis 1993; 167: 1184–1188

Eidelberg D, Sotrel A, Vogel H, et al. Progressive polyradiculopathy in acquired immune deficiency syndrome. Neurology 1986; 36: 912–916

Emanuel D, Cunningham I, Jules-Elysee K, et al. Cytomegalovirus pneumonia after bone marrow transplantation successfully treated with the combination of ganciclovir and high-dose intravenous immune globulin. Ann Intern Med 1988; 109: 777–782

Fiala M, Singer E J, Graves M C, et al. AIDS dementia complex complicated by cytomegalovirus encephalopathy. J Neurol 1993; 240: 223–231

Fletcher C, Sawchuk R, Chinnock B, et al. Human pharmacokinetics of the antiviral drug DHPG. Clin Pharmacol Ther 1986; 40: 281–286

Gillespie S M, Chang Y, Lemp G, et al. Progressive multifocal leukoencephalopathy in persons infected with human immunodeficiency virus, San Francisco, 1981–1989. Ann Neurol 1991; 30: 597–604

Gozlan J, Salord J M, Roullet E, et al. Rapid detection of cytomegalovirus DNA in cerebrospinal fluid of AIDS patients with neurologic disorders. J Infect Dis 1992; 166: 1416–1421

Hawley D A, Schaefer J F, Schulz D M, Muller J. Cytomegalovirus encephalitis in acquired immunodeficiency syndrome. Am J Clin Pathol 1983; 80: 874–877

Hayashi S, Norbeck D W, Rosenbrook W, et al. Cyclobut-A and cyclobut-G, carbocyclic oxetanocin analogs that inhibit the replication of human immunodeficiency virus in T cells and monocytes and macrophages in vitro. Antimicrob Agents Chemother 1990; 34: 287–294

Hengge U R, Brockmeyer N H, Malessa R, et al. Foscarnet penetrates the blood–brain barrier: rationale for therapy of cytomegalic encephalitis. Antimicrob Agents Chemother 1993; 37: 1010–1014

Hierons R, Janota I J, Corsellis J A N. The late effects of necrotising encephalitis of the temporal lobes and limbic areas: a clinico-pathological study of 10 cases. Psychol Med 1978; 8: 21–42

Holland N R, Power C, Mathews V P, et al. CMV encephalitis in acquired immunodeficiency syndrome (AIDS). Neurology 1994; 44: 507–514

Houff S A, Major E O, Katz D A, et al. Involvement of JC virus-infected mononuclear cells from the bone marrow and spleen in the pathogenesis of progressive multifocal leukoencephalopathy. N Engl J Med 1988; 318: 301–305

Jabs D A, Enger C, Bartlett J G. Cytomegalovirus retinitis and acquired immunodeficiency syndrome. Arch Ophthalmol 1989; 107: 75–80

Kalayjian R C, Cohen M L, Bonomo R A, Flanigan T P. Cytomegalovirus ventriculoencephalitis in AIDS. Medicine 1993; 72: 67–77

Karahalios D, Breit R, Dal Canto M C, Levy R M. Progressive multifocal leukoencephalopathy in patients with HIV infection: lack of impact of early diagnosis by stereotactic brain biopsy. J Acquired Immunodeficiency Syndromes 1992; 5: 1030–1038

Kupperman B D, Petty J G, Richman D D, et al. Correlation between CD4+ counts and prevalence of cytomegalovirus retinitis and human immunodeficiency virus-related noninfectious retinal vasculopathy in patients with acquired immunodeficiency syndrome. Am J Ophthalmol 1993; 115: 575–582

Laskin O L, Cederberg D M, Mills J, et al. Ganciclovir for the treatment and suppression of serious infections caused by cytomegalovirus. Am J Med 1987; 83: 201–207

Levy R M, Bredesen D E, Rosenblum M L. Neurological manifestations of the acquired immunodeficiency syndrome (AIDS): experience at UCSF and review of the literature. J Neurosurg 1985; 62: 475–495

Luer W, Poser S, Weber T, et al. Chronic HIV encephalitis. I. Cerebrospinal fluid diagnosis. Klin Wochenschr 1988; 66: 21–25

Mahieux F, Gray F, Fenellon G, et al. Acute myeloradiculitis due to cytomegalovirus as the initial manifestation of AIDS. J Neurol Neurosurg Psychiatr 1989; 52: 270–274

Miller R G, Storey J R, Greco C M. Ganciclovir in the treatment of progressive AIDS-related polyradiculopathy. Neurology 1990; 40: 569–574

Moskowitz L B, Gregorios J B, Hensley G T, Berger J R. Cytomegalovirus-induced demyelination associated with acquired immune deficiency syndrome. Arch Pathol Lab Med 1984; 108: 873–877

Newsome D A, Green W R, Miller E D, et al. Microvascular aspects of acquired immune deficiency syndrome retinopathy. Am J Ophthalmol 1984; 98: 590–601

Novak O S, Truilillo J R, Rivera V M, et al. Ganciclovir in the treatment of CMV infection in AIDS patients with neurologic complications. Neurology 1989; 39 (suppl): 379–380

Oxbury J M, MacCallum F O. Herpes simplex virus encephalitis: clinical features and residual damage. Postgrad Med J 1973; 49: 387–389

Padgett B L, Walker D L, Zu Rhein G M, Eckroade R J. Cultivation of papova-like virus from human brain with progressive multifocal leukoencephalopathy. Lancet 1971; 1: 1257–1260

Peters M, Timm U, Schurmann D, et al. Combined and alternating ganciclovir and foscarnet in acute and maintenance therapy of human immunodeficiency virus-related cytomegalovirus encephalitis refractory to ganciclovir alone. Clin Invest 1992; 70: 456–458

Portegies P, Algra P R, Hollak C E, et al. Response to cytarabine in progressive multifocal leukoencephalopathy in AIDS. Lancet 1991; i: 680–681

Post M J, Hensley G T, Moskowitz L B, Fischl M. Cytomegalic inclusion virus encephalitis in patients with

AIDS: CT, clinical, and pathologic correlation. AJR 1986; 146: 1229–1234

Power C, Holland N R, Mathews V P, et al. CMV encephalitis in AIDS: distinction from HIV dementia. Neurology 1992; 42: 211 (abstr)

Reed E C, Bowden R A, Dandliker P S, et al. Treatment of cytomegalovirus pneumonia with ganciclovir and intravenous cytomegalovirus immunoglobulin in patient with bone marrow transplants. Ann Intern Med 1988; 109: 783–788

Rhodes R H, Ward J M, Walker D L, Ross A A. Progressive multifocal leukoencephalopathy and retroviral encephalitis in acquired immunodeficiency syndrome. Arch Pathol Lab Med 1988; 112: 1207–1213

Richardson E P. Progressive multifocal leukoencephalopathy. In: Vinken P J, Bruyn G W, editors. Handbook of clinical neurology. Amsterdam: Elsevier, 1970: 485–499

Rowley A H, Whitley R J, Lakeman F D, Wolinsky S M. Rapid detection of herpes-simplex-virus DNA in cerebrospinal fluid of patients with herpes simplex encephalitis. Lancet 1990; 335: 440–441

Sawyer J, Ellner J. To biopsy or not to biopsy in suspected herpes simplex encephalitis. Med Decis Making 1988; 8: 95–101

Schmidbauer M, Budka H, Ulrich W, Ambros P. Cytomegalovirus (CMV) disease of the brain in AIDS and connatal infection: a comparative study by histology, immunocytochemistry and in situ DNA hybridization. Acta Neuropathologica 1989; 79: 286–293

Shepp D H, Dandiker P S, de Miranda P, Burnette T C. Activity of 9-(2-hydroxy-1-(hydroxymethyl)ethoxymethyl) guanine in the treatment of cytomegalovirus pneumonia. Ann Intern Med 1985; 103: 368–373

Snider W D, Simpson D M, Nielsen S, et al. Neurological complications of acquired immune deficiency syndrome: analysis of 50 patients. Ann Neurol 1983; 14: 403–418

Snoeck R, Sakuma T, De Clercq E, et al. (S)-1-(3-hydroxy-2-phosphonylmethoxpropyl) cytosine, a potent and selective inhibitor of human cytomegalovirus replication. Antimicrob Agents Chemother 1988; 32: 1839–1844

Soong S-J, Watson N E, Caddell G R, et al. Use of brain biopsy for diagnostic evaluation of patients with suspected herpes simplex encephalitis: a statistical model and its clinical implications. J Infect Dis 1991; 163: 17–22

Studies of Ocular Complications of AIDS Research Group, AIDS Clinical Trials Group. Mortality in patients with the acquired immunodeficiency syndrome treated with either foscarnet or ganciclovir for cytomegalovirus retinitis. N Engl J Med 1992; 326: 213–220

Tashiro K, Doi S, Moriwaka F, Maruo Y, et al. Progressive multifocal leukoencephalopathy with magnetic resonance imaging verification and therapeutic trials with interferon. J Neurol 1987; 234: 427–429

Telenti A, Marshall W F, Aksamit A J, et al. Detection of JC virus by polymerase chain reaction in cerebrospinal fluid from two patients with progressive multifocal leukoencephalopathy. Eur J Clin Microbiol 1992; 11: 253–254

Telenti N, Aksamit A J, Proper J, Smith T F. Detection of JC virus DNA by polymerase chain reaction in patients with progressive multifocal leukoencephalopathy. Infect Dis 1990; 162: 858–861

Tornatore C, Berger J R, Houff S A, et al. Detection of JC virus DNA in peripheral lymphocytes from patients with and without progressive multifocal leukoencephalopathy. Ann Neurol 1992; 31: 454–462

Van Landingham K E, Marsteller H B, Ross G W. Relapse of herpes simplex encephalitis after conventional acyclovir therapy. JAMA 1988; 259: 1051–1053

van Loon A M, van der Logt J T M, Heessen F W A, et al. Diagnosis of herpes simplex virus encephalitis by detection of virus-specific immunoglobulins A and G in serum and cerebrospinal fluid by using an antibody-capture enzyme-linked immunosorbent assay. J Clin Microbiol 1989; 27: 1983–1987

Vinters H V, Kwok M K, Ho H W, et al. Cytomegalovirus in the nervous system of patients with the acquired immune deficiency syndrome. Brain 1989; 112: 245–268

Weber T, Turner R W, Ruf B, et al. JC virus detected by polymerase chain reaction in cerebrospinal fluid of AIDS patients with progressive multifocal leukoencephalopathy. In: Berger J R, Levy R L, editors. Neurological and neuropsychological complications of HIV infection. Proceedings from Satellite Meeting of the International Conference on AIDS, Monterey, Canada 1990, 110

Whiteley R J, Soong S-J, Linneman C, et al. Herpes simplex encephalitis: clinical assessment. JAMA 1982; 247: 317–320

Whiteman M L H, Post M J, Berger J R, et al. Progressive multifocal leukoencephalopathy in 47 HIV-seropositive patients: neuroimaging with clinical and pathological correlation. Radiology 1993; 187: 233–240

Whitley R, Arvin A, Prober C, et al. Predictors of morbidity and mortality in neonates with herpes simplex virus infections. New Engl J Med 1991; 324: 450–454

Winston D J, Ho W G, Lin C H, et al. Intravenous immune globulin for prevention of cytomegalovirus infection and interstitial pneumonia after bone marrow transplantation. Ann Intern Med 1987; 106: 12–18

Wolf D G, Spector S A. Diagnosis of human cytomegalovirus central nervous system disease in AIDS patients by DNA amplification from cerebrospinal fluid. Infect Dis 1992; 166: 1412–1415

Zurlo J J, O'Neill D, Polis M A, et al. Lack of clinical utility of cytomegalovirus blood and urine cultures in patients with HIV infection. Ann Intern Med 1993; 118: 12–17

Zu Rhein G M, Chou S-M. Particles resembling papova viruses in human cerebral demyelinating disease. Science 1965; 148: 1477–1479

10. Opportunistic infections – bacteria

NEUROSYPHILIS IN HIV INFECTION

Epidemiology

In Great Britain and Canada, the incidence of primary and secondary syphilis had declined since 1978. In the USA, in contrast, there has been a resurgence of syphilis since 1985, particularly among inner city African-American and Hispanic populations (Fig. 10.1). By 1987 it had reached levels not seen since 1950 (Hook 1989). This change appeared to occur despite changes in sexual practice in the homosexual population in the face of the AIDS epidemic. In fact, the incidence of syphilis among homosexual men has dropped in the past decade, while the incidence of syphilis continues to rise, particularly among African-Americans and Hispanics and disproportionately among females (Centers for Disease Control 1988a). This increase in primary and secondary syphilis has been attributed to several causes, including the 'sex for drugs' phenomenon

linked to the use of cocaine, the widespread use of spectinomycin rather than penicillin for treatment of gonorrhoea (spectinomycin is not effective against syphilis) and the shifting of resources from syphilis control to AIDS (Hook & Marra 1992, Mann et al 1992). The use of illicit drugs, prostitution or contact with a prostitute have all been associated with rising syphilis incidence (Centers for Disease Control 1988b). It also emerged that prior syphilis was a risk factor for the development of AIDS (Greenblatt et al 1988). There was therefore much epidemiological interest in the interaction of the two diseases. The role of sexually transmitted diseases (STDs) as co-factors for HIV transmission is strongest for the diseases that cause genital ulceration: syphilis, herpes, chancroid.

Darrow et al (1987) in a prospective study found evidence that men with serological evidence of prior syphilis had an almost four-fold increased risk of HIV seroconversion (odds ratio 3.6; CI 1.9–6.2). The evidence from Africa

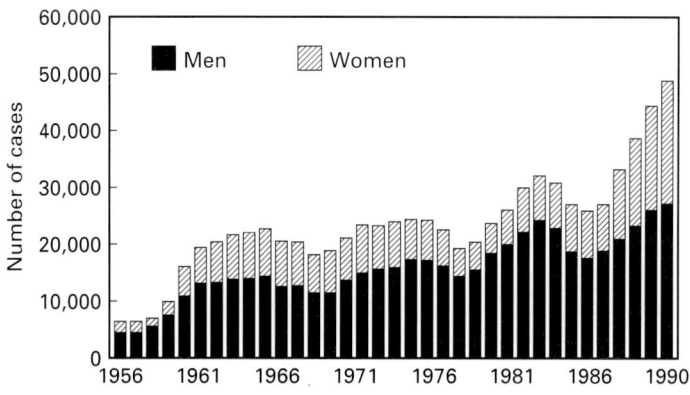

Fig. 10.1 Number of cases of primary and secondary syphilis in the USA. (Reproduced from Hook & Marra 1992.)

suggests that the mechanism relates to the effect of genital ulceration on the efficiency of HIV transmission, but both illnesses may be coincidentally related through sexual behaviour patterns. The practical point is that patients with serological evidence of recently acquired HIV or syphilis should always be tested for the other pathogen.

To this has been added clinical concern that the course or manifestations of neurosyphilis might be altered in the presence of immunodeficiency, with implications for serological diagnosis and adequacy of treatment. Katz and Berger (1989) found a surprisingly high rate of neurosyphilis in a hospitalized population and estimated that 1.5% of all patients with AIDS would have neurosyphilis. Other reports (Johns et al 1987, Spence & Abrutyn 1987, Tramont 1987, Hook 1989) have suggested an increased frequency or virulence for neurosyphilis in patients co-infected with HIV. To date, however, a careful epidemiological survey has yet to be completed.

Clinical features

In the pre-antibiotic era, neurological complications of secondary and tertiary syphilis were seen in 6.5% of untreated patients as identified in the Oslo study of the natural history of untreated syphilis (Clark & Danbolt 1955). The clinical spectrum of AIDS-related neurosyphilis appears to be no different from that in HIV-negative patients, although some have suggested that the course may be accelerated in the setting of cellular immunodeficiency. Thus, the interval between syphilis infection and neurological manifestations (Fig. 10.2) may be shorter than usual. Musher feels that the 'neurological involvement caused by syphilis in HIV-infected patients is entirely consistent with early neurosyphilis or neuro-recurrence as classically described in the pre-penicillin era' (Musher 1991). In fact, in Musher's series (1991), five of 16 patients treated for syphilis developed neurosyphilis within 6 months of therapy, though one could argue in each case that antibiotic treatment had been suboptimal. Apart from scattered case reports, most people feel that cutaneous involvement is no more progressive or severe in patients co-infected with HIV. In one large study of patients with syphilis seen at an

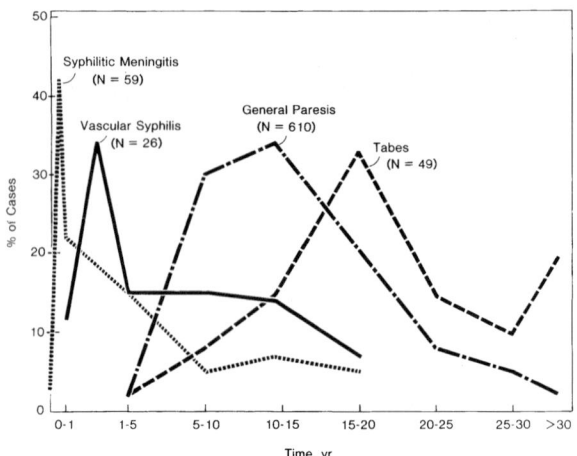

Fig. 10.2 Timing of neurological complications of neurosyphilis. (© American Medical Association 1985. Reproduced from Simon 1985 with permission of the American Medical Association.)

STD clinic, no significant differences in the manifestations of syphilis were found, contrasting HIV-positive and HIV-negative patients. Most of these patients, however, had a relatively high CD4 count (Hutchinson et al 1991).

The clinical features of syphilis are usually divided into stages: primary, secondary, latent and tertiary. Latent syphilis is usually subdivided into an early latent or infectious phase (CDC 1 year, WHO 2 years syphilis duration) or late latent or non-infectious. Primary syphilis lesions develop at the site of inoculation, with an incubation period averaging 21 days (range 10–90 days). The typical chancre is a single, rounded, painless lesion with a raised border and a rubbery or hard consistency. Chancres are found most commonly on the glans and foreskin in heterosexual men, the external genitalia in women, and the perianal and rectal areas in homosexual men. Chancres may also occur in the mouth or on the lips. During the secondary stage of syphilis, there is haematogenous dissemination of *Treponema pallidum* with fever, malaise and generalized lymphadenopathy. A variety of dermatological signs are seen, including typically non-pruritic 'coppery' rashes, condylomata lata and painless ulcerations on mucous membranes. Tertiary syphilis develops in one-third of untreated patients and includes gummatous disease and cardiovascular involvement with

Table 10.1 Clinical presentations of neurosyphilis

	1932–1942 Number (%)	1965–1980 Number (%)
Symptomatic		
Seizures	4 (<1)	59 (18)
Neuro-ophthalmological	20 (3)	56 (17)
Meningovascular	103 (13)	42 (13)
General paresis (dementia)	203 (26)	26 (8)
Tabes dorsalis	203 (26)	9 (3)
Other	34 (4)	20 (6)
Asymptomatic	219 (28)	123 (37)
Total	782	335

(After Hotson 1981)

Table 10.2 Definition of asymptomatic neurosyphilis

No neurological symptoms or signs
Positive CSF VDRL
Serum RPR $\geq$ 1:16 and reactive FTA/ABS
CSF cell count $\geq$ 20 WBC/mm^3 or protein concentration $\geq$ 50 mg%

aortitis. Neurosyphilis tends to develop during the secondary or tertiary stages. Neurological involvement in syphilis can be divided into asymptomatic and symptomatic neurosyphilis (Table 10.1) and comprises a diverse group of neurological syndromes affecting the neuraxis at several different levels, including eye, meninges, brain parenchyma, spinal cord and peripheral nerves.

Asymptomatic neurosyphilis

This represents the stage during late latent infection where cerebrospinal fluid (CSF) abnormalities are present without specific neurological signs. Asymptomatic neurosyphilis is thought to be a harbinger of symptomatic neurosyphilis because early work from the pre-penicillin era suggested that symptomatic neurosyphilis did not develop in patients who had normal CSF during latent infection (Moore 1922, Mills 1927, Moore & Hopkins 1930). It is unclear whether the designation 'asymptomatic neurosyphilis' has the same prognostic value now. An added complication, as discussed below, is the frequency of CSF abnormalities in HIV-infected individuals without syphilis. The CSF abnormalities in asymptomatic neurosyphilis include lymphocytic pleocytosis, elevated protein, elevated immunoglobulin G, IgG index and the presence of oligoclonal bands. Some authors require a positive CSF VDRL to characterize this stage; others include patients without a positive CSF VDRL who have prominent pleocytosis or protein elevation. In a comparative study of intravenous penicillin and ceftriaxone (ACTG 145), a useful working de-

finition of possible asymptomatic neurosyphilis was employed, as listed in Table 10.2. Holtom et al (1992) screened 312 HIV-infected individuals and identified 71 (22.8%) with reactive serum rapid-plasma-reagin tests (RPRs) and micro-haemagglutination assays (MHA-TPs). Thirty-three (47%) underwent CSF analysis and 13 had abnormal CSF profiles, either with reactive CSF VDRL in three of 33 and non-reactive in 10 of 33. Thus, CSF VDRL-positive asymptomatic neurosyphilis is found in 1% of a general outpatient population of HIV-infected adults. By broadening the definition to include CSF VDRL-negative patients with reactive serum RPRs and abnormal CSF profiles, as many as 30% can be classified as having asymptomatic neurosyphilis. The true figure cannot be estimated as this latter criterion is distorted by the tendency for HIV-infected patients to have an abnormal CSF anyway.

Syphilitic meningitis

This typically occurs in association with secondary syphilis during the first 12 months of infection. The presentation is typical of many forms of meningitis with fever, headache, meningismus and cranial nerve involvement. In the HIV-infected individual, particularly with a CD4 count below 200, the differential includes opportunistic infections, including, most importantly, cryptococcal meningitis. There appears to be a predilection to affect cranial nerves VII and VIII with facial paresis and hearing loss (Burke & Schaberg 1985). Ocular involvement can accompany syphilitic meningitis with the development of anterior uveitis or iritis or, less commonly, posterior uveitis. Optic neuritis (Fig. 10.3) is an uncommon manifestation, more typically developing in late neurosyphilis as a manifestation of tabes dorsalis.

Syphilitic involvement of the spinal cord is

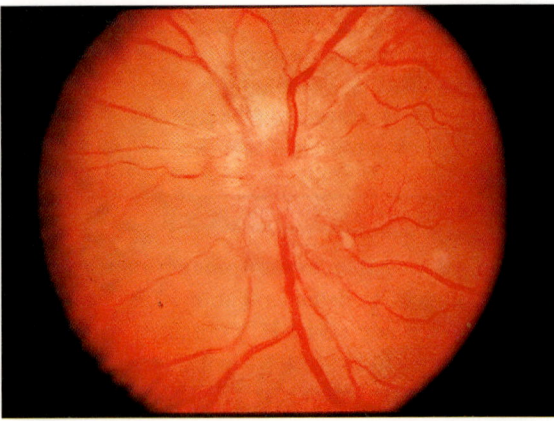

Fig. 10.3 Severe optic neuropathy with optic pallor in an HIV-negative patient with treated neurosyphilis. (Courtesy of Dr David Knox, Wilmer Institute, Johns Hopkins University.)

Table 10.4   Ocular involvement in neurosyphilis

Pupillary defect
   Argyll-Robertson pupil
   Afferent pupillary defect
Conjunctivitis
Uveitis
Chorioretinitis
Optic neuritis
Papillitis
Extraocular paresis
Superior orbital fissure syndrome
Retinal artery/vein occlusion

relatively rare, accounting for only 5% or less of cases of neurosyphilis. In the past, tabes dorsalis represented the most common form of spinal cord involvement in syphilis; however, today syphilitic meningomyelitis is the most common manifestation (Berger 1992). Syphilitic meningomyelitis usually develops relatively early after initial infection, sometimes developing in association with the other manifestations of syphilitic meningitis. Although the full range of presentations is not well defined, myelopathy can develop either abruptly or gradually, typically with a thoracic level spastic paraparesis, bowel and bladder involvement, and sensory loss. Berger (1987) has extensively reviewed the different manifestations of syphilitic involvement of the spinal cord (Table 10.3). A rare cause of spinal cord compression is syphilitic pachymeningitis, which may be attributed to epidural compression by gumma or by

Table 10.3   Syphilis of the spinal cord

Syphilitic meningomyelitis
Syphilitic spinal pachymeningitis
   Spinal cord gumma
   Syphilitic hypertrophic pachymeningitis
Spinal vascular syphilis
Syphilitic poliomyelitis
Tabes dorsalis
Miscellaneous
   Syringomyelia
   Syphilitic aortic aneurysm

(Reproduced from Berger 1983 with permission of Marcel Dekker Inc.)

hypertrophic pachymeningitis. In 31 cases of spinal syphilis, the onset of myelopathy ranged from a few months to 25 years (Adams & Merritt 1944, Merritt et al 1946).

Ocular manifestations of syphilis

A variety of different ocular manifestations of syphilis have been reported (Table 10.4). Syphilitic uveitis affecting either anterior or posterior compartments often accompanies syphilitic meningitis, while optic neuritis, a less common manifestation, usually develops with late neurosyphilis, often accompanying tabes dorsalis. Syphilitic uveitis typically presents with visual blurring, pain and photophobia. A 1933 study by Moore identified 249 cases of syphilitic iritis from over 10 000 syphilitic patients at Johns Hopkins. In 111 cases, iritis accompanied secondary syphilis, in 29 the iritis was a recurrence after inadequate treatment, and in the remaining 109 iritis was a late feature. The late type appeared on average 9 years after infection, and often proved chronic. The breakdown of ocular lesions was iritis in 89, keratoiritis in 79, neuroretinitis in 27 (Fig. 10.4), iridocyclitis in 18, iritis papulosa in 16, interstitial keratitis in 14, lenticular opacities in eight, corneal ulcers, hypopyon and optic atrophy in five each, and rare examples of perforated cornea, detached retina, episcleritis and panophthalmitis. The early iritis was often unilateral and relapse was unusual. Overall 10–20% were left with visual impairment. Spinal fluid findings revealed no association between iritis and asymptomatic neurosyphilis.

The situation in AIDS may be different. Thus Katz et al (1993) in studying 46 patients with

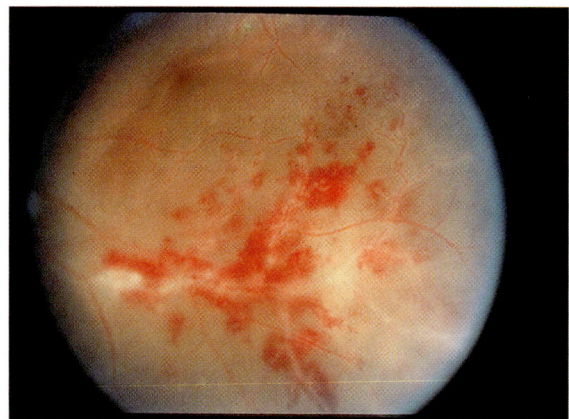

Fig. 10.4 Syphilitic choroidoretinitis (Forster's retinitis) in an HIV-positive patient. (Courtesy of Dr David Knox, Wilmer Institute, Johns Hopkins University.)

CSF VDRL-positive neurosyphilis compared 13 with AIDS, 11 with HIV infection, and 22 HIV-seronegative individuals. Ophthalmic involvement was particularly common in both HIV-infected groups, and was diagnosed in 36% of HIV-seropositive individuals and 46% of those with AIDS compared with only 14% of the seronegative individuals. Among the combined group of HIV-infected individuals, ophthalmic abnormalities included optic neuritis or papillitis in three, conjunctivitis in two, pupillary abnormalities in four, and uveitis or chorioretinitis in one. Ophthalmic disease was associated with syphilitic meningitis in five HIV-seropositive patients and with meningovascular syphilis in four. This study demonstrates that 42% of HIV-infected patients with CSF VDRL-positive neurosyphilis may have ophthalmic involvement, providing an important corollary to a previous study that demonstrated that 85% of patients with ophthalmic syphilis also had neurosyphilis (Levy et al 1989). In a review of 17 patients with syphilitic uveitis, 12 were found to be HIV seropositive (Becerra et al 1989). In this series, none of the patients had symptoms of syphilitic meningitis and only three patients had rash. In 11 patients, uveitis was bilateral, 10 had posterior uveitis, four optic neuropathies and four disc oedema. Three patients had a neuroretinitis and two had branch retinal vein occlusions. Serum RPRs ranged from 1:8 to 1:8152 and in all patients CSF analysis was abnormal, six having

reactive CSF VDRL, 10 increased protein and eight pleocytosis. In 11 of the 12 patients, visual acuity improved with penicillin. By contrast, in the five HIV-negative individuals with syphilitic uveitis, only one had posterior uveitis and optic nerve involvement, while all had anterior uveitis (three bilateral, two unilateral). None had a positive CSF VDRL, one of five had increased CSF protein and one of five had CSF pleocytosis. The study suggests that ocular syphilis is not only more progressive when it occurs with HIV infection, but that nervous system involvement is more frequent.

Meningovascular syphilis

Meningovascular syphilis typically occurs 2–10 years after primary infection and presents as ischaemia or stroke affecting the brain or spinal cord (Fig. 10.5). Typically endarteritis of small- and medium-sized vessels is found and angiography may show multiple areas of beading of the cerebral arteries. Stroke in meningovascular syphilis should be considered in the diagnosis of

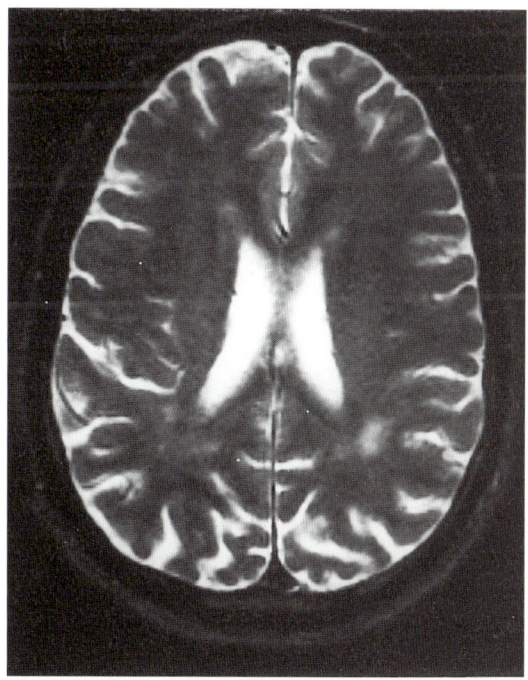

Fig. 10.5 T2-weighted MRI showing small infarct due to meningovascular syphilis in an HIV-infected patient.

stroke in a young person. It has been suggested that HIV-infected individuals may show more rapid progression to meningovascular syphilis because of their profound cellular immunodeficiency (Musher 1991). In this article, Musher makes the point that in the pre-penicillin era, early neurosyphilis (asymptomatic neurosyphilis, syphilitic meningitis or meningovascular syphilis) was relatively rare, and during the era of arsphenamine therapy it was found only in inadequately treated individuals. In a subsequent survey, Musher et al (1990) identified 40 cases of neurosyphilis co-occurring with HIV infection (Table 10.5). Five patients had asymptomatic neurosyphilis, 24 acute syphilitic meningitis and 11 meningovascular syphilis, while only one displayed one of the late manifestations of neurosyphilis – general paresis. None had tabes dorsalis. Johns et al (1987) reported two HIV-infected patients with meningovascular syphilis, one developing within 4 months of primary infection, suggesting an accelerated course of syphilitic infection. Both patients developed infarctions of the basis pontis, visualized on magnetic resonance imaging (MRI). Thus early stages of neurosyphilis with prominent meningeal and vascular involvement appear more common. Musher et al (1990) in a review of the literature found 23 cases of acute syphilitic meningitis. Nine had meningitic features (headache, fever, neck stiffness) and five of them and 13 others had cranial nerve palsies (usually cranial nerves II or VIII). They also located 11 reports of meningovascular syphilis with strokes and computed tomographic (CT) features of cerebral infarction. A case of syphilitic spinal cord involvement has been recorded in which a paraparesis recovered to a large extent after a full course of penicillin (Berger 1992).

Table 10.5   Neurosyphilis in 40 HIV-positive patients

Asymptomatic neurosyphilis	5
Acute syphilitic meningitis	
Meningitis	9
Cranial nerve dysfunction	13
Polyradiculopathy	1
Meningovascular syphilis	11
General paresis	1

(Reproduced from Musher 1991 with permission of The University of Chicago Press)

Late manifestations of neurosyphilis typically occur 5–40 years after initial infection and involve nervous system parenchyma. In the pre-penicillin era, tabes and general paresis occurred in 7–10% of untreated and 1–2% of treated individuals with an average incubation period of 25 years. Both forms are uncommon today, both in HIV-infected and uninfected individuals. The principal features of general paresis are of a chronic dementia syndrome with prominent personality change and seizures. Tabes dorsalis results from involvement of the dorsal roots, dorsal root ganglia and posterior columns of the spinal cord. Patients develop sensory ataxia, pupillary abnormalities (Argyll Robertson pupils), with light near dissociation of pupillary reflexes and lower-extremity hyporeflexia or areflexia. In severe cases, the profound loss of proprioception in the lower extremities produces traumatic joint involvement with the development of Charcot joints. Bowel and bladder incontinence may develop, as well as the classical, albeit relatively uncommon, symptom of tabetic 'lightning' pains. Optic atrophy can develop in tabes dorsalis. Optic nerve disease in HIV-infected individuals with syphilis includes optic perineuritis, characterized by optic disc oedema, normal visual acuity and fields, an enlarged blind spot and normal pupils. Retro-bulbar neuritis and papillitis have also been reported in syphilis (Winward et al 1989). Syphilitic perineuritis frequently accompanies syphilitic meningitis.

Unusual manifestations of neurosyphilis include gummatous disease of the central nervous system (CNS), which may involve brain or spinal cord. There are case reports of biopsy-proven intracerebral gummas in HIV-infected individuals, which have caused confusion with other more common intracranial mass lesions such as toxoplasmosis (Berger et al 1992). Other uncommon manifestations include syphilitic polyradiculopathy (Lanska et al 1988), a case of rapidly progressive polyradiculopathy occurring in an HIV-positive individual with a recent history of secondary syphilis treated with intramuscular penicillin appearing 2.5 months after secondary syphilis. This case appears similar to descriptions in the pre-penicillin era of 'syphilitic amyotrophic meningomyelitis' with cases of progressive areflexic paraparesis (Martin 1925).

In retrospective (Katz & Berger 1989) and prospective (Berger 1991) studies, Berger et al have outlined the spectrum of neurosyphilis in HIV infection. In the first retrospective study, 12 patients with HIV infection and positive CSF VDRL were identified. Three were classified with asymptomatic neurosyphilis (one had retinitis at the time), three syphilitic meningitis, five with meningovascular syphilis and one with general paresis. The mean CSF white blood cell count was 132 and all had elevated CSF proteins with a mean value of 106. Five of six patients showed improvements in pleocytosis and protein elevations with treatment, but none had reversion of CSF VDRL to non-reactive. Five of 10 CT scans were abnormal, revealing cerebral atrophy (1), multiple infarctions (2), meningeal enhancement and lobar haemorrhage (1) and a small nodular enhancing lesion (1). In the prospective study, Berger (1991) reviewed 163 asymptomatic HIV-positive individuals and 63 neurologically symptomatic patients. Three of the asymptomatic and one of the neurologically symptomatic subjects had a reactive CSF VDRL test and another subject had a penicillin-responsive myelopathy (with non-reactive CSF VDRL). Thus, among neurologically asymptomatic HIV-positive subjects, the rate of asymptomatic neurosyphilis was 1.8% overall and 4.2% in subjects with a history of syphilis or reactive serum FTA.

Musher et al (1990) reviewed 40 cases with HIV infection and syphilis. Thirty-nine patients presented with asymptomatic neurosyphilis, syphilitic meningitis with or without cranial nerve involvement, or meningovascular syphilis. Eighteen had AIDS, seven AIDS-related complex and 13 asymptomatic HIV infection. Sixteen of these patients had previously been treated for syphilis, five developing early neurosyphilis within 6 months of therapy (one received two doses of procaine penicillin, four only a single dose of procaine penicillin).

Laboratory diagnosis

Serological tests for syphilis

At present, isolation of *T. pallidum* is not practical for clinical purposes. *T. pallidum* can be cultured in rabbits or guinea pigs, but animal inoculation is laborious and expensive. Polymerase chain reaction (PCR) to detect *T. pallidum* DNA is under development and may eventually facilitate diagnosis and monitoring of response to therapy (Hook & Marra 1992). Serological testing includes quantitative non-treponemal or reaginic tests (Venereal Disease Research Laboratory (VDRL) or the rapid-plasma-reagin (RPR) test) or specific treponemal tests (fluorescent treponemal antibody absorption (FTA-ABS) and the microhaemagglutination assay (MHA-TP)). Both the RPR and VDRL tests can be quantified by performing serial two-fold dilutions, and blood RPR levels usually peak during the secondary or early latent stages of syphilis, subsequently declining with treatment or spontaneously (Hook & Marra 1992). Diagnosis of neurosyphilis is not clear cut because the serum RPR or VDRL may be negative or of low titre in up to a quarter of patients with late neurosyphilis (although the serum FTA should always remain positive). Because of laboratory variation, changes in RPR or VDRL titres of less than two serial dilutions are not clinically relevant. Table 10.6 indicates the definitions of serological response, failure and relapse.

Davis and Schmitt (1989) compared CSF VDRL and CSF FTA-ABS. Forty-eight of 1665 (3%) CSF samples had positive CSF FTA-ABS. Thirty-eight patients had clinical details available and a CSF VDRL test performed. Four had reactive CSF VDRL. Fifteen were thought to have active neurosyphilis: 11 general paresis, one meningovascular syphilis, one acute syphilitic meningitis, and two both general paresis and meningo-

Table 10.6 Serological definitions of response to syphilis therapy

Response	Four-fold or greater decline in RPR titre, sustained during follow-up
Serofast	No change in titre during follow-up and no signs of progressive infection
Relapse	An initial four-fold decline in serum RPR titre followed by four-fold or greater titre rise
Reinfection	As for relapse, but with history of re-exposure
Failure	Four-fold increase in serum RPR titre without an initial response, persistence of titre $\geq$ 1:64, and/or development of clinical disease

(After Dowell et al 1992)

vascular syphilis. The sensitivity of the CSF VDRL in diagnosing neurosyphilis was 27% with 100% specificity. Only 39% of patients with a reactive CSF FTA-ABS had active neurosyphilis, suggesting that this test is overly sensitive and is less specific.

In conclusion, non-reactive serum FTA-ABS rules out syphilis infection (Simon 1985), and reactive serum FTA-ABS with non-reactive CSF FTA-ABS makes active neurosyphilis unlikely.

In HIV infection there has been great concern that standard serology may be unreliable, with frequent false negatives or false positives. There have been scattered case reports in which non-treponemal antibody responses measured with RPR or VDRL are negative despite biopsy-proven active secondary syphilis (Hicks et al 1987). Haas et al (1990) examined syphilis serology in 109 homosexual men with a documented history of treated syphilis. None of the HIV-negative individuals lost treponemal seroreactivity, whereas 7% of asymptomatic HIV seropositives and 38% of those with symptomatic HIV infection did. This suggests that treponemal tests fail to identify previous syphilis infection, particularly in immune-suppressed HIV-seropositive patients. Biologically false positive reaginic tests for syphilis are more common in HIV-infected persons, although the biologically false positive reaction rate is still low: 11% in a series from Rompalo et al (1992) in Baltimore City STD Clinics. Biological false positive RPRs in this series were twice as common in women than men and were also associated with a history of injection drug use. Other potential causes of false positive RPRs include pregnancy, chronic liver disease, multiple blood transfusions, bacterial endocarditis and tuberculosis. Potential causes of false positive treponemal tests include systemic lupus erythematosus, Lyme disease and malaria. Haas et al (1990) showed that the MHA-TP reactivity may be lost with progression of HIV infection. This suggests that the MHA-TP should not be used to exclude syphilis in HIV-infected patients.

In the vast majority of HIV-infected individuals, syphilis serology will reliably reflect the activity and response to treatment, even at low levels of CD4+ cells. In fact, HIV infection may be associated with higher RPR or VDRL titres because of polyclonal activation (Hutchinson et al 1991) or the presence of cross-reacting antiphospholipid antibodies (Dowell et al 1992). Dowell et al (1992) point out that 88% of their patients with latent syphilis had an RPR $\geqslant$ 1:16 compared with the serological experience in HIV negatives where only 4% had titres this high (Fiumara 1979). Most HIV-infected patients with neurosyphilis have positive serological tests; however, the development of RPR seropositivity may be delayed or blunted (Bolan 1990, Haas et al 1990, Gregory 1991, Johnson et al 1991). In general, mean VDRL antibody titres are higher in HIV-infected persons (Musher 1991) because polyclonal B cell activation in HIV infection may lead to an increased production of antibodies against previously encountered antigens.

Cerebrospinal fluid changes in syphilis

In the pre-penicillin era, CSF abnormalities were common with pleocytosis or protein abnormalities occurring in up to 20% of patients with primary syphilis and up to 70% with secondary syphilis, falling to 30% during latent syphilis. CSF abnormalities found during secondary syphilis will resolve in nearly 70% of patients (Stokes et al 1944, Hahn & Clark 1946). Of relevance in the management of HIV-infected patients with syphilis is that early studies in the pre-penicillin era showed that neurosyphilis was more likely to develop in patients with the most abnormal CSF studies (Moore & Hopkins 1930). In the pre-AIDS era, symptomatic neurosyphilis develops in 4–9% of patients with untreated syphilis (Moore & Hopkins 1930, Hook & Marra 1992), but there are no reliable data to estimate the incidence of neurosyphilis in HIV-infected persons.

The largest series to use isolation techniques included both HIV-positive and HIV-negative patients. Using rabbit inoculation, Lukehart et al (1988) isolated *T. pallidum* from 12 of 40 CSF samples in patients with untreated primary and secondary syphilis. In four of the 12 from whom *T. pallidum* was isolated, there were no other laboratory abnormalities. Patients in whom *T. pallidum* was recoverable were more likely to have positive CSF VDRL, suggesting an association between treponemal load and VDRL

Table 10.7   CSF abnormalities in HIV-positive patients with neurosyphilis

	Cells	Protein	Glucose	VDRL
No. of patients with abnormalities				
No. tested	27/37	26/32	11/30	30/37
Median	173	125	37	1:4
Range	8–2800	46–1000	11–42	WR 1:16

WR, weakly reactive.
(Reproduced from Musher 1991 with permission of The University of Chicago Press.)

positivity. Musher et al (1990) reviewed the range of CSF abnormalities in neurosyphilis in 40 HIV-infected patients (Table 10.7). Other studies have shown that CSF VDRL is positive in between 30 and 70% of patients with neurosyphilis, depending on the diagnostic criteria, and a positive CSF VDRL, by definition, indicates neurosyphilis. The use of the FTA-ABS test on the CSF is prone to false positive reactions because of its sensitivity and potential carry-over of serum reactivity from red cell contamination of CSF.

Prospective CSF studies (Berger 1991) in some HIV-infected groups reveal serological and historical evidence of syphilis in 40–50% with a diagnosis of CSF VDRL positive neurosyphilis in 3–5% of HIV-seropositive individuals.

The major difficulty in interpretation of the CSF abnormalities in an HIV-infected patient with syphilis is whether to attribute the abnormalities to CNS invasion with *T. pallidum* or HIV. CSF abnormalities are very frequent with HIV infection, representing early CNS infection. Thus 65% of asymptomatic HIV seropositives will have either a CSF lymphocytosis, protein elevation or increased IgG percentage (McArthur et al 1988). Unless the CSF VDRL is positive, there is at this point no definitive method of attributing the abnormalities to either syphilis or HIV. Hopefully, as PCR techniques become more reliable, this confusion will dissipate. McArthur et al (1989) assessed whether previous syphilis infection was associated with an increased CNS HIV-1 infection as measured by the frequency of CSF abnormalities. Eighty-eight men were studied, none of whom had neurosyphilis, opportunistic infections or HIV-related CNS disease. All had negative CSF VDRL and negative RPR or RPR

titres <1/4 indicating adequate treatment of their past syphilis. There was no evidence that those with previous syphilis (serum FTA positive) had any increase in CSF abnormalities. The implication is that adequately treated syphilis does not lead to increased HIV activation, at least not in the early stages (all patients had CD4 counts over 500/mm^3).

Traumatic lumbar puncture should not result in a false positive CSF VDRL in a patient with serum VDRL of 1:256 or less unless the CSF is visibly bloody (Izzat et al 1971).

Detection of *T. pallidum* antigens or of *T. pallidum* DNA by PCR will hopefully permit a more precise diagnosis of neurosyphilis by identifying CNS invasion where CSF VDRL is negative. These advances may assist in the diagnosis and management of syphilis (Stamm et al 1988, Burstain et al 1991, Wicher et al 1992).

Treatment

Adequacy of syphilis treatment in HIV

One incompletely answered question is whether traditional syphilis treatment is less effective in patients co-infected with HIV. The optimal treatment of primary, secondary or tertiary syphilis in HIV infection remains controversial, and many would advocate increasing the penicillin dose for early syphilis or treating presumptive neurosyphilis when CSF abnormalities are present, even with negative CSF VDRL (Davis 1990). Frederick et al (1988) showed the persistence of cutaneous lesions for more than 3 months in seven of 16 HIV-infected patients with failure of VDRL titre to decrease in the first 6 months after treatment. Lukehart et al (1988) found that a single dose of procaine penicillin did sterilize the CSF in HIV-seronegative individuals, but failed to eliminate recoverable *T. pallidum* (by rabbit inoculation) from CSF in four patients co-infected with HIV and in one HIV-positive patient who received three doses of intramuscular procaine penicillin. McMillan et al (1990) studied 20 HIV-positive homosexual men who had previously been treated for syphilis (19 received i.m. procaine penicillin 600 mg daily for 14 days; one received doxycycline for 21 days). The CD4 counts ranged from 13 to 541. Recrudescence of syphilis was seen only in the one patient who had been treated with doxycycline. Terry et al (1988) examined homosexual men with a history of treated syphilis with positive serum RPR and documented HIV seroconversion and HIV-seroprevalent men. After HIV seroconversion in eight homosexual men with a history of treated syphilis, no change in the serological markers of syphilis was noted, suggesting that reactivation of syphilis did not occur. In HIV seropositive men with syphilis, serological responses were comparable to those seen in HIV-seronegative individuals with seroreversion.

Measuring response to treatment

After treatment of neurosyphilis, CSF pleocytosis and protein may decrease during a period of 2–6 months; however, CSF VDRL may remain positive for 1–2 years after treatment (Hahn et al 1956).

In a historical cohort study of all cases of infectious syphilis followed in Alberta, Canada from 1981 to 1987, 1090 patients were originally seen and 882 were treated with the recommended antibiotic regime for syphilis (602 primary syphilis, 161 secondary syphilis, 38 early latent syphilis) (Romanowski et al 1991). Homosexual men accounted for about 17% of the total cases, but HIV serostatus was unknown. At the end of 36 months, 63% showed seroreversion, the proportion being highest in those with primary syphilis. By 24 months, 97% of patients with primary syphilis had a four-fold (two serial dilutions) reduction in RPR titre. For those with secondary syphilis, 80% of patients achieved a six-fold (three serial dilutions) or greater decrease by 6 months. Serological response was not affected by sex, age, race or sexual orientation, but was dependent on pre-treatment titre. Individuals with first infection were more likely to serorevert than those reinfected. The higher the initial titre, the less likely seroreversion was to occur in both primary and secondary syphilis. The specific treponemal tests were less likely to serorevert, particularly for patients with early latent or secondary syphilis. The study challenged previous

expectations that adequate treatment of primary or secondary syphilis was followed by a four-fold decrease in serum RPR by 3 or 4 months and an eight-fold decrease by 6 or 8 months with negative RPR after the first year. Romanowski showed that with successful treatment for primary and secondary syphilis there is at least a four-fold decrease in RPR titre by 12 months. Response is delayed in early latent syphilis. Seroreversion of treponemal tests was noted in 24% of patients after 2–3 years of follow-up. Fiumara (1980) has shown that after adequate treatment for primary and secondary syphilis in non-AIDS patients, seroreversion of serum RPR should occur by 12 months for primary and 24 months for secondary syphilis.

Current treatment guidelines

There has been much discussion of what constitutes adequate chemotherapy in HIV-infected patients. One issue that has been overlooked in many discussions of treatment relates to compliance and the follow-up after treatment. If compliance with therapy or for follow-up for serological testing is likely to be problematic, inpatient supervised treatment may be the only certain way to ensure delivery of adequate amounts of antibiotic. Because benzathine penicillin does not achieve treponemicidal levels in the CSF, it should not be used for treatment of neurosyphilis. Table 10.6 lists some of the commonly used serological definitions for assessment of treatment response. Lukehart et al (1988) isolated treponemes from some HIV-seropositive individuals after courses of benzathine penicillin. At present it is probably advisable to use 2.4 million units of procaine penicillin daily for 10–14 days with oral probenecid or intravenous penicillin for 10 days. Ceftriaxone 2 G daily for 2–10 days has been proposed as an alternative and a comparative trial of standard i.v. penicillin and i.v. ceftriaxone is underway in the USA (ACTG 145). Follow-up after treatment of syphilis or neurosyphilis needs to be extra vigilant in the setting of HIV infection. We endorse previous recommendations of checking serum RPR titres monthly for 12 months after treatment as well as CSF analysis if titre rises (Hook 1989) (Tables 10.8 and 10.9). If the CSF

VDRL remains positive after 1–2 years, retreatment is indicated. The HIV epidemic has brought syphilis back as a major health problem, and neurosyphilis back to the neurological clinic (Hook & Marra 1992). Fig. 10.6 sets out a schema for management of the patient with positive syphilis serology.

BORRELIA

A single case of Lyme disease in the presence of HIV infection has been reported. It is not yet known if this is more than coincidence (Garcia-Monco et al 1989).

CLOSTRIDIA

Injection drug users are at risk of contracting *Clostridium botulinum* and *Clostridium tetani*. Botulism presents with cranial nerve dysfunction and descending paralysis. EMG studies show

Table 10.8   Treatment of syphilis

Primary, secondary or early latent (<12 months)

Benzathine penicillin 2.4 mU i.m. × 1
or doxycycline 100 mg b.i.d. × 14 days
Repeat serology at 1, 2, 3, 6, 9 months; 12 months if HIV+ :
if four-fold rise in titre – CSF analysis, neurosyphilis treatment
Routine lumbar puncture not recommended unless stage uncertain

---

Late latent (>12 months)

CSF analysis if:
   neurological symptoms and signs
   treatment failure
   serum RPR >1:32
   evidence of active syphilis, e.g. aortitis, iritis
   non-penicillin treatment planned
Benzathine penicillin 2.4 mU i.m. × 3
or doxycycline 100 mg b.i.d. × 28 days
Repeat serology at 6 months and 12 months:
if serofast or if rising titre – neurosyphilis treatment

Table 10.9   Treatment of neurosyphilis

Aqueous penicillin 2–4 mU every 4 hours i.v. for 10–14 days
or Procaine penicillin 2.4 mU i.m. each day + probenecid 500 mg q.i.d. for 10–14 days
Repeat CSF every 6 months until cell count normal
If CSF cell count not decreasing at 6 months or abnormal at 2 years – retreatment

---

(After Centers for Disease Control 1989)

presynaptic blockade with an incremental muscle action potential to repetitive nerve stimulation with additional signs of denervation in some cases. The toxin can be detected early on in faeces, serum or wounds. Botulinum antitoxin is used in treatment.

Tetanus results from disinhibition of alpha and gamma neurones. Patients present with back stiffness, worsened by stimulation, trismus and risus sardonicus. The diagnosis which is clinical, is suspected from the presentation and a history of inadequate vaccination. Treatment is with human tetanus immunoglobulin, supportive care, benzodiazepines or neuromuscular blockade.

TUBERCULOSIS

Worldwide, 1.7 billion people are infected with *Mycobacterium tuberculosis*, and each year 8 million people develop active tuberculosis (TB), which is fatal in 3 million. Fifteen million people in the USA are estimated to have latent TB. The WHO estimates that 4.4 million people worldwide are co-infected with TB and HIV, of whom 121 000 are in the USA.

People co-infected with TB and HIV develop active TB at an annual rate of 8% (compared with a 10% life-time risk of active TB in an HIV-seronegative individual) (Selwin et al 1989). TB including involvement of the nervous system is now recognized as a complication of AIDS. Indeed, the AIDS pandemic has led to an increase of TB in countries such as the USA where it had been on the decline, and it is particularly common in Africa. From 1953, when national reporting of TB began in the USA, until about 1984 there was a steady year-on-year decrease in the incidence of TB of about 5%. Since 1985 the trend has reversed and TB is on the increase (22 201 cases in 1985, at least 24 905 in 1990). The greatest increases have been reported from centres such as New York, and the major impact has fallen on the Blacks and Hispanics (56%) in the 24–44 years age group. The relationship to AIDS is clear-cut. In a study of 217 seropositive and 303 seronegative intravenous drug users (IVDU) enrolled in a methadone programme, positive skin tests at entry showed a parallel exposure to *M. tuberculosis*, but active TB developed in 14% of the HIV-positive but none of the HIV-negative cohort

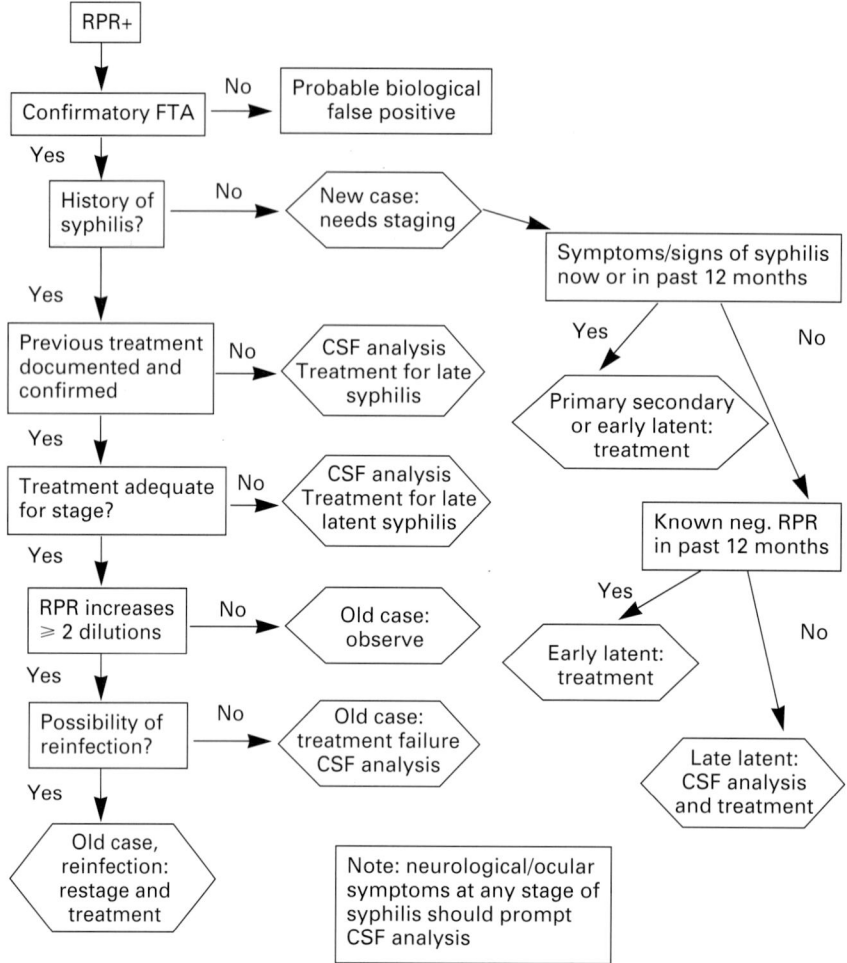

Fig. 10.6　Scheme for management of positive syphilis serology.

(Selwin et al 1989). It has been suggested that HIV-positive individuals should be skin tested and those who are positive (>5 mm induration) should receive prophylaxis with isoniazid. Those who are negative should not receive BCG vaccination because of the risks with a live vaccine in immunocompromised individuals.

The prevalence of TB in HIV-infected patients depends on the exposure as well as on the severity of immunosuppression. There are large differences in exposure. For example, Haitian immigrants in Florida have a skin test positivity rate of up to 91% compared with 22% for IVDU in New York and 1.5% for mainly non-Hispanic medical students (Pitchenik & Fertel 1992). Seen from the other standpoint some 30–40% of TB cases are

seropositive for HIV in New York, with wide variations elsewhere depending on town and racial case-mix. Overall about 3–8% of HIV-positive people in developed countries will develop active TB (Barnes et al 1991).

In some developing countries, 50% of the adult population has been infected by tubercle bacilli (Sudre et al 1992). Rising incidence associated with the AIDS epidemic has been reported from a number of African states.

The increase in cases is of particular concern as multi-drug resistant TB is on the increase and this carries a case fatality rate of 70–90% (Dooley et al 1992).

Extrapulmonary TB in a patient with HIV infection is AIDS defining, and extrapulmonary (with or without pulmonary) TB is more common in HIV-positive than HIV-seronegative individuals. Pitchenik and Fertel (1992) reviewed the literature to quote figures of 62% for extrapulmonary infection in HIV-positives contrasting with 17.5% for the total national reporting database in the USA.

The infection with *M. tuberculosis* is a reactivation of a latent focus and the risk of such reactivation in AIDS approaches 50% in some estimates (Shafer et al 1991). This reflects the importance of cellular immunity in the control of TB.

Neurological complications

TB of the meninges results from the rupture of small subependymal foci. The meninges become thickened and opaque and cranial nerves and roots can be affected as they penetrate the meninges, which contain caseating granulomata. The other mechanism of symptom production is the direct effect of a granuloma in the brain parenchyma or an endarteritis with ischaemic foci.

Immunosuppression need not be severe and in one series (Dube et al 1992) CD4 counts varied from 7 to 251/mm^3. This has been contrasted with the situation in cryptococcal infection where CD4 counts tend to be lower. Bishburg et al (1986) found 10 patients with CNS involvement amongst 52 cases of TB from a population of approximately 420 patients with AIDS.

TB meningitis is usually preceded by a period of malaise, fatigue and headache. A review of 26 HIV-related cases by Shafer et al (1991) and of 15 cases by Dube et al (1992) demonstrated that most patients had confusion and/or headache. Less than half had neck stiffness, but 11 from the combined series had focal signs such as a hemiparesis or cranial nerve lesion. By the time meningitis has developed, fever is to be expected. The CSF in the two studies showed a pleocytosis in all but five instances with predominantly a lymphocytosis of up to 1000/mm^3. Cases with normal cell counts tended to have miliary infection with positive blood cultures. The protein was normal or up to 1000 mg/dl. CSF cultures were positive in cases with and without a pleocytosis. CT scans with contrast had been carried out in all

save two of Shafer's patients revealing meningeal enhancement in five. Dube reported focal lesions in nine of his 15 cases either on CT or MRI. Several patients had hydrocephalus. At least two cases had normal scans. Berenguer et al (1992) reported mass lesions in eight of 10 cases, with ring enhancement on CT in five (Fig. 10.7). Interestingly, 52 HIV-infected patients with no evidence of CNS TB had scans and four of these had enhancing brain lesions which responded to anti-TB treatment (Shafer et al 1991). Clearly this suggests that HIV-infected patients who develop TB at any site should probably have a cranial CT scan (or MRI). It also means that ring-enhancing lesions (Bishburg et al 1986) may be due to TB if they do not respond to anti-*Toxoplasma* treatment or the patient has pulmonary TB.

The clinical presentation does not appear to differ in a major way from that seen in non-AIDS patients. Dube et al (1992) addressed this issue directly comparing 15 patients with culture-proven meningitis resulting from *M. tuberculosis* who were HIV-positive or had AIDS, with 16 from the same institution who were not HIV

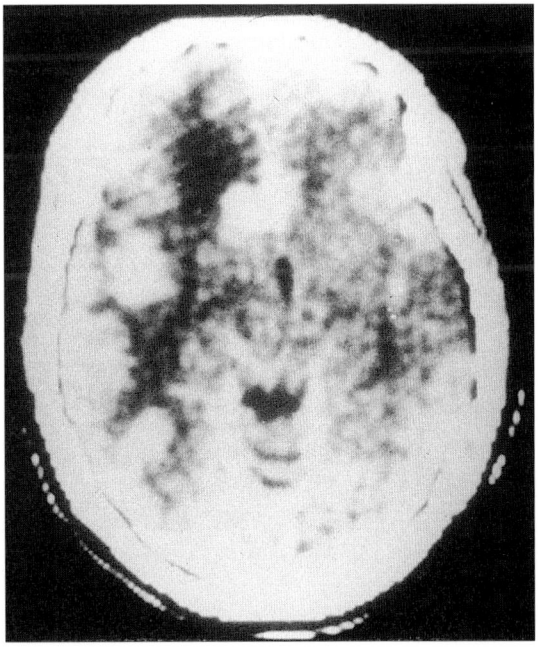

Fig. 10.7   CT scan showing enhancing tuberculomas. (Reproduced from Williams 1989.)

infected. There were no differences in the incidence of the major symptoms of headache, confusion and fever. Physical signs were equally common in the two groups (papilloedema, focal findings and depressed consciousness), except for the presence of neck stiffness, which was less common in the HIV-infected cases. This difference was barely significant, however (47% instead of 80%, $p = 0.06$), and in the context of a large number of comparisons in a small number of cases may well be fortuitous. CSF findings were similar in the two groups, except for the opening pressure, which was lower in the HIV cases (7–24 cm CSF compared with 9–55 cm, $p = 0.03$). This might reflect a somewhat blunted meningeal response to infection in the immunocompromised, and support the difference in neck stiffness, but the cellular response did not confirm this, being just as active. In cryptococcal infection with more advanced immunosuppression there is a tendency for HIV-related cases to show less CSF reaction than non-HIV cases (Dismukes 1988).

Neuroimaging revealed a significant difference in the incidence of mass lesions. Nine of 15 HIV-infected patients but only two of 14 non-HIV patients had scans showing such lesions ($p<0.01$). Such lesions are sometimes large enough to behave as space-occupying abscesses (Bishburg et al 1986) (Fig. 10.7). Others have reported similar findings. Vertebral and spinal cord abscesses (Doll et al 1987) have also been described (Fig. 10.8) (see also Chapter 5, Fig. 5.3). MRI shows enhancing lesions when the meningitis is accompanied by tuberculomas as in non-HIV-related TB meningitis (Fig. 10.9).

Diagnosis depends on a high risk of suspicion, the chest radiograph and the CSF findings with reduced glucose level. In the absence of pulmonary TB, ring-enhancing lesions in the brain in a febrile patient will usually be treated as possible *Toxoplasma* infection. When there is no response to *Toxoplasma* treatment a biopsy will be indicated, which will reveal the caseating tuberculous lesion. In the presence of active pulmonary infection, and a negative *Toxoplasma* antibody test,

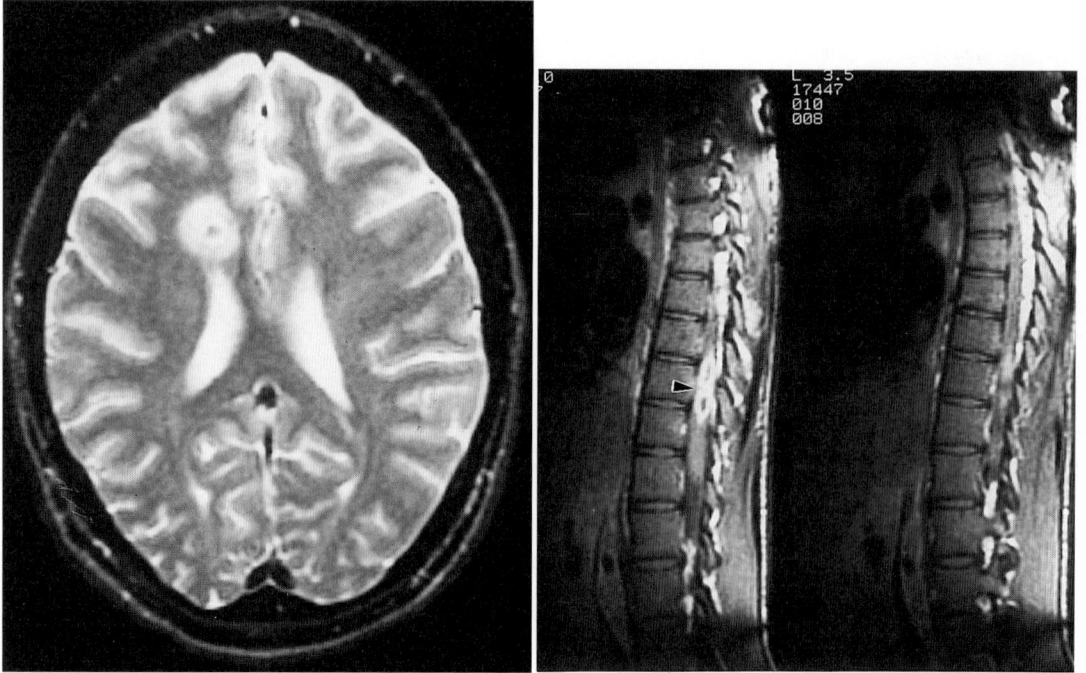

A   B

Fig. 10.8   Neuroimaging in a case with tuberculous abscesses. **A** T2-weighted MRI showing frontal lobe abscess.
B Sagittal T2 images of the thoracic cord showing high signal from a spinal abscess (arrowed). **C** Axial MRI showing ring nature of the thoracic lesion (arrowed). **D** CT myelogram showing cord swelling with lack of contrast behind the cord.

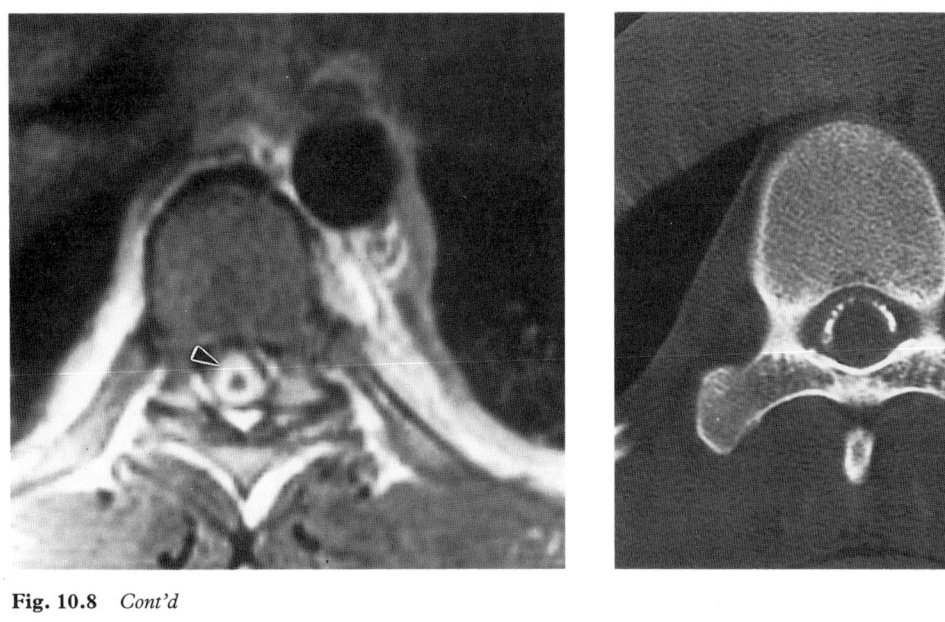

C

D

Fig. 10.8   *Cont'd*

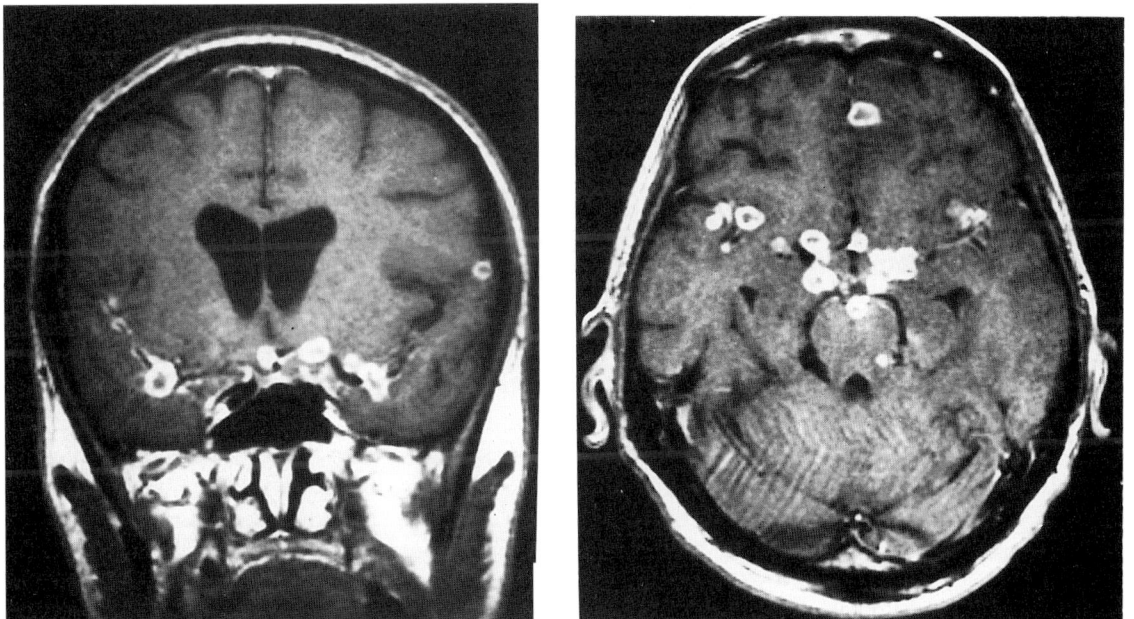

A

B

Fig. 10.9   Cranial MRI in a case of TB meningitis in an HIV-negative patient. **A** Coronal and **B** axial T1 images show numerous enhancing basal tuberculomas. (Courtesy of Dr Richard Johnson.)

focal neurological and/or brain imaging findings would be sufficiently suspicious of CNS tubercle to limit treatment to standard anti-tuberculous therapy.

Kramer et al (1990) found that the diagnosis of pulmonary TB in HIV-infected patients was delayed in 48%. The reason seemed to be the failure to consider the diagnosis and to pursue investigation with adequate sputum samples. Sputum samples were positive in 61%, stools in 42% (probably due to swallowed sputum rather than gut infection) and blood cultures in 38%. Modern culture techniques permit a bacterial diagnosis in as early as 3 weeks. Earlier diagnosis of neurological involvement may become possible with the use of PCR to detect the organism's genome in the CSF.

Treatment with standard quadruple regimes is successful, though the mortality remains higher than in non-AIDS patients. A diagnostic reduction in fever can be expected within a week in 85% of pulmonary cases (Kramer et al 1990), and a therapeutic trial may point to the diagnosis ahead of bacteriological confirmation. Mortality after discharge from hospital depends primarily on the CD4 count (Stoneburner et al 1992), but rates of drug resistance as high as 30% are being reported from some areas (Chawla et al 1992). Initial treatment is with isoniazid 300 mg daily, rifampicin up to 600 mg/day, pyrazinamide 20–30 mg/kg/day and ethambutol 15–25 mg/kg. Monno et al (1991) suggest that where in vitro drug resistance is a problem, rifabutin (450 mg/day) may be successful. Pyrazinamide should be given for the first 2 months, or longer if resistance or allergy develops to isoniazid or rifampicin. Non-compliance is a problem in some AIDS patients and supervised ambulatory treatment may be necessary. Zidovudine can be continued, but ketoconazole inhibits the absorption of rifampicin, and the two should not be prescribed together. Minor changes in liver function tests (LFTs) should not be allowed to cause cessation of first-line anti-TB drugs. As noted, treatment is usually successful, but after a course of 9 months or more with culture conversion, isoniazid should probably be continued lifelong, because of the risk of relapse in the immunocompromised. Obstruction of CSF pathways due to meningitis may cause hydrocephalus with declining conscious level. Such a deterioration whilst on drug treatment is therefore an indication for repeat imaging in case a ventricular shunt is needed. This would only be likely in the first days or weeks of tuberculous meningitis. Later deterioration suggests relapse, a second opportunistic infection or additional pathology.

MYCOBACTERIUM AVIUM INTRACELLULARE

Atypical mycobacteria such as members of the *Mycobacterium avium* complex are the most common cause of systemic bacterial infection in AIDS patients, and have been identified in 50% of AIDS autopsies (Armstrong et al 1985). Before the AIDS epidemic, infection was rarely disseminated, and the main victims of pulmonary infection were patients with other lung diseases.

In HIV-infected patients *Mycobacterium avium intracellulare* (MAI) may also affect the gut, skin, lymph nodes and CNS. Extrapulmonary MAI, unless in the skin or cervical or hilar lymph nodes, is AIDS defining in the absence of other causes of immunodeficiency. The infection with MAI appears to be environmentally acquired rather than by person-to-person contact. Involvement of the bowel mucosa is common with poorly formed granulomas and large numbers of organisms. This is thought to be a primary infection and is more common in younger individuals. The route of entry may be the bowel from ingestion of contaminated water or food.

Clinical features

Pulmonary infection, though common, is accompanied by varied and non-specific chest radiographic findings, and there are usually only mild respiratory symptoms. The usual clinical problem is of pyrexia and malaise accompanying disseminated infection in the late stages of immunosuppression. Most affected patients have had a diagnosis of AIDS for many months prior to presentation with disseminated MAI, and CD4 counts are usually less than 100 cells/ml (Modilevsky et al 1989). Indeed, MAI is probably the most common cause of fever of unknown origin in AIDS patients in the West (*M. tuberculosis* would be in Africa). In patients with disseminated infection, the organism can be detected in blood cultures (90%), stool and sputum samples (60%), bronchoalveolar lavage fluid (35%) and CSF (11%). Biopsies of bone marrow, lymph nodes and bowel all yield the organisms in 75–85% (Pitchenik & Fertel 1992). The diagnosis of disseminated infection requires more than sputum or stool cultures, and in such cases blood cultures and marrow examination would be advised. Treatment is difficult as standard drug regimens are ineffective. The morbidity and mortality are less than with TB, and there is no comparable public health risk. In some situations when sputum cultures are not accompanied by serious symptoms, it may be appropriate to follow events closely without specific drug therapy. When systemic symptoms are thought to be due to disseminated infection, a regimen of four or five drugs should be tried. Amikacin, clofazimine, ethambutol and rifampicin may be combined (Young 1988) with rifabutin and clarithromycin. As infection in AIDS appears to relate to failure of macrophage function, there may in the future be a role for recombinant granulocyte-macrophage colonystimulating factor. Despite the presence of MAI in the CSF in cases of disseminated infection, neurological problems are rare. Meningitis and encephalopathy have been described (Zakowski et al 1982).

NOCARDIA

Nocardia are branching soil bacteria that enter the body by inhalation. Pulmonary infection is thus the rule, but a third of patients develop CNS infection. A pure meningitis is extremely rare (Byrne et al 1979), but multiple multilocular abscesses may develop in immunocompromised individuals (Levy & Bredesen 1988). The patients develop headache, mental changes and focal signs, and the differential diagnosis is with *Toxoplasmosis*. Both conditions produce multiple ring-enhancing mass lesions on CT or MRI. Biopsy in the face of deterioration on anti-*Toxoplasmosis* treatment is the way to make the diagnosis. Antimicrobial treatment is problematical and drainage or excision of abscesses should be attempted if the patient's general condition permits. Intravenous third-generation cephalosporins are probably the best choice as they produce high CSF penetration (see also p. 130).

LISTERIA

Listeria monocytogenes is a Gram-positive rod of wide distribution in nature. It is found in soil, silage and sewerage. It was named after Lord Lister, and at one time was incorrectly thought to be responsible for infectious mononucleosis. Human infections were rarely diagnosed before 1950. One to 5% of the general population are colonized at any one time, with low rates of faecal carriage. Infection is usually seen in the context of a degree of immunodeficiency as, for example, encountered in pregnancy and the puerperium, malignancy or in renal transplant recipients. Examination of several outbreaks has revealed that most infection stems from the ingestion of contaminated food. Soft cheeses contaminated with unpasteurized milk have predominated, and HIV-infected patients should be advised to avoid such food products.

Meningitis and encephalitis may occur, but despite the theoretical risks, the incidence in AIDS has been surprisingly low (Gould et al 1987, Mascola et al 1988). Tumour necrosis factor is part of the endogenous defence against *Listeria* (Nakane et al 1988) so perhaps its production in HIV-infected brain is paradoxically protective? Alternatively, it may simply be a matter of suppression of *Listeria* by antibiotics given, for example, for *Pneumocystis* prophylaxis (Mascola et al 1988). There are no special features to the meningitis, which may cause only headache, fever and confusion. The organisms are best sought in blood cultures, not always being detectable in the CSF, which shows a predominantly polymorphonuclear pleocytosis.

Parenchymal involvement by *Listeria* can cause encephalitis or abscess formation. Focal deficit is to be expected in this case. Brainstem involvement is rare (Kennard et al 1979), but should always prompt consideration of listerial rhombencephalitis. This is perhaps the human equivalent of 'circling' disease in sheep, in whom listerial encephalitis causes repetitive turning behaviour.

Optimum treatment has not been defined, but ampicillin, a combination of gentamicin and penicillin, or trimethoprim-sulphamethoxazole all have their advocates.

REFERENCES

Adams R D, Merritt H H. Meningeal and vascular syphilis of the spinal cord. Medicine (Baltimore) 1944; 23: 181–214

Armstrong D, Gold J W M, Dryjanski J, et al. Treatment of infections in patients with the acquired immunodeficiency syndrome. Ann Intern Med 1985; 103: 738–743

Barnes P F, Bloch A B, Davidson P T, Snider D E. Tuberculosis in patients with acquired immunodeficiency virus infection. New Engl J Med 1991; 324: 1644–1650

Becerra L I, Ksiazek S M, Savino P J, et al. Syphilitic uveitis in human immunodeficiency virus-infected and non-infected patients. Ophthalmology 1989; 96: 1727–1730

Berenguer J, Moreno S, Laguna F, et al. Tuberculous meningitis in patients with the human immunodeficiency virus. N Engl J Med 1992; 326: 668–672

Berger J R. Syphilis of the spinal cord. In: Davidoff R A, editor. Handbook of the spinal cord. New York: Marcel Dekker, 1983: 491–538

Berger J R. Neurosyphilis in human immunodeficiency virus type 1-seropositive individuals. Arch Neurol 1991: 48: 700–702

Berger J R. Spinal cord syphilis associated with human immunodeficiency virus infection: a treatable myelopathy. Am J Med 1992; 92: 101–103

Berger J R, Waskin H, Pall L, et al. Syphilitic cerebral gumma with HIV infection. Neurology 1992; 42: 1282–1287

Bishburg E, Sunderam G, Reichman L B, Kapila R. Central nervous system tuberculosis with the acquired immunodeficiency syndrome and its related complex. Ann Intern Med 1986; 105: 210–213

Bolan G. Syphilis in HIV-infected hosts. In: Cohen P T, Sande M A, Volberding P A, editors. The AIDS knowledge base. Waltham, MA: The Medical Publishing Group, 1990

Burke J M, Schaberg D R. Neurosyphilis in the antibiotic era. Neurology 1985; 35: 1368–1371

Burstain J M, Grimprel E, Lukehart S A, et al. Sensitive detection of Treponema pallidum by using the polymerase chain reaction. J Clin Microbiol 1991; 29: 62–68

Byrne E, Brophy B P, Perrett L V. Nocardia cerebral abscess; new concepts in diagnosis, management and prognosis. J Neurol Neurosurg Psychiatr 1979; 42: 1038–1045

Centers for Disease Control. Syphilis and congenital syphilis: United States: 1985–1988. MMWR 1988a; 37: 486–490

Centers for Disease Control. Relationship of syphilis to drug use and prostitution: Connecticut and Philadelphia, Pennsylvania. MMWR 1988b; 37: 755–764

Centers for Disease Control. Sexually transmitted disease treatment guidelines. MMWR 1989; 38 (suppl 8): 1–13

Chawla P K, Klapper P J, Kamholz S L, et al. Drug resistant tuberculosis in an urban population at risk for human immunodeficiency virus infection. Am Rev Respir Dis 1992; 146: 280–284

Clark E G, Danbolt N. The Oslo study of the natural history of untreated syphilis: an epidemiologic investigation based on a re-study of the Boeck-Bruusgaard material: a review and appraisal. J Chron Dis 1955; 2: 311–344

Darrow W W, Echenberg D F, Jaffe H W, et al. Risk factors for human immunodeficiency virus (HIV) in homosexual men. Am J Public Health 1987; 77: 479–483

Davis L E. Neurosyphilis in the patient infected with human immunodeficiency virus (editorial). Ann Neurol 1990; 27: 211–212

Davis L E, Schmitt J W. Clinical significance of cerebrospinal fluid tests for neurosyphilis. Ann Neurol 1989; 25: 50–55

Dismukes W E. Cryptococcal meningitis in patients with AIDS. J Infect Dis 1988; 157: 624–628

Doll D, Yarbro J W, Phillips K, Klott C. Mycobacterial spinal cord abscess with an ascending polyneuropathy. Ann Intern Med 1987; 106: 333–334

Dooley S W, Jarvis W R, Martone W J, Snider D E. Tuberculosis in patients with acquired immunodeficiency virus infection. Ann Intern Med 1992; 117: 257–259

Dowell M E, Ross P G, Musher D M, et al. Response of latent syphilis or neurosyphilis to ceftriaxone therapy in persons infected with human immunodeficiency virus. Am J Med 1992; 93: 481–488

Dube M P, Holtom P D, Larsen R A. Tuberculous meningitis in patients with and without human immunodeficiency virus infection. Am J Med 1992; 93: 520–524

Fiumara N J. Serologic responses to treatment of 128 patients with late latent syphilis. Sex Trans Dis 1979; 6: 243–246

Fiumara N J. Treatment of primary and secondary syphilis: serological response. JAMA 1980; 243: 2500–2502

Frederick W R, Delapenha R, Barnes S, et al. Secondary syphilis and HIV infection (abstract 1175). Proceedings and abstracts of the 28th Interscience Conference on Antimicrobial Agents and Chemotherapy. Washington, DC: Am Soc Microbiol, 1988

Garcia-Monco J C, Frey H M, Fernandez Villar B, et al. Lyme disease concurrent with human immunodeficiency virus infection. Am J Med 1989; 87: 325–328

Gould I A, Belok L C, Handwerger S. Listeria monocytogenes: a rare cause of opportunistic infection in the acquired immunodeficiency syndrome (AIDS) and a new cause of meningitis in AIDS. A case report. AIDS Res 1987; 2: 231–234

Greenblatt R M, Lukehart S A, Plummer F A, et al. Genital ulceration as a risk factor for human immunodeficiency virus infection. AIDS 1988; 2: 47–50

Gregory N. Clinical problems of syphilis in the presence of HIV. Clin Dermatol 1991; 9: 71–74

Haas J S, Bolan G, Larsen S A, et al. Sensitivity of treponemal tests for detecting prior treated syphilis during human immunodeficiency virus infection. J Infect Dis 1990; 162: 862–866

Hahn R D, Clark E G. Asymptomatic neurosyphilis: a review of the literature. Am J Syph, Gon Ven Dis 1946; 30: 305–316

Hahn R D, Cutler J C, Curits A C, et al. Penicillin treatment of asymptomatic central nervous system syphilis. Arch Dermatol 1956; 74: 367–377

Hicks C B, Benson P M, Lupton G, Tramont E C. Seronegative secondary syphilis in a patient infected with the human immunodeficiency virus (HIV) with Kaposi sarcoma: a diagnostic dilemma. Ann Intern Med 1987; 107: 492–495

Holtom P D, Larsen R A, Leal M E, Leedom J M. Prevalence of neurosyphilis in human immunodeficiency virus-infected patients with latent syphilis. Am J Med 1992; 93: 9–12

Hook E W. Syphilis and HIV infection. J Infect Dis 1989; 160: 530–534

Hook E W, Marra C M. Acquired syphilis in adults. New Engl J Med 1992; 326: 1060–1069

Hotson J R. Modern neurosyphilis: a partially treated chronic meningitis. West J Med 1981; 135: 191–200

Hutchinson C M, Rompalo A M, Reichart C A, Hook E W. Characteristics of patients with syphilis attending Baltimore STD clinics: multiple high-risk subgroups and interactions with human immunodeficiency virus infection. Arch Intern Med 1991; 151: 511–516

Izzat N N, Bartruff K J, Glicksman J M, et al. Validity of the VDRL test on cerebrospinal fluid contaminated by blood. Br J Ven Dis 1971; 47: 162–164

Johns D R, Tierney M, Felsenstein D. Alteration in the natural history of neurosyphilis by concurrent infection with the human immunodeficiency virus. New Engl J Med 1987; 316: 1569–1572

Johnson P R, Graves S R, Stewart L, et al. Specific syphilis serologic tests may become negative in HIV infection. AIDS 1991; 5: 419–423

Katz D A, Berger J R. Neurosyphilis in acquired immunodeficiency syndrome. Arch Neurol 1989; 46: 895–898

Katz D A, Berger J R, Duncan R C. Neurosyphilis – a comparative study of the effects of infection with human immunodeficiency virus. Arch Neurol 1993; 50: 243–249

Kennard C, Howard A J, Scholtz C, Swash M. Infection of the brain stem by *Listeria monocytogenes*. J Neurol Neurosurg Psychiatr 1979; 42: 931–933

Kramer F, Modilevsky T, Waliany A R, et al. Delayed diagnosis of tuberculosis in patients with human immunodeficiency virus infection. Am J Med 1990; 89: 451–456

Lanska M J, Lanska D J, Schmidley J W. Syphilitic polyradiculopathy in an HIV-positive man. Neurology 1988; 38: 1297–1301

Levy J H, Liss R A, Maguire A M. Neurosyphilis and ocular syphilis in patients with concurrent human immunodeficiency virus infection. Retina 1989; 9: 175–180

Levy R M, Bredesen D E. Central nervous system dysfunction in acquired immunodeficiency syndrome. In: Rosenblum M L, Levy R M, Bredesen D E, editors. AIDS and the nervous system. New York: Raven Press, 1988: 29–63

Lukehart S A, Hook E W, Baker-Zander S A, et al. Invasion of the central nervous system by *Treponema pallidum*: implications for diagnosis and treatment. Ann Intern Med 1988; 109: 855–862

Mann J M, Tarantola D J M, Netter T W. AIDS in the world. Cambridge, MA: Harvard University Press, 1992

Martin J P. Amyotrophic meningo-myelitis (spinal progressive muscular atrophy of syphilitic origin). Brain 1925; 48: 153–182

Mascola L, Lieb L, Chiu J, et al. Listeriosis: an uncommon opportunistic infection in patients with acquired immunodeficiency syndrome. Am J Med 1988; 84: 162–164

McArthur J C, Alwood K, Fox R, et al. Effect of previous syphilis infection on CSF abnormalities in HIV-1 infected individuals. V Int Conf AIDS 1989 (abstr)

McArthur J C, Cohen B A, Farzedegan H, et al. Cerebrospinal fluid abnormalities in homosexual men with and without neuropsychiatric findings. Ann Neurol 1988; 23: S34–S37

McMillan A, Young H, Peutherer J F. Influence of human immunodeficiency virus infection on treponemal serology, in patients who have been treated for syphilis. J Infect 1990; 21: 95–103

Merritt H H, Adams R D, Solomon H C. Neurosyphilis. New York: Oxford University Press, 1946

Mills C H. Routine examination of the cerebrospinal fluid in syphilis: its value in regard to more accurate knowledge, prognosis, and treatment. Br Med J 1927; 2: 527–532

Modilevsky T, Sattler F R, Barnes P F. Mycobacterial disease in patients with human immunodeficiency syndrome virus infection. Arch Intern Med 1989; 149: 2201–2205

Monno L, Carbonara S, Costa D, et al. Emergence of drug-resistant *Mycobacterium tuberculosis* in HIV-infected patients. Lancet 1991; 337: 852

Moore J E. Studies in asymptomatic neurosyphilis. II. The classification, treatment, and prognosis of early asymptomatic neurosyphilis. Bull Johns Hopkins Hosp 1922; 33: 231–246

Moore J E. Syphilitic iritis. A study of 249 patients. Am J Ophthalmol 1933; 14: 110–126

Moore J E, Hopkins H H. Asymptomatic neurosyphilis. XI. The prognosis of early and late asymptomatic neurosyphilis. JAMA 1930; 95: 1637–1641

Musher D M. Syphilis, neurosyphilis, penicillin, and AIDS. J Infect Dis 1991; 63: 1201–1206

Musher D M, Hamill R J, Baughn R D. Effect of human immunodeficiency virus (HIV) infection on the course of syphilis and on the response to treatment. Ann Intern Med 1990; 113: 872–881

Nakane A, Minagawa T, Kato K. Endogenous tumour necrosis factor (cachectin) is essential to host resistance against *Listeria monocytogenes* infection. Infect Immun 1988; 56: 2563–2569

Pitchenik A E, Fertel D. Tuberculosis and nontuberculous mycobacterial disease. Med Clin North Am 1992; 76: 121–171

Romanowski B, Sutherland R, Fick G H, et al. Serologic response to treatment of infectious syphilis. Ann Intern Med 1991; 114: 1005–1009

Rompalo A M, Cannon R O, Quinn T C, Hook E W. Association of biologic false-positive reactions for syphilis with human immunodeficiency virus infection. J Infect Dis 1992; 165: 1124–1126

Selwin P A, Hartel D, Lewis V A, et al. A prospective study of the risk of tuberculosis among intravenous drug users with human immunodeficiency syndrome virus infection. N Engl J Med 1989; 320: 545–550

Shafer R W, Kim D S, Weiss J P, Quale J M. Extrapulmonary tuberculosis in patients with human immunodeficiency virus infection. Medicine 1991; 70: 384–397

Simon R P. Neurosyphilis. Arch Neurol 1985; 42: 606–616

Spence M R, Abrutyn E. Syphilis and infection with the human immunodeficiency virus. Ann Intern Med 1987; 107: 587

Stamm L V, Dallas W S, Ray P H, Bassford P J. Identification, cloning, and purification of protein antigens of *Treponema pallidum*. Rev Infect Dis 1988; 10 (suppl 2): S403–S407

Stokes J H, Beerman H, Ingraham N R. Modern clinical syphilology: diagnosis, treatment, case study. Philadelphia: WB Saunders, 1944

Stoneburner R, Laroche E, Prevots R, et al. Survival in a cohort of human immunodeficiency virus-infected tuberculous patients in New York City. Arch Intern Med 1992; 152: 2033–2037

Sudre P, ten Dam G, Kochi A. Tuberculosis: a global overview of the situation today. Bull WHO 1992; 70: 149–159

Terry P M, Page M L, Goldmeier D. Are serological tests of value in diagnosing and monitoring response to treatment of syphilis in patients infected with human immunodeficiency virus? Genitourin Med 1988; 64: 219–222

Tramont E C. Syphilis in the AIDS era. New Engl J Med 1987; 316: 1600–1601

Wicher K, Noordhoek G T, Abbruscato F, Wicher V. Detection of *Treponema pallidum* in early syphilis by DNA amplification. J Clin Microbiol 1992; 30: 497–500

Williams I, Mindel A, Weller I V D. AIDS pocket picture guide. Philadelphia: Lippincott, 1989: 84

Winward K E, Hamed L M, Glaser J S. The spectrum of optic nerve disease in human immunodeficiency virus infection. Am J Ophthalmol 1989; 107: 373–380

Young L S. *Mycobacterium avium* complex infection. J Infect Dis 1988; 157: 863–867

Zakowski P, Fliegel S, Berlin G W, Johnson L. Disseminated *Mycobacterium avium-intracellulare* infection in homosexual men dying of acquired immunodeficiency. JAMA 1982; 248: 2980–2982

11. Opportunistic infections – parasites

TOXOPLASMOSIS

Prior to 1980, cerebral toxoplasmosis was a rarely encountered complication of immunosuppression, for example in renal transplant recipients. With the AIDS epidemic it has become a frequent cause of encephalitis, and a *Toxoplasma* abscess is the most common cause of a cerebral mass lesion in adult patients with AIDS (Navia 1986, Holliman 1988).

Central nervous system (CNS) infection with

Toxoplasma gondii, an obligate intracellular protozoan, causes necrotic abscesses that are often multifocal and scattered throughout the cerebral hemispheres with a predilection for the basal ganglia (Figs 11.1 and 11.2). The infection is caused by the reactivation of latent organisms encysted within the brain as opposed to the 'true' opportunistic infection of cryptococcosis. Frequently, the abscesses contain both tissue cysts (bradyzoites) and the active organisms (tachyzoites) in an area with prominent macrophage infiltration (Fig. 11.3). *T. gondii* is spread by ingestion of oocysts or tissue cysts in undercooked meat. The oocysts are excreted in the faeces of cats, the definitive hosts. Ingestion leads to disseminated infection of the new host, perhaps manifested as a glandular-fever-like illness with lifelong encystment in any tissue (Fig. 11.4). T helper cells and activated macrophages are

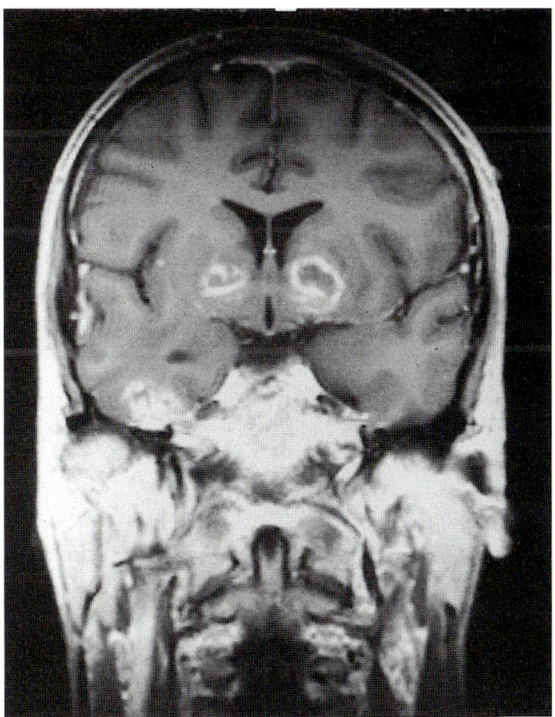

Fig. 11.1   MRI T1-weighted images showing ring-enhancing lesions due to toxoplasmosis in the basal ganglia.

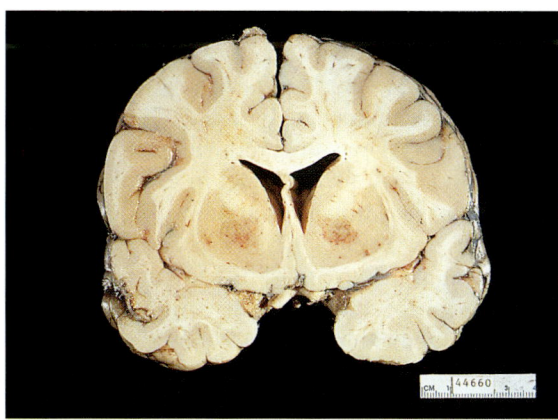

Fig. 11.2   Coronal brain slice showing necrotic *Toxoplasma* abscesses in the basal ganglia.

171

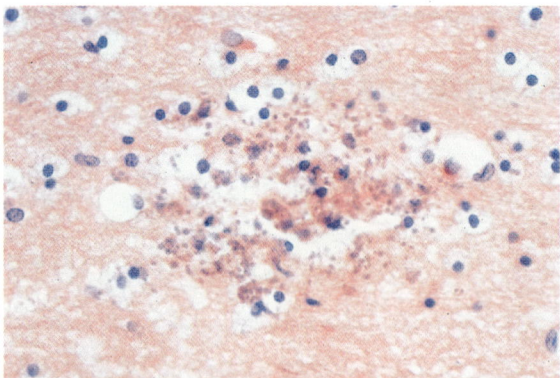

Fig. 11.3 *Toxoplasma* tachyzoites in an area of macrophage inflammation.

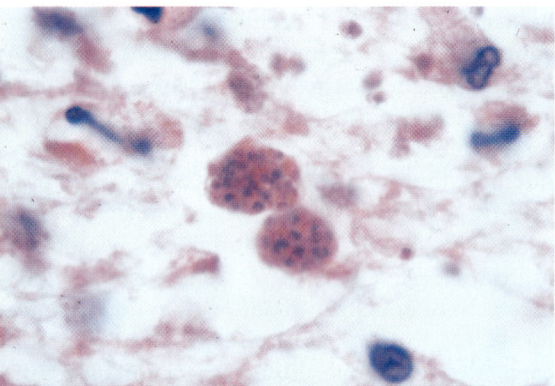

Fig. 11.4 *Toxoplasma* cysts in the brain.

involved in the containment and elimination of the parasite; the advent of AIDS therefore leads to failure of suppression and the development of pathological infection at sites of encysted organisms, e.g. in the brain. Exposure levels vary widely between communities dependent on their dietary habits. Seroprevalence studies show high levels of exposure in adults in France, Germany and central Africa when compared with those found in the UK and USA, for example. In France as many as 90% of the adult population have serum IgG antibodies to *Toxoplasma*, whilst the figures for the UK and USA are less than 50% (Holliman 1990). Disease in AIDS patients is virtually always a reactivation, with 97% showing IgG but few IgM antibodies. About 25% of patients with AIDS in Berlin and Paris will develop *Toxoplasma* encephalitis, compared with an incidence of 10% in some parts of the USA. The estimated proba-

bility of developing cerebral toxoplasmosis is 28% for antibody-positive individuals (Grant et al 1990). Surveillance data from the Centers for Disease Control (CDC) show that toxoplasmosis occurred in 2.68% of the first 23 307 patients with AIDS in the USA (Levy et al 1988). However, in some regions toxoplasmosis is seen much more frequently, in up to 20% of patients, possibly because of referral patterns or geographical differences in *T. gondii* primary exposure.

Toxoplasmosis typically presents with the development of fever (about 30–40%), headache, altered mentation, seizures and focal neurological

Table 11.1 Clinical features of cerebral toxoplasmosis

Headache
Fever
Confusion
Hemiparesis, other focal signs
Posterior fossa syndrome
Seizures
Raised intracranial pressure

Table 11.2 Signs and symptoms of cerebral toxoplasmosis

Variable	Number	%
Symptoms		
Headache	63	55
Confusion	60	52
Fever	54	47
Lethargy	49	43
Seizures	33	29
Poor coordination/gait	29	25
Focal weakness	25	22
Nausea or vomiting	20	17
Visual disturbance	17	15
Incontinence	8	7
Neck stiffness	4	3
Signs		
Focal signs	79	69
Hemiparesis	45	39
Ataxia	34	30
Cranial nerve palsies	32	28
Sensory deficits	14	12
Aphasia	9	8
Hemianopsia	8	7
Temperature > 38.4°C	54	47
Abnormal level of consciousness	48	42
Mildly decreased	31	27
Minimal response	13	11
Obtunded	4	3
Psychomotor retardation	44	38
Meningismus	11	10
Behavioural disturbance	5	4

(Reproduced from Porter & Sande 1992 with permission of The New England Journal of Medicine)

signs (Table 11.1) developing over a few days (Navia et al 1986). The examination usually reveals an obtunded and/or confused patient who is obviously unwell. Focal signs commonly take the form of a progressive hemispheric syndrome with aphasia or hemiparesis, or the features of posterior fossa lesions with dysarthria and ataxia (Table 11.2). Neck stiffness is found in only about 10%. Despite the propensity for toxoplasmosis to develop subacutely and to cause focal neurological deficits, the clinical features are not sufficiently specific to allow distinction from primary CNS lymphoma, the other major process associated with intracranial mass lesions in AIDS.

In both conditions (toxoplasmosis and lymphoma), imaging studies demonstrate multiple contrast-enhancing mass lesions (Fig. 11.5). Areas of oedema usually surround *Toxoplasma* lesions, sometimes producing mass effect and shift of surrounding structures (Fig. 11.6). *Toxoplasma* abscesses are more typically small 'ring' lesions (Fig. 11.9), whereas lymphoma

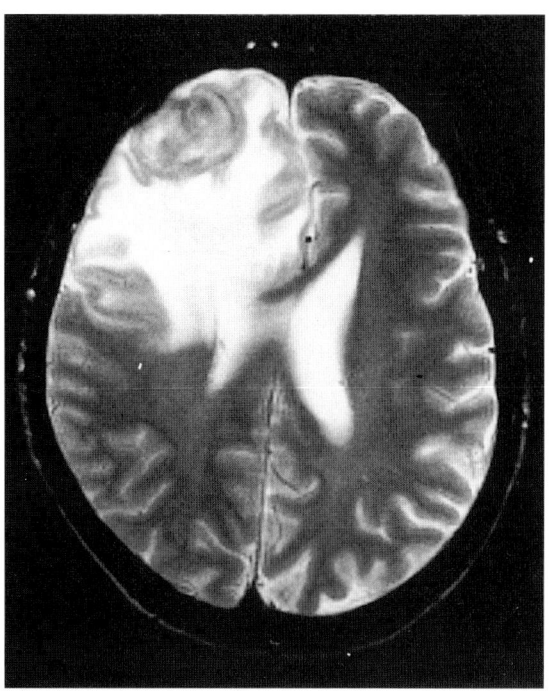

Fig. 11.6   Marked oedema around a frontal *Toxoplasma* abscess on T2-weighted MRI.

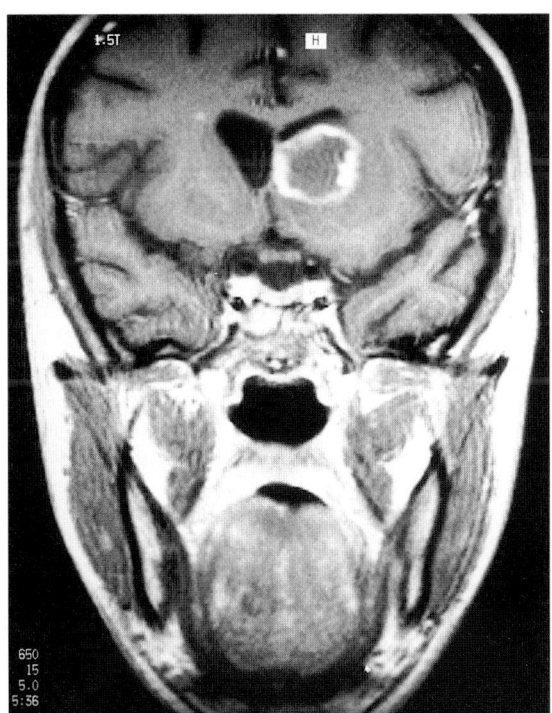

Fig. 11.5   Single lesion on MRI (T1 with gadolinium) abutting the ventricle due to toxoplasmosis, but difficult to distinguish from a lymphoma.

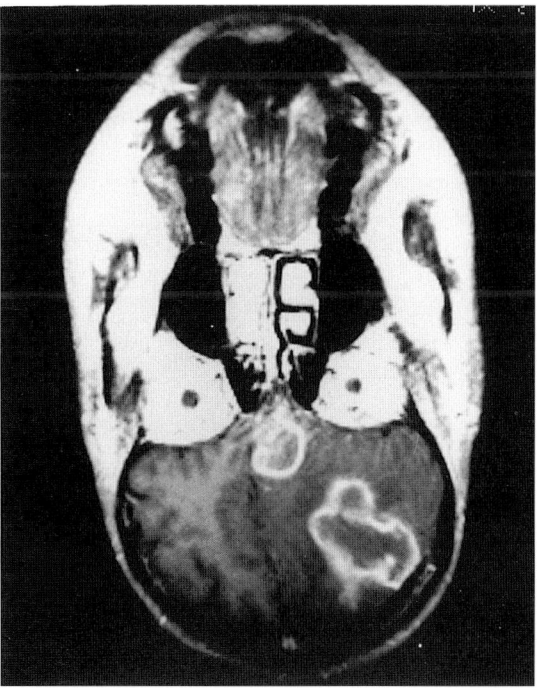

Fig. 11.7   Multiple ring-enhancing *Toxoplasma* abscesses.

Table 11.3   Radiological findings in 103 patients with toxoplasmosis

	%
Appearance	
Contrast-enhancing lesions	91
Ring enhancement	82
Mild oedema	22
Mass effect	55
Location	
Basal ganglia	48
Frontal	48
Parietal	37
Occipital	19
Temporal	18
Cerebellar	15
Centrum semiovale	10
Thalamus	10
Number of lesions	
1	27
2	22
3	21
≥ 4	26

(Reproduced from Porter & Sande 1992 with permission of The New England Journal of Medicine)

lesions are larger with more heterogeneous enhancement. The abscesses show an unexplained predilection for the basal ganglia (Fig. 11.1). Other areas affected, in order of frequency, include frontal, parietal and occipital lobes, and occasionally the cerebellum (Table 11.3). Contrast magnetic resonance imaging (MRI) is more sensitive than computed tomography (Fig. 11.8), frequently showing lesions that are not identifiable even on contrast CT (Levy et al 1985, 1986). Enhancement when the lesion is small may be 'solid' rather than of 'ring' pattern (Fig. 11.9). MRI may reveal second lesions when CT suggests a single mass (Fig. 11.10). Unfortunately, neither the number of discrete CT or MRI lesions, their location, nor their radiological characteristics allows for reliable differentiation of toxoplasmosis from lymphoma or other

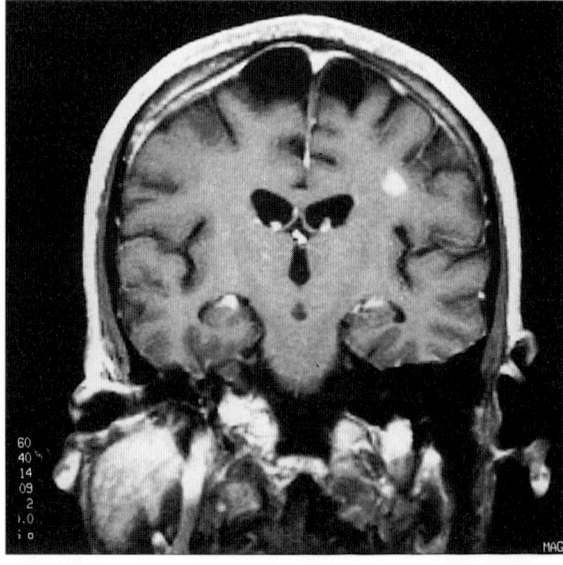

Fig. 11.9   Small *Toxoplasma* abscess with 'solid'-looking enhancement on T1 MRI.

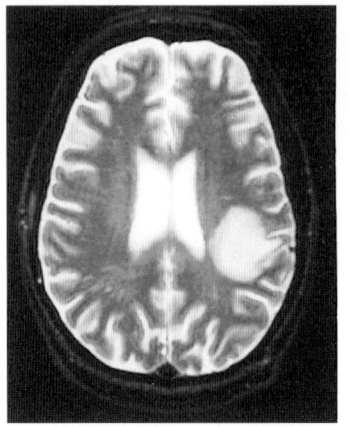 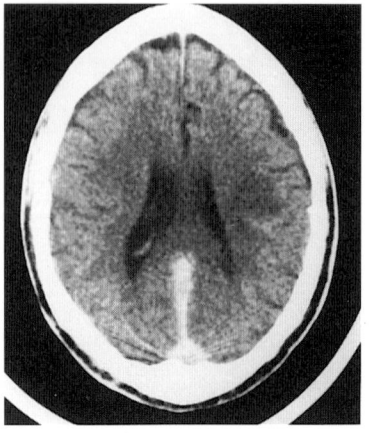

Fig. 11.8   Comparison of sensitivity of cranial MRI and CT. T2-weighted MRI (left) shows a large area of oedema in the left parietal lobe. A corresponding enhanced CT scan defines the area less definitely.

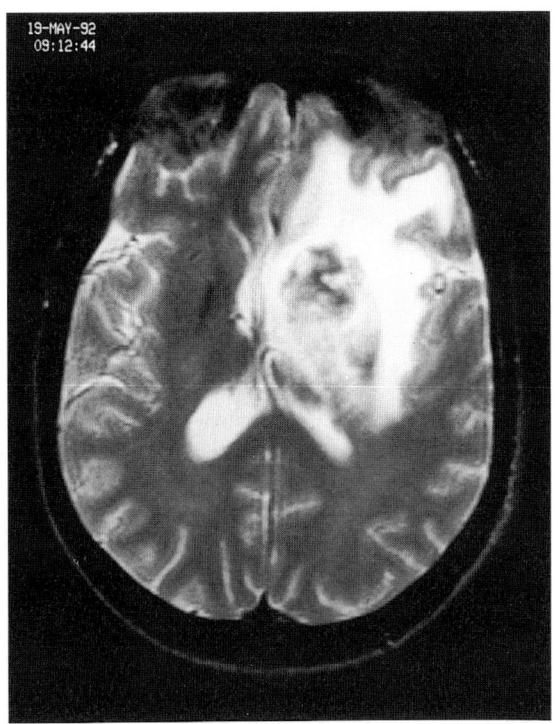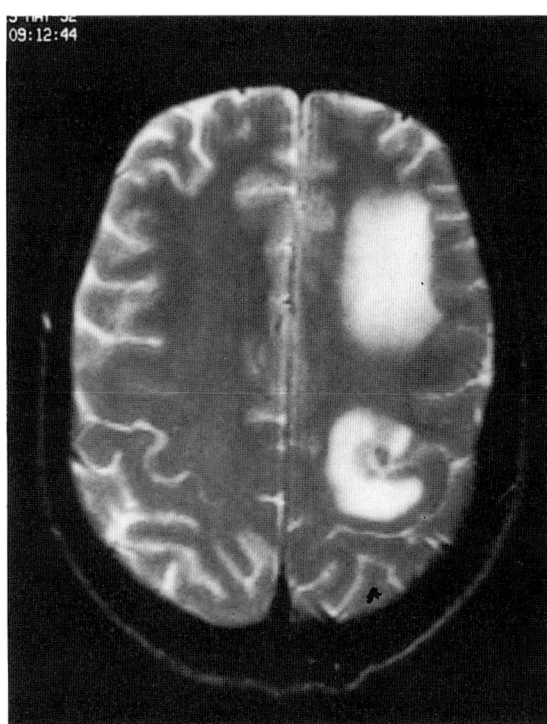

A   B

Fig. 11.10   Though this lesion looks single on one 'slice' (**A**), there are in fact two abscesses (**B**).

causes of brain abscess. Cerebrospinal fluid (CSF) is usually abnormal, with elevated protein and pleocytosis. However, because of the mass effect associated with *Toxoplasma* abscesses, lumbar puncture often has to be deferred to avoid herniation. Serological testing is not diagnostic; however, because this is a reactivated infection, 85% or more of patients with toxoplasmosis have detectable anti-*Toxoplasma* IgG. Negative serologies may reflect false negatives because of the tests' insensitivity. Israelski et al (1993) found 117 of 1073 HIV-positive individuals to be seropositive for toxoplasmosis. Five out of 13 seropositive patients who progressed to AIDS also developed cerebral toxoplasmosis, but none of 183 seronegative individuals did, despite progression to AIDS. Measurement of intrathecal synthesis of anti-*Toxoplasma* antibody has been suggested as a useful diagnostic test, but in practice CSF cannot always be safely obtained from patients with large mass lesions. When it can be safely studied, polymerase chain reaction (PCR) may be helpful. Schoondermark-van de Ven et al (1993) found *T. gondii* using primers against the B1 gene in 13 of

20 patients with presumed cerebral toxoplasmosis. CSF samples from nine seropositive for *Toxoplasma* patients without CNS disease were negative. In a separate study Ostergaard et al (1993) found *Toxoplasma* positive CSF by PCR in all five patients with cerebral infection and one false positive.

The diagnosis in practice depends on the suspicious clinical picture and on compatible neuroimaging by CT (Fig. 11.11) or MRI (Fig. 11.7). The role of brain biopsy in the management of patients with AIDS and intracranial mass lesions has changed over the past few years, as experience has accumulated with empirical *Toxoplasma* therapy. In the early days of the epidemic, brain biopsy was routinely recommended for the diagnosis of cerebral toxoplasmosis, a reaction to the lack of specificity of serology and imaging. Needle biopsy occasionally proved inconclusive, however, and open biopsy carried a real risk of deterioration in these sick patients. Furthermore, the diagnosis might remain uncertain after biopsy, though the advent of PCR improves detection of the organism

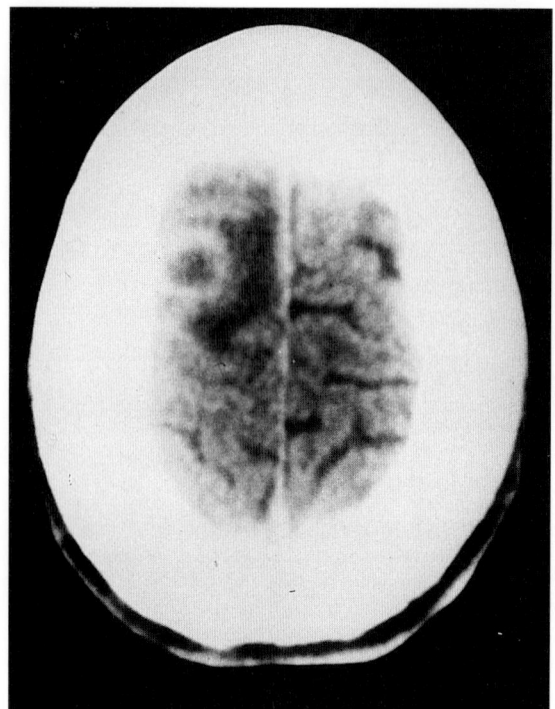

Fig. 11.11 CT scan showing a ring-enhancing *Toxoplasma* abscess in the frontal lobe.

ical diagnosis for several reasons. First, the biopsy may miss the lesion or sample only the necrotic core of the abscess. Second, therapy has often been started at the time of biopsy, making it difficult to recognize the tachyzoites histologically. Last, routine haematoxylin and eosin staining is insensitive, and immunoperoxidase staining should be used (Luft et al 1984, Moskowitz et al 1984). A recent report of 31 stereotactic biopsies from Vienna (Alesch et al 1993) revealed that 35% of cerebral lesions were due to toxoplasmosis. Many of these patients had had 2 weeks of anti-*Toxoplasma* treatment, but had deteriorated clinically or failed to improve clinically or on a CT scan. The implication is that response may be delayed.

Rarely an encephalitic process is seen without abscess formation. The clinical picture resembles herpes encephalitis (Carrazana et al 1989) or even HIV dementia (Arendt et al 1991). Neuroimaging may be normal and the only clues lie in the positive blood serology, evidence in the CSF of intrathecal production of anti-*Toxoplasma* IgG, and in the response to treatment.

Toxoplasma myelitis

There have been several case reports of *Toxoplasma* myelitis in AIDS. Some of the cases were recognized only after cord biopsy or at postmortem examination. Most had cord enlargement with contrast-enhancing intramedullary lesions (Herskovitz et al 1989, Harris et al 1990, Kayser et al 1990, Overhage et al 1990).

Toxoplasma chorioretinitis

T. gondii can affect the eyes, presenting with a painful, inflamed eye, with sudden change in visual acuity. Inflammation in the anterior chamber and vitreous are usually evident and retinal haemorrhages and exudates can develop. Response to pyrimethamine and sulphadiazine is usually good.

Treatment of cerebral toxoplasmosis (Fig. 11.12)

Prompt initiation of treatment with pyrimeth-

(Holliman et al 1990). Unfortunately the technique at present does not distinguish between quiescent cysts and an active disease process. The search continues for primers to detect the RNA of the active tachyzoite. At present, empirical therapy for toxoplasmosis is started for patients with AIDS presenting with contrast-enhancing intracranial mass lesions. Cimino et al (1991), using Bayesian analysis, showed that a mass lesion was more likely to be due to toxoplasmosis if there was enhancement on CT scanning and if, in addition, *Toxoplasma* antibody titres were greater than 1:64. Biopsy can be reserved for individuals who (a) fail a 2-week trial of empirical toxoplasmosis therapy; (b) have atypical presentations, e.g. single large lesions developing over several months; or (c) would tolerate biopsy and radiation therapy if a lymphoma were found. Stereotactic CT or MRI-guided biopsy is, in general, preferable to open biopsy, and allows for precise biopsy of deep-seated lesions with minimal morbidity. In cerebral toxoplasmosis, biopsies can fail to provide a definitive patholog-

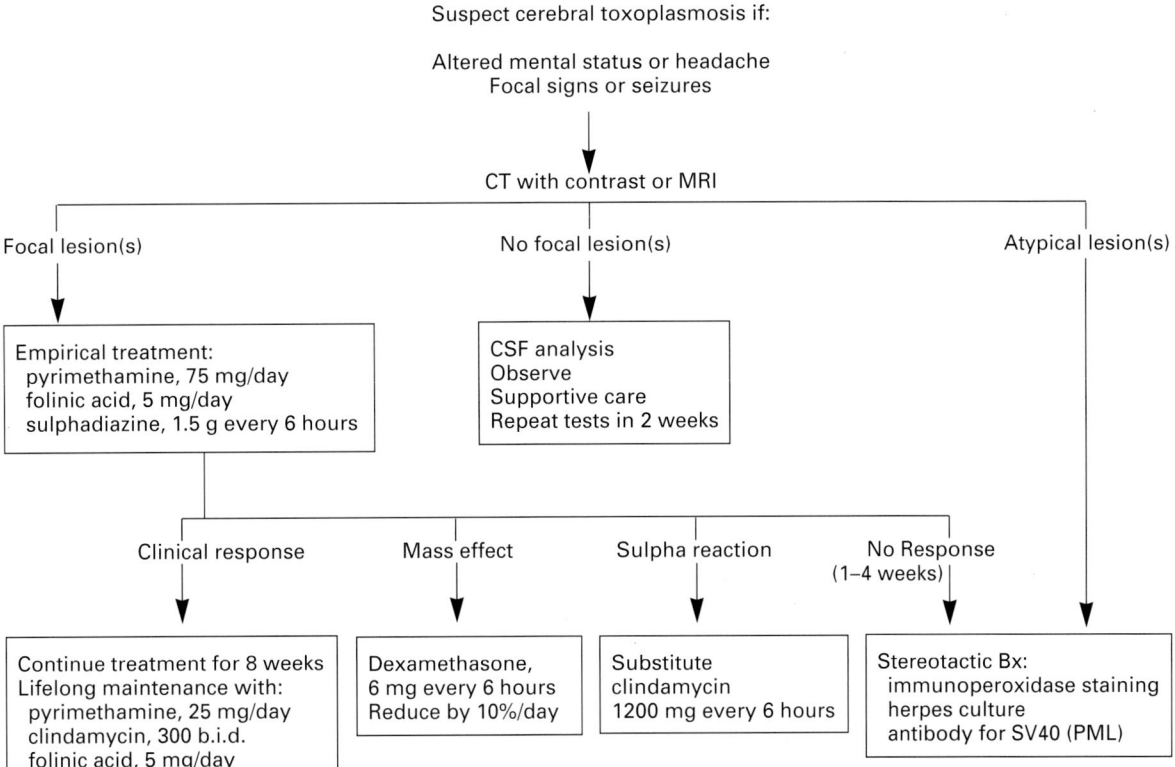

Fig. 11.12   Treatment of cerebral toxoplasmosis.

amine and sulphadiazine (Table 11.4) will lead to clinical and radiological improvement in 80% of cases within 1–4 weeks (Navia et al 1986, McArthur 1987) (Fig. 11.13). MRI monitoring may be more sensitive than CT to early response. A change in enhancement may precede reduction in size and prove to be a useful pointer (personal observations). Sulphamethoxazole, sulphadiazine

and dapsone inhibit dihydropteroate synthetase (Kovacs et al 1989). Adverse reactions, including fever, itchy macular rash, stomatitis, headache, leucopenia and chemical hepatitis, are common with sulphamethoxazole, probably related to the hydroxylamine metabolite. Stevens-Johnson syndrome is rare. Desensitization can be performed, although it is complicated and somewhat lengthy. Mild adverse reactions can be managed symptomatically. The adverse effects of dapsone include rash, nausea, haemolysis, methaemoglobinaemia and, rarely, production of a demyelinating peripheral neuropathy. Trimethoprim, pyrimethamine and trimetrexate inhibit dihydrofolate reductase in vitro.

Pyrimethamine is administered orally in a loading dose of 150 mg, and continued at 75 mg daily with 5 mg folinic acid to prevent anaemia. Sulphadiazine is given orally in a dose of 1.5 g every 6 hours. Clindamycin can be substituted for the sulphonamide at a dose of 600 mg every

Table 11.4   Treatment regimen for cerebral toxoplasmosis (4–6 weeks)

Pyrimethamine	150 mg loading dose, 75 mg thereafter
Sulphadiazine	2–8 g daily in divided doses oral or i.v.
Folinic acid	5 mg daily
Alternatives	Clindamycin 600 mg q.d.s. (risk of rash and pseudomembranous colitis), dapsone, atovaquone, azithromycin
Monitor	Blood count. If mild marrow suppression, reduce pyrimethamine. If severe, stop pyrimethamine and sulphadiazine, continue folinic acid and switch to clindamycin

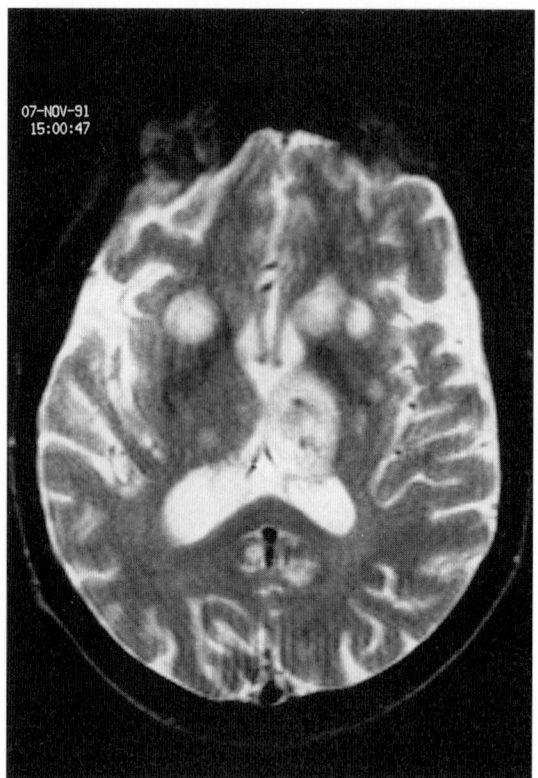
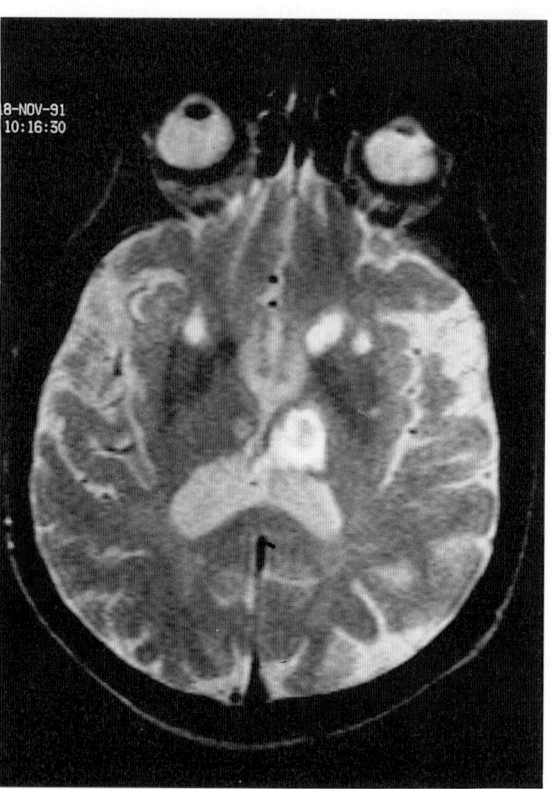

A   B

Fig. 11.13   Response of multiple abscesses to treatment. T2-weighted MRI **A** before and **B** after treatment.

6 hours either orally or intravenously and appears to have equivalent efficacy (Rolston & Hoy 1987). After 6 weeks of induction therapy, maintenance therapy (Table 11.5) of pyrimethamine 25 mg daily with folinic acid and a second agent, either sulphadiazine or clindamycin 300 mg every 6 hours, needs to be continued life-long. Alternative agents that are currently under study include atovaquone and azithromycin. Corticosteroids should be avoided for at least two reasons. First, they will cause additional immune suppression. Second, any mass lesion may show non-specific improvement after steroids, thus masking any effect of the antimicrobial drugs.

Table 11.5   Maintenance regimen after cerebral toxoplasmosis, lifelong

Pyrimethamine	25–50 mg daily
Sulphadiazine	1–3 g daily
Folinic acid	5–50 mg daily
Alternatives	Fansidar/clindamycin/dapsone

However, in patients with large mass lesions with prominent shift and potential for herniation, dexamethasone should be used in doses of 4–10 mg every 6 hours. Of 114 patients treated initially with pyrimethamine, sulphadiazine and leucovorin, six died during the initial episode (Porter & Sande 1992). Between 90 and 95% of those who eventually improved clinically had done so by 2 weeks and all had improved by day 42. Over 95% of patients responded radiologically by 2 weeks (Figs 11.13 and 11.14). Decreased survival was associated with depressed level of consciousness, history of Kaposi's sarcoma or *Pneumocystis carinii pneumonia* (PCP) as an AIDS-defining illness, temperature greater than 38.4°C and blood lymphocyte count ≤ 24%. Multivariate analysis, however, showed only that a history of PCP and a blood lymphocyte count of ≤ 24% were independent predictors of decreased survival. Relapses occurred in 10% of those receiving maintenance pyrimethamine and sulphadiazine and 22% of those receiving pyrimeth-

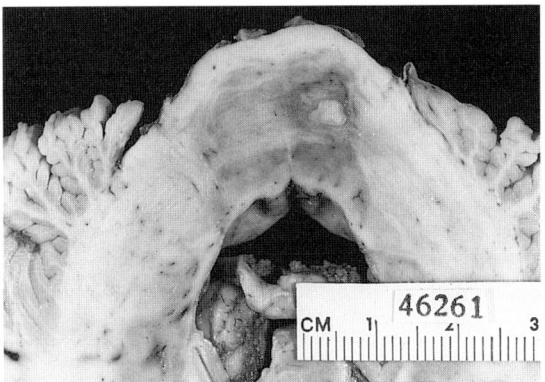

Fig. 11.14 Resolved cerebral toxoplasmosis. Previously treated, now partially calcified pontine *Toxoplasma* abscess. Patient died 2 years after treatment.

amine and clindamycin, but no significant difference in mean relapse-free survival was seen between the two treatment groups. Sixteen per cent had negative serum anti-*Toxoplasma* IgG antibodies (assay by ELISA).

Kovacs (1992) gave atovaquone to eight patients with cerebral toxoplasmosis who were intolerant of standard therapies. They received 750 mg of atovaquone q.i.d. Five patients improved with no recurrence of toxoplasmosis (follow-up 16–60 weeks). One died of other AIDS-related complications after 6 weeks with no evidence of recurrent toxoplasmosis. The two other patients suffered relapses at 10 and 32 weeks respectively. Apart from a rash in one patient, no major side-effects were attributed to the drug. A current trial (ACTG 237) is comparing atovaquone plus pyrimethamine with atovaquone plus sulphadiazine for *Toxoplasma* encephalitis. Another trial (ACTG 156) compares azithromycin and pyrimethamine.

Prophylaxis

Primary prophylactic therapy can be instituted in *Toxoplasma*-seropositive individuals with CD4 counts less than 200. The optimal regimen has not been determined and a community-based trial of pyrimethamine and clindamycin is under way. In a retrospective study comparing trimetho-prim/sulphamethoxazole with aerosolized pentamidine, as secondary prophylaxis for PCP, no patient in the trimethoprim/sulphamethoxazole group developed toxoplasmosis after 3 years of follow-up, while one-third of those in the aerosolized pentamidine group developed toxoplasmosis after a mean period of 15 months (Carr et al 1992).

In another controlled trial comparing aerosolized pentamidine or trimethoprim/sulphamethoxazole for primary prophylaxis (Schneider et al 1992), 215 HIV-positive patients with a CD4 count <200 received either monthly aerosolized pentamidine, daily 80 mg trimethoprim and 400 mg of sulphamethoxazole, or 160 mg trimethoprim and 800 mg sulphamethoxazole. Three patients died of toxoplasmosis in the pentamidine group, while none died of this cause among those who received trimethoprim/sulphamethoxazole (Wormser et al 1991, Zangerle & Allerberger 1991). In a controlled trial of trimethoprim/sulphamethoxazole versus aerosolized pentamidine for secondary prophylaxis in 310 adults with recent PCP, patients received 160 mg of trimethoprim and 800 mg of sulphamethoxazole daily or aerosolized pentamidine (Hardy et al 1992). Four cases of toxoplasmosis were seen in those randomly assigned to trimethoprim/sulphamethoxazole compared with six receiving aerosolized pentamidine. A controlled French study compared dapsone 50 mg/day plus pyrimethamine 50 mg/week and folinic acid to aerosolized pentamidine for primary prophylaxis of both PCP and toxoplasmosis in 349 HIV-seropositive individuals with a CD4 count less than 200. The dapsone/pyrimethamine regimen showed a highly significant protective effect with only 15 cases compared with 29 in the aerosolized pentamidine group. Seven of 15 cases occurred after discontinuation of dapsone/pyrimethamine. All occurred in *T. gondii*-seropositive individuals. The principal side-effects were rash and haematological toxicity. Girard et al (1993) reported toxoplasmosis in 32 of 176 patients on pentamidine but in only 19 of 173 patients on dapsone and pyrimethamine. Those who were seropositive for toxoplasmosis had a 2.37 times higher incidence if on pentamidine. The numbers who defaulted on treatment were higher for dapsone and pyrimethamine, however. As atovaquone is effective in the treatment of PCP, though not as reliable as bactrim (Girard et al 1993), it may prove a useful alternative.

Recommendations

Primary prophylaxis should be given to *T. gondii*-seropositive individuals with a CD4 count less than 200. Current regimens of trimethoprim/sulphamethoxazole for PCP prophylaxis (Recommendations 1992) should provide the additional protection against toxoplasmosis. For patients unable to tolerate sulpha medications, dapsone with pyrimethamine 50 mg/weekly with folinic acid is recommended.

Management plan

Patients with a short history of change in mental state, focal deficit, seizures or headache, whether or not they are febrile, warrant imaging to detect *Toxoplasma* abscesses. Serology can help indicate whether the diagnosis is unlikely, or possible. MRI is more sensitive than CT. Multiple ring-enhancing mass lesions with surrounding oedema are typically found. Aggressive treatment with pyrimethamine and sulphonamide, or clindamycin in those revealing allergy to sulpha drugs, should be started on suspicion, and steroids avoided if possible. Lack of clinical and radiological response should prompt reconsideration of the diagnosis and consideration of a brain biopsy. Success should be followed by long-term pyrimethamine and low-dose sulphonamide or clindamycin. Neurologically normal subjects with serological evidence of prior exposure to *Toxoplasma* with CD4 counts at or below 200 should be offered prophylaxis.

OTHER PARASITES

Rare cases have been documented of cerebral infection in AIDS patients by *Acanthamoeba*, *Trypanasoma* and *Pneumocystis*.

Amoeba

Free-living amoebae are rare causes of meningo-encephalitis in man. An acute amoebic meningo-encephalitis is usually due to *Naegleria* and affects otherwise healthy children and young adults who have been in recent contact with brackish water. The illness is an acute pyogenic meningitis with trophozoites in the CSF and in areas of haemorrhagic necrosis in the brain. By contrast, *Acanthamoeba* produces a subacute or chronic meningitis or brain abscess in immunosuppressed patients. Three examples in AIDS have been reported (Gonzalez et al 1986, Wiley et al 1987, Gardner et al 1991).

A primary focus of infection, for example in the skin, may be apparent. The neurological illness is often of insidious onset with headache, fever and focal signs related to abscess formation. Scans reveal multiple necrotic areas or abscesses. The CSF is unhelpful as trophozoites are not usually seen or cultured. Any pleocytosis is non-specific. The differential diagnosis includes toxoplasmosis and tuberculosis. The diagnosis is unlikely to be made without biopsy. Extensive demyelination associated with the trophozoites suggests that *Acanthamoeba* produces cytokines, but the necrotic areas and abscesses depend on a granulomatous giant cell encephalitis. A necrotizing thromboangiitis with amoebae in the vessel wall can also be seen (Gardner et al 1991). There are no drugs of proven efficacy though 5-fluorocytosine and sulphonamides have some in vitro or experimental basis.

REFERENCES

Alesch F, Armbruster Ch, Vole D, Budka H. Stereotactic biopsy of cerebral lesions in AIDS: the Vienna experience. Clin Neuropathol 1993; 12 (suppl 1): S15

Arendt G, Hefter H, Figge C, et al. Two cases of cerebral toxoplasmosis in AIDS patients mimicking HIV-related dementia. J Neurol 1991; 238: 439–442

Carr A, Tindall B, Brew B J, et al. Low-dose trimethoprim-sulfamethoxazole prophylaxis for toxoplasmic encephalitis in patients with AIDS. Ann Intern Med 1992; 117: 106–111

Carrazana E J, Rossitch Jr E, Schachter S. Cerebral toxoplasmosis masquerading as herpes encephalitis in a patient with the acquired immunodeficiency syndrome. Am J Med 1989; 86: 730–732

Cimino C, Lipton R B, Williams A, et al. The evaluation of patients with human immunodeficiency virus-related disorders and brain mass lesions. Arch Intern Med 1991; 151: 1381–1384

Gardner H A R, Martinez A J, Visvesvara G S, Sotrel A. Granulomatous amebic encephalitis in an AIDS patient. Neurology 1991; 41: 1993–1995

Girard P M, Landman R, Gaudebout C, et al. Dapsone pyrimethamine compared with aerosolized pentamidine as primary prophylaxis against *Pneumocystis carinii* pneumonia and toxoplasmosis in HIV infection. New Eng J Med 1993; 328: 1514–1520

Gonzalez M M, Gould E, Dickinson G, et al. Acquired immunodeficiency syndrome associated with *Acanthamoeba* infection and other opportunistic infections. Arch Pathol Lab Med 1986; 110: 749–751

Grant I H, Gold J M W, Rosenblum M, et al. *Toxoplasma gondii* serology in HIV-infected patients: the development of central nervous system toxoplasmosis in AIDS. AIDS 1990; 4: 519–521

Hardy W D, Feinberg J, Finkelstein D M, et al. A controlled trial of trimethoprim sulfamethoxazole or aerosolized pentamidine for secondary prophylaxis of *Pneumocystis carinii* pneumonia in patients with the acquired immunodeficiency syndrome. AIDS Clinical Trial Group Protocol 021. N Engl J Med 1992; 327: 1842–1848

Harris T M, Smith R R, Edwards M K. Toxplasmic myelitis in AIDS: gadolinium-enhanced MR. J Comput Assist Tomogr 1990; 14: 809–811

Herskovitz S, Siegel S E, Schneider A T, et al. Spinal cord toxoplasmosis in AIDS. Neurology 1989; 39: 1552–1553

Holliman R E. Toxoplasma and the acquired immune deficiency syndrome. J Infect 1988; 16: 121–128

Holliman R E. Serological study of the prevalence of toxoplasmosis in asymptomatic patients infected with human immunodeficiency virus. Epidemiol Infect 1990; 105: 415–418

Holliman R E, Johnson J D, Savva D. Diagnosis of cerebral toxoplasmosis in association with AIDS using polymerase chain reaction. Scand J Infect Dis 1990; 22: 243–244

Israelski D M, Chmiel J S, Poggensee L, et al. Prevalence of toxoplasma infection in a cohort of homosexual men at risk of AIDS and toxoplasma encephalitis. J AIDS 1993; 6: 414–418

Kayser C, Campbell R, Sartorious C, Bartlett M. Toxoplasmosis of the conus medullaris in a patient with hemophilia A-associated AIDS. Case report. J Neurosurg 1990; 73: 951–953

Kovacs J A. Efficacy of atovaquone in treatment of toxoplasmosis in patients with AIDS. The NIAID-Clinical Center Intramural AIDS Program. Lancet 1992; 340: 637–638

Kovacs J A, Allergra C J, Beaver J, et al. Characterization of de novo folate synthesis of *Pneumocystis carinii* and *Toxoplasma gondii*: potential for screening therapeutic agents. J Infect Dis 1989; 160: 312–320

Levy R M, Bredesen D E, Rosenblum M L. Neurological manifestations of the acquired immunodeficiency syndrome (AIDS): experience at UCSF and review of the literature. J Neurosurg 1985; 62: 475–495

Levy R M, Janssen R S, Bush T J, et al. Neuroepidemiology of acquired immunodeficiency syndrome. J AIDS 1988; 1: 31–40

Levy R M, Rosenbloom S, Perrett L V. Neuroradiologic findings in AIDS: a review of 200 cases. AJR 1986; 147: 977–983

Luft B J, Brooks R G, Conley F K, et al. Toxoplasmic encephalitis in patients with acquired immune deficiency syndrome. JAMA 1984; 252: 913–917

McArthur J C. Neurologic manifestations of AIDS. Medicine (Baltimore) 1987; 66: 407–437

Moskowitz L B, Hensley G T, Chan J C, et al. Brain biopsies in patients with acquired immune deficiency syndrome. Arch Pathol Lab Med 1984; 108: 368–371

Navia B A, Petito C K, Gold J W, et al. Cerebral toxoplasmosis complicating the acquired immune deficiency syndrome: clinical and neuropathological findings in 27 patients. Ann Neurol 1986; 19: 224–238

Ostergaard L, Nielsen A K, Black F T. DNA amplification on cerebrospinal fluid for diagnosis of cerebral toxoplasmosis among HIV-positive patients with signs or symptoms of neurological disease. Scand J Infect Dis 1993; 25: 227–237

Overhage J M, Greist A, Brown D R. Conus medullaris syndrome resulting from *Toxoplasma gondii* infection in a patient with the acquired immunodeficiency syndrome. Am J Med 1990; 89: 814–815

Porter S B, Sande M A. Toxoplasmosis of the central nervous system in acquired immunodeficiency syndrome. N Engl J Med 1992; 327: 1643–1648

Recommendations for prophylaxis against *Pneumocystis carinii* pneumonia for adults and adolescents infected with human immunodeficiency virus. MMWR 1992; 41(RR-4): 1–11

Rolston K V, Hoy J. Role of clindamycin in the treatment of central nervous system toxoplasmosis. Am J Med 1987; 83: 551–554

Schneider M M E, Hoepelman A I M, Schattenkerk J K M E, et al. Dutch AIDS Treatment Group. A controlled trial of aerosolized pentamidine or trimethoprim-sulfamethoxazole as primary prophylaxis against *Pneumocystis carinii* pneumonia in patients with human immunodeficiency virus infection. N Engl J Med 1992; 327: 1838–1841

Schoondermark-van de Ven E, Galama J, Kraaijeveld C, et al. Value of polymerase chain reaction for the detection of *Toxoplasma gondii* in cerebrospinal fluid from patients with AIDS. Clin Infect Dis 1993; 16: 661–666

Wiley C A, Safrin R E, Davis C E, et al. *Acanthamoeba* meningoencephalitis in a patient with AIDS. J Infect Dis 1987; 155: 130–133

Wormser G P, Horowitz H W, Duncanson F P, et al. Low dose intermittent trimethoprim-sulfamethoxazole for prevention of *Pneumocystis carinii* pneumonia in patients with human immunodeficiency virus infection. Arch Intern Med 1991; 151: 688–692

Zangerle R, Allerberger F. Effect of prophylaxis against *Pneumocystis carinii* on toxoplasma encephalitis. Lancet 1991; 337: 1232

12. Neoplasms

NEOPLASMS IN AIDS: NEUROLOGICAL ASPECTS

As many as one in six people with AIDS in the West will develop a malignancy. Intriguingly these are cancers that appear to develop because of the chronic and profound defects in immune surveillance associated with HIV infection. Viruses and other co-factors, in addition to HIV, may induce malignant transformation directly or indirectly. HIV-positive individuals are at substantially higher risk of developing non-Hodgkin's lymphoma (100 times), or Kaposi's sarcoma (40 000 times) and these two malignancies account for 95% of cancers in AIDS. Cervical dysplasia and condylomata acuminata (genital warts) occur more frequently in HIV-positive individuals and human papilloma virus (HPV) is responsible for most cases of cervical carcinoma, which occurs with increased frequency in HIV-positive women. Other cancers have been found in HIV-infected individuals, for example squamous cell carcinoma of the skin and vulva, although it is not clear that there is a truly increased incidence (Rabkin et al 1991).

KAPOSI'S SARCOMA

Kaposi's sarcoma (KS) was described in 1872 by Moritz Kaposi, a Hungarian dermatologist, as a malignant tumour of the arteries, veins and heart. Prior to AIDS, KS was rare in the USA, affecting mainly the elderly, and was more common among people of Mediterranean and Jewish origins. In the past 30 years, a higher incidence was noted in east and central Africa with two patterns of disease: a rapidly fatal early childhood form with prominent lymph node dissemination, and an adult form affecting males with clusters of indolent cutaneous nodules, usually on the legs. In some races KS is related to HLA-DR5. Immunosuppression, for example after renal transplantation, causes an increased incidence with a mean latency of over 12 months (Qunibi et al 1988). KS is at least six times more common among homosexual men than other HIV exposure groups and some investigators have speculated that these epidemiological differences indicate the action of a second sexually transmitted agent (Jacobson et al 1990). Environmental factors or other infectious agents may play a role in the development of KS and there is evidence that oral–faecal contact may play a role. In the USA, a declining proportion of KS as the first AIDS-defining illness was noticed initially (Rutherford et al 1989) and more recent analyses from the Multicenter AIDS Cohort Study (MACS) show a downward trend in the incidence of KS after 1988 (Munoz et al 1993). This downward trend may in part reflect the fact that non-KS AIDS diagnoses present first in severely immunocompromised patients. Alternatively, antiretrovirals may have a protective role and changes in sexual behaviour may have reduced the exposure to the hypothesized agent for KS (Jacobson et al 1990).

Homosexual men with AIDS have as much as a 25% risk of developing cutaneous or systemic KS. KS in AIDS is usually nodular in form and the raised lesions are often purple, violet or dark brown, although they can be non-pigmented or plaque-like. They are generally 0.5–2.0 cm in diameter and develop in typical sites: the lower legs, palate and medial canthus of the eye. Usually the lesions are painless, but large lesions can be very painful, and in the groin can coalesce to produce lymphatic obstruction and lymph-oedema. Visceral involvement develops in most cases, although it may be silent. Infiltration of the gastrointestinal tract causes bleeding and infiltration of the lungs producing progressive pulmonary failure or haemorrhage. Endoscopy may reveal endobronchial or gastric lesions that are amenable to biopsy.

Neurological involvement is relatively rare. Peripheral nerves can be directly affected by local infiltration producing neuralgic pain or motor deficits. Rarer still, metastatic lesions have developed in the brain. These behave like other brain metastases, with contrast-enhancing lesions at the grey–white matter junction. In the series of Levy et al (1985), three of 366 AIDS patients with neurological complications had CNS KS. The lesions were vascular with areas of haemorrhage and necrosis, and presented in one patient with hemiparesis (Gorin et al 1985) and in a second with dizziness. CNS involvement with KS is distinctly unusual, however, with no cases recognized in other neurological referral series (McArthur 1987) or series of patients with KS (Snider et al 1983, Welch et al 1984, Koppel et al 1985). CNS KS lesions can bleed, producing coma or a stroke-like illness. Microscopically, CNS KS shows the spindle cell proliferation typical of KS with frequent haemorrhage and haemosiderin pigmentation.

The diagnosis of KS can be easily confirmed with a punch skin biopsy, although the clinical features are sufficiently characteristic that tissue is not needed in most cases. Occasionally, capillary angiomas and benign naevi cause diagnostic confusion.

Treatment of KS depends on the site and extent of involvement. Small cutaneous lesions can be watched carefully and, if enlarging or causing cosmetic concerns, treated with intralesional vincristine or liquid nitrogen. Both treatments usually cause some regression and depigmentation of the lesions. More widespread cutaneous involvement or visceral involvement may require radiotherapy or chemotherapy (Hill 1987). Alpha-interferon has been used for treatment of widespread disease, and high doses $(20 \, \text{mU/m}^2)$ may induce and maintain remissions, particularly in individuals with CD4+ counts above 200 (Mitsuyasu et al 1986, Vadhan-Raj et al 1986).

Chemotherapy for KS includes a variety of different regimens (Odajnyk & Muggia 1985, Volberding 1987). The major limitations to all of these regimens, apart from specific toxicities, have been marrow suppression and the development of opportunistic infections. The more widespread use of haematopoietic growth factors and of effective prophylactic medications may improve treatment responses in the future. Vincristine is a component of many of the regimens and the development of a toxic sensorimotor neuropathy can be anticipated. The agent produces a neuropathy by disrupting axonal transport by binding to tubulin, the microtubule subunit protein. This agent produces stereotypic sensory symptoms after a few weeks of treatment, beginning with acral paraesthesias, often affecting fingers before toes. Signs are delayed and sensory loss is usually mild and distal. Motor impairment is common, sometimes predominantly affecting the upper limbs (Casey et al 1973), with hypo-reflexia or areflexia sometimes the first manifestations (McLeod & Penny 1969). Schaumburg et al (1983) have described trigeminal sensory symptoms, including jaw pain in some patients. In our experience with vincristine used for the treatment of KS or lymphoma in AIDS, the neuropathy leaves permanent residua, even after withdrawal of drug or dose reduction, although the severity of the paraesthesias may lessen with time.

SYSTEMIC LYMPHOMA IN AIDS

Epidemiology

The development of non-Hodgkin lymphomas (NHL) in homosexual men was first reported in 1982 and malignant lymphomas have been found to occur in AIDS almost 60 times more often than in the normal population (Beral et al 1991). The definition of AIDS was expanded in 1985 to include HIV-positive patients with high-grade B cell NHL and in 1987 intermediate-grade lymphomas were added as an index diagnosis.

The incidence of NHL has been rising in the USA, in part because of the association with

AIDS, but there also appear to be increasing numbers of non-AIDS-related CNS lymphoma (Eby et al 1988, Biggar & Rabkin 1992). An increased frequency in patients with renal or cardiac transplants on immunosuppressive medication has also been seen (Remick et al 1990). In the USA, the incidence of systemic lymphoma is 10.2 in men and 7.5 in women per 100 000 (age-adjusted 1973–1974 figures) (Ries et al 1991). NHL incidence has increased approximately 3% annually throughout the world during the past 30 years. The reasons for the increase in incidence are uncertain. In AIDS, the risk of NHL has been projected to increase as severely immunodeficient individuals live longer (Pluda et al 1990). Over 4000 cases are anticipated in the USA in 1994.

Data from a cohort of more than 1000 individuals with advanced HIV disease in a multicentre prospective observational study of zidovudine recipients identified NHL in 2.3% (rate 1.6/100 person-years of therapy) (Moore et al 1991). The development of NHL was associated with a prior diagnosis of KS, cytomegalovirus (CMV) disease or oral hairy leukoplakia (Cox proportional hazard analysis). Acyclovir use did not appear to be protective. In a second study in a small cohort of HIV-positive individuals receiving antiretroviral drugs, eight (14.5%) of 55 patients developed NHL 13–35 months (median 24 months) after starting antiretroviral therapy. The estimated probability of developing lymphoma was 28.6% by 30 months of treatment and 46.4% by 36 months of treatment (Pluda et al 1990).

AIDS-related NHL increases with age and HIV is not present in the tumour genome. There is little variation by risk group or region and immunodeficiency alone appears to be the major causative factor with no environmental component (unlike KS). Among 4337 patients in the USA reported through June 1990, 61% had immunoblastic NHL, 20% small non-cleaved lymphoma and 19% primary CNS lymphoma. Small non-cleaved cell lymphoma is often called Burkitt's or Burkitt-like lymphoma. In a population-based study initiated in 1989 by NCI, all cases of intermediate- or high-grade NHL were identified by the Cancer Surveillance Program. As of September 1991, 55 HIV-positive NHL patients, 239 HIV-negative HDL and 181 HIV-positive and HIV-negative neighbourhood control subjects had been included. In this series, 82% of HIV-positive NHL were high-grade B cell types vs. 40% of HIV-negative NHL. Epstein-Barr virus (EBV) titres greater than 1:1280 were found in 82% of HIV-positive NHL vs. 50% of HIV-negative NHL. Geometric mean titres of EBV, EBV-VCA and HHV-6 antibodies were similar among the groups (Levine et al 1992).

Clinical features

AIDS-related lymphomas are mostly high-grade large-cell immunoblastic tumours that present as aggressive extranodal tumours with extensive disease and a propensity for CNS metastasis. Extranodal presentation is common in HIV-associated NHL. Table 12.1 shows common sites of involvement. In one series, 43% of patients had extranodal and nodal involvement and 31% had only extranodal disease (Kaplan et al 1989). In another series, 42% had CNS disease and 33% bone marrow involvement (Ziegler et al 1984). The most common extranodal sites include bone marrow, brain, meninges, gastrointestinal tract and liver. Unusual sites of systemic involvement have included the rectum, heart and biliary tract. Systemic lymphoma may metastasize to the leptomeninges when the clinical picture is one of multiple cranial nerve palsies, or raised intracranial pressure or both. Involvement of the cavernous sinuses with progressive extraocular palsies is not uncommon. CNS metastasis occurs in about 50% of systemic lymphoma. Imaging shows hydrocephalus with basilar meningeal enhancement and sometimes with cavernous sinus lesions (Fig. 12.1). The CSF may contain lymphoma cells (Fig. 12.2), and a low glucose

Table 12.1 Common sites of involvement in systemic lymphoma in AIDS ($n = 100$)

Nodal	39
Digestive tract	27
CNS	15
Bone marrow	9
Respiratory tract	3
Spleen	2
Other	5

(Reproduced from Ioachim et al 1991 with permission of W B Saunders Company)

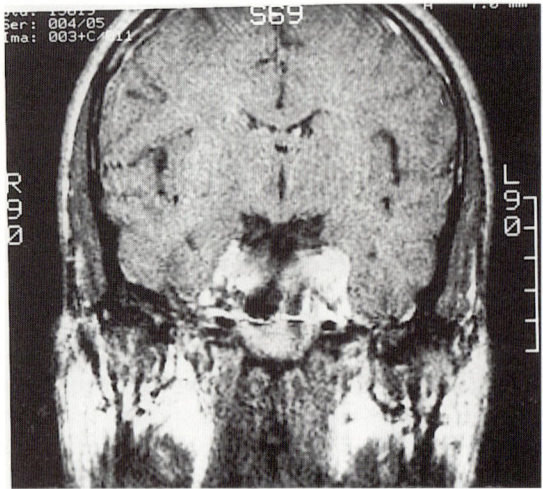

Fig. 12.1   T1-weighted MRI showing enhancing mass of systemic lymphoma in the region of the cavernous sinuses.

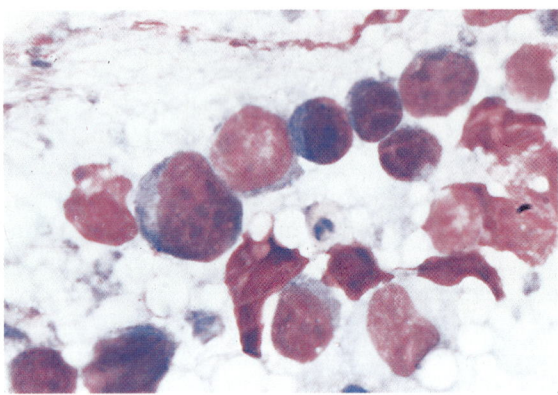

Fig. 12.2   Cytology specimen showing large, pleomorphic darkly staining lymphoma cells.

level. Epidural deposits can be a rare cause of spinal cord compression or of root symptoms (Leger et al 1989). The differential diagnosis of the cord lesion includes epidural abscess, tuberculoma and viral myelitis due to herpes zoster or simplex and requires magnetic resonance imaging (MRI) or myelography. The appearance of root lesions also requires imaging to distinguish lymphoma from CMV polyradiculitis. In this context CSF cytology is more likely to be positive or the diagnosis is made by biopsy at the time of surgical decompression.

Aetiopathogenesis

The aetiopathogenesis of NHL appears to require EBV latent infection and prolonged immunodeficiency. Using polymerase chain reaction (PCR) and in situ hybridization of NHL tissue, EBV was present in 68% of HIV-positive NHL compared with 15% of HIV-negative NHL. In another series, the EBV genome is found in about 65% of immunoblastic lymphomas and 20% of Burkitt-type tumours (Hamilton-Dutoit et al 1991). HIV-positive NHLs were genotypically monoclonal without t(14:18) and no serological differences in EBV or HHV-6 were identified as markers for the development of HIV-positive NHL (Levine et al 1992).

Profound cellular immunodeficiency is a prerequisite for the development of HIV-positive NHL and most cases develop with CD4 counts less than 100. In 11 homosexual men with HIV-positive NHL, the median CD4+ count within 6 months of diagnosis was 12 (range 5–40). The HIV-infected monocyte may play a critical role both by harbouring HIV by releasing interleukin-6, a B cell-stimulating lymphokine. B cell proliferation driven by EBV or cytokines from HIV-infected monocytes may allow the opportunity for genetic errors. These might take the form of activated oncogenes (c-myc, ras), or loss of suppressor genes with inactivation of p53 (Gaidano & Della-Favera 1992, Fig. 12.3) An alternative theory for the malignant transformation is that antiviral therapies might induce DNA damage leading to increased susceptibility to the development of lymphoma (Broder 1992). However, the high incidence of lymphoma was detected in AIDS before the advent of antiviral therapy. A simple overall lack of host 'cancer surveillance' due to immunosuppression cannot be the explanation as there is no excess of most other tumours.

Treatment

Response to chemotherapy has generally been poor compared with non-HIV-associated NHLs (Levine et al 1984, Knowles et al 1988, Lowenthal et al 1988, Kaplan et al 1989). Combination chemotherapy regimens for non-

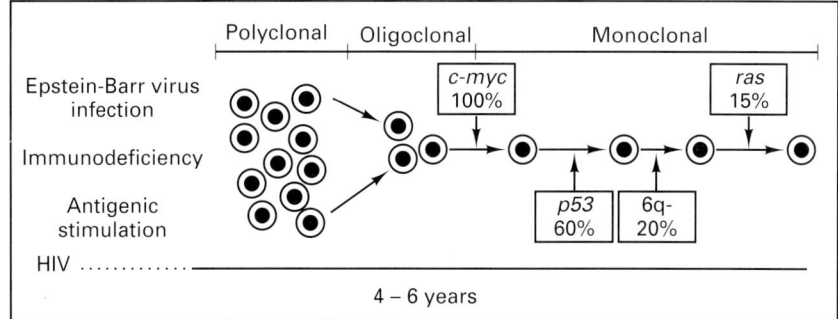

Fig. 12.3 A genetic model for development of lymphoma in AIDS with roles for both antigenic stimulation (HIV, EBV) and multiple genetic lesions. (Reproduced from Gaidano & Della-Favera 1992.)

HIV-associated NHLs have had complete remission rates of 80–90% and 2-year survivals of about 60% (Urba et al 1990). In HIV infection, however, these regimens have been far less successful with treatment response rates ranging from 32% to 56% and median survival times from 4 to 7 months (Kaplan & McGrath 1991). The poor response and short survival partly reflect the underlying immunodeficiency and partly reflect an inability to deliver adequate doses of chemotherapy because of limited bone marrow reserve. The most common causes of death are uncontrolled lymphoma and opportunistic infections. Some patients may have prolonged survival, usually those with the following characteristics: large cell histology, CD4 count of >100 before treatment, no previous AIDS-defining illnesses, no extranodal involvement and lack of systemic symptoms (Kaplan & McGrath 1991). Kaplan and others have developed approaches using reduced doses of the standard MBACOD regimens (methotrexate, bleomycin, doxorubicin, cyclophosphamide, vincristine and dexamethasone) (Levine et al 1991). The advantage of this regimen is that haematological toxicity is reduced with fewer episodes of febrile neutropenia. The use of haematopoietic growth factors such as G-CSF (granulocyte colony stimulating factor) or GM-CSF (granulocyte macrophage colony stimulating factor) reduces the need for chemotherapy interruptions and episodes of febrile neutropenia (Kaplan et al 1991). Because about one-third of patients with HIV-associated NHL die from opportunistic infections, a full range of prophylaxis should be used, including prophylaxis against *Pneumocystis carinii* pneumonia (PCP), candidiasis, *Mycobacterium avium intracellulare* (MAI) and toxoplasmosis. Treatment of lymphomatous meningitis requires intrathecal methotrexate 10–15 mg/week given via repeated lumbar puncture or via an Ommaya reservoir (Levine et al 1991). This is administered for 2–3 weeks after the CSF cytologies have normalized.

Prevention may prove possible with limitation of B cell stimulation through an attack on EBV or lymphokines (Biggar & Rabkin 1992).

PRIMARY CNS LYMPHOMA

Epidemiology

Primary CNS lymphoma (PCNSL) has been recognized as an AIDS-defining feature of HIV infection since 1987 (Centers for Disease Control 1987) and not uncommonly is the presenting illness. The CDC data up to 1989 include 548 cases of primary brain lymphoma, which represents an increased incidence of 1000-fold compared with that expected in the population. The experience of most clinics accords with these figures with an estimated incidence of 5% in AIDS (So et al 1986, Formenti et al 1989). Almost all PCNSLs are B cell-derived with 60% of HIV-associated PCNSLs small cell, non-cleaved lymphoma and 30% large cell immunoblastic (Rosenblum et al 1988). Rare angiocentric T cell tumours are encountered in the form of lymphoid granulomatosis, with areas of inflam-

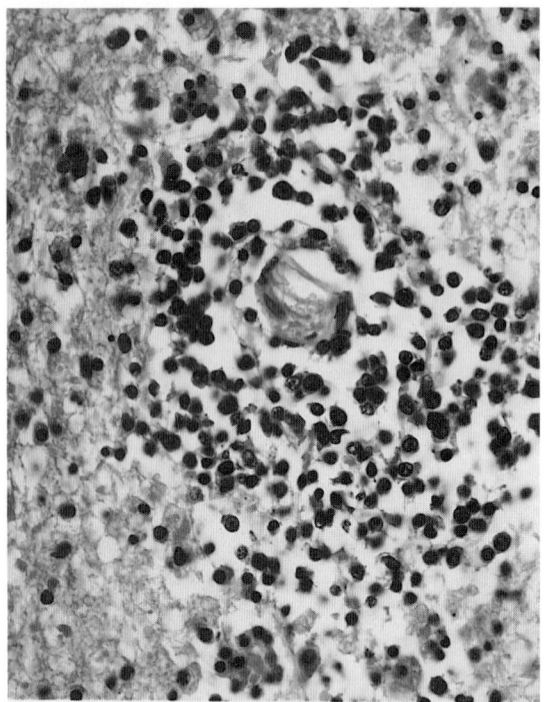

Fig. 12.4 Microscopic appearance of primary CNS lymphoma showing typical perivascular collection of pleomorphic lymphoma cells.

Table 12.2 Clinical presentation of cerebral lymphoma in 55 patients

Feature	%
Confusion, memory loss	53
Hemiparesis, dysphasia	31
Seizures	20
Cranial nerve palsy	18

(Reproduced from Baumgartner et al 1990 with permission of Journal of Neurosurgery)

mation, thrombosis and necrosis (Vinters & Anders 1987, Anders et al 1989). The presentation is similar to PCNSL, with multifocal lesions scattered throughout the brain parenchyma. Supratentorial tumours outnumber posterior fossa masses by 9–10 to 1. The lesions are characterized by a mixed inflammatory infiltrate of lymphocytes, histiocytes, plasma cells and atypical mononuclear cells (Fig. 12.4). Bizarre mononuclear cells and mitotic figures portend a poor prognosis. The majority of cells are T lymphocytes, mostly CD8+. Lymphomatoid granulomatosis may evolve into NHL in some patients.

Clinical features

Most cases of PCNSL present with headache, mental change, seizures and focal deficits (Table 12.2). Rather non-specific complaints of lethargy, memory loss and confusion are common, but by the time of diagnosis half also have focal signs and symptoms. The differential diagnosis of focal

problems such as a hemiplegia includes progressive multifocal leucoencephalopathy (PML), toxoplasmosis, abscess, infarct and haemorrhage. PML is suggested by the absence of seizures, headache, fever, and depressed consciousness. Infarcts and haemorrhages are suspected with an acute onset. The distinction between lymphoma and abscess is far more difficult as the symptoms and signs can overlap (Marks et al 1989).

Primary cerebral lymphoma is also difficult to differentiate from toxoplasmosis on neuroimaging (Table 12.3). Most tumours are multicentric at autopsy, and imaging reveals multiple lesions in 60–80% (Fig. 12.5). Large solitary mass lesions should suggest PCNSL. On computed tomographic (CT) scans (Figs 12.5 and 12.6) the lesion is of low or less commonly of high density, has mass effect, and usually enhances (Poon et al 1989). In some lesions, a small haemorrhagic component can be seen, with hyperattenuation on CT, and this appears to be useful in differentiating PCNSL from toxoplasmosis (Dina 1991). The pattern of enhancement is somewhat different from that seen in non-AIDS patients where the lesion is more often hyperdense, and is virtually always single (Poon et al 1989). Most non-AIDS lymphomatous lesions were either hyper- or isodense, round or oval masses with solid contrast enhancement and surrounding oedema. Another difference lies in the nature of

Table 12.3 Primary CNS lymphoma: radiological features

58 lesions in 32 patients
41% multiple; 1.5–7 cm
47% peripheral cortical
36% central grey (14 caudate)
Enhancement: ring 36%, homogeneous 31%

(After Dina 1991)

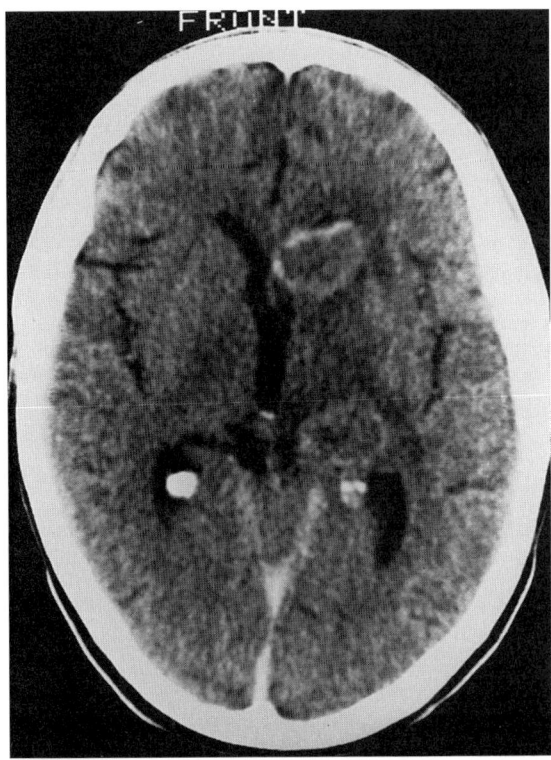

Fig. 12.5   Multiple enhancing lymphomas on contrast CT.

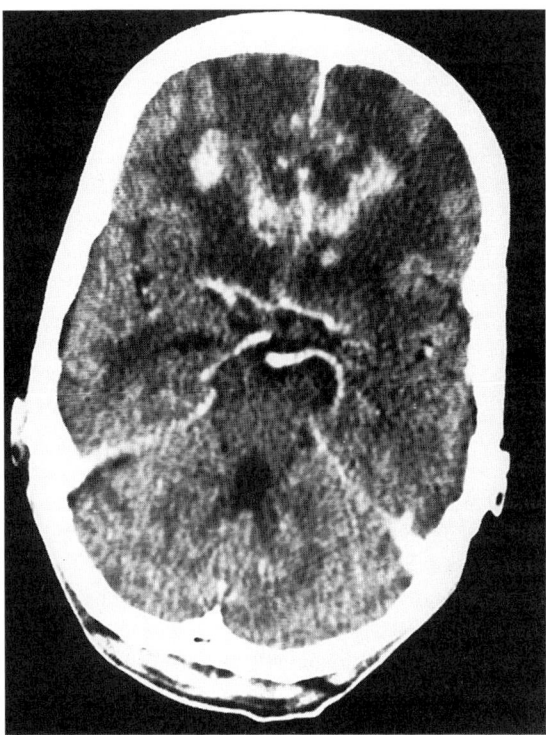

Fig. 12.6   CT scan with contrast showing 'butterfly' lymphoma in the frontal lobes on CT.

enhancement which is usually irregular in non-AIDS cases but is often of ring pattern in AIDS, particularly in lesions >1 cm. This produces a real problem in differentiation from *Toxoplasma* abscesses whose enhancement is also usually of ring pattern (Fig. 12.7). Unusual patterns of

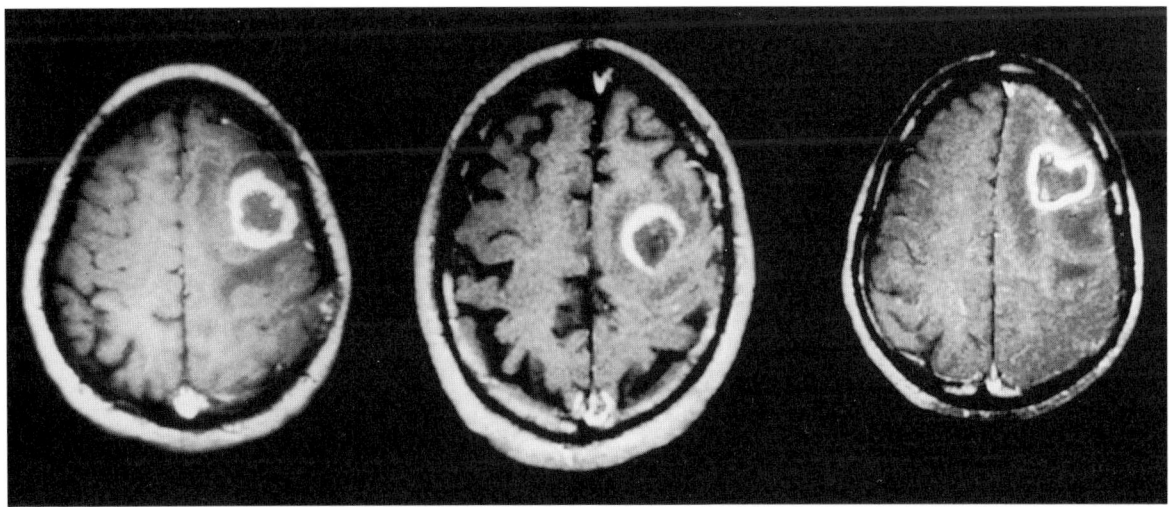

Fig. 12.7   Examples of lymphoma (centre) and toxoplasmosis (left and right) indistinguishable on imaging. Both types of lesion show ring enhancement (T1 MRI) and associated oedema.

enhancement can be seen, including gyral or ventricular (Dina 1991). MR pictures are of variable intensity on T2-weighted images (Fig. 12.8), and usually of low intensity on T1. Enhancement is usually peripheral. Most lesions are located in cerebral lobes or central grey matter, but some 10% are in the posterior fossa (Fig. 12.9).

A periventricular spread (Fig. 12.10) is particularly suggestive of lymphoma and helpful in the differentiation from toxoplasmosis (Dina 1991). In one series, 50% of biopsy-proven PCNSLs had periventricular lesions with subependymal spread or ventricular encasement in 38%. In contrast, only 3% of toxoplasmosis lesions are periventricular, and none showed subependymal spread or ventricular encasement. Another differentiating point is spread across the corpus callosum, which would be very rare with an infectious cause of an enhancing mass lesion.

Recently, Macapinlac et al (1993) have shown that thallium-201 SPECT scanning can differentiate lymphoma from abscesses in AIDS in keeping with findings in non-AIDS patients. The radioisotope is taken up by neoplastic cells and produces a 'hot spot', whereas infection remains cold (Fig. 12.11). FDG-PET also appears to make the distinction between infection and lymphoma (Hoffman et al 1993).

Doubt can still remain, however, and interpretation of either CT or MRI is especially liable to error in lymphoma (Heimans et al 1990). A recent report has highlighted this difficulty with a group of cases of lymphoma without enhancement on CT (DeAngelis 1993). Examination of the CSF only reveals tumour cells in about 5% of cases (McArthur 1987) and lumbar puncture is not without risk so this non-invasive means to a diagnosis is rarely helpful. Biopsy (Sherman et al 1991) is currently the only reliable way to make the diagnosis and the usual policy is to biopsy lesions likely to be lymphomas on imaging criteria soon after presentation. Cases that could possibly be toxoplasmosis receive anti-*Toxoplasma* therapy for up to 2 weeks as a therapeutic diagnostic trial. Failure of clinical and radiological response is then an indication for brain biopsy because PCNSL is the most common cause of a mass lesion that does not respond to anti-*Toxoplasma* treatment.

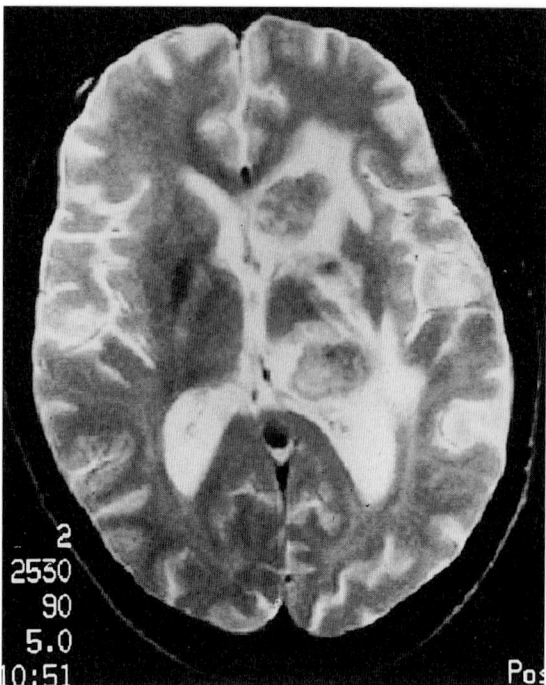

Fig. 12.8   Multiple mass lesions on MRI (T1) due to lymphomas.

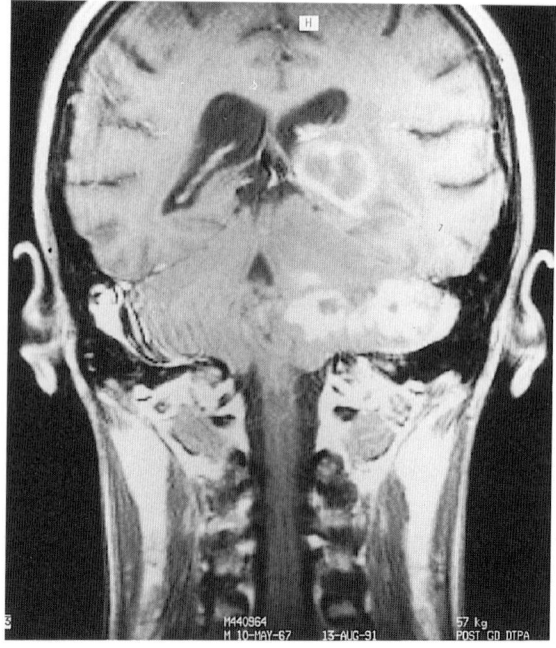

Fig. 12.9   Multiple lymphomas affecting the basal ganglia and posterior fossa on T1-weighted MRI.

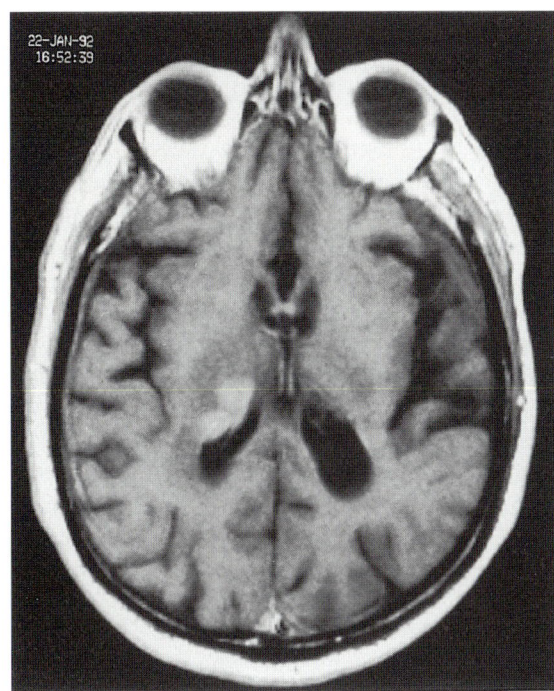

Fig. 12.10 T1-weighted MRI showing lymphoma affecting the ventricular wall.

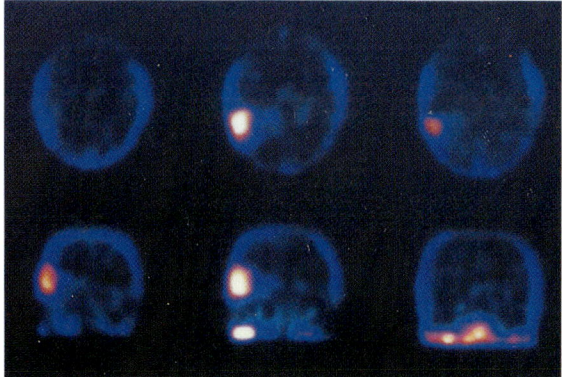

Fig. 12.11 Thallium brain scan showing hot spot of tracer concentration in a biopsy-proven case of lymphoma. (Courtesy of Prof. P.Ell and Dr D. da Costa, Institute of Nuclear Medicine, Middlesex Hospital.)

In most patients presenting with PCNSL, there is no need to perform screening for systemic NHL. There have been cases of dual development of separate tumours, but these are rare. Similarly, it is most unusual for a systemic NHL to present with brain masses in the absence of nodal or extranodal involvement. Bone marrow sampling and chest/abdomen CT scanning are therefore not necessary.

Biopsy confirmation of PCNSL can be achieved using stereotactic CT- or MRI-guided brain biopsy, or for larger lesions requiring decompression, open craniotomy. Stereotactic CT- or MRI-guided biopsy is a safe technique which can be used to obtain tissue from enhancing lesions. Two types of stereotactic frames are in widespread use: the Brown-Roberts-Wells system or the Leksell frame. The neurosurgical techniques have been described elsewhere (Levy et al 1992); the imaging coordinates of the lesion are used to localize then guide the needle approach to the lesion and the aspiration of tissue for microhistological and cytopathological examination. For lymphoma diagnosis, a panel of monoclonal antibodies including common leucocyte antigen (LCA), pan-T cell antibody (UCHL-1), and pan B antibody (L26) are used in addition to haematoxylin and eosin staining. Recently, a dioxigenin-labelled probe for EBV RNA transcripts has been developed for research applications, which is highly sensitive for PCNSL (MacMahon et al 1991).

The haemorrhagic complications of stereotactic biopsy can be minimized by avoiding aspirin or aspirin-containing compounds for 7 days preoperatively, and by excluding thrombocytopenia and coagulopathies. In the largest series to date, with 50 biopsies performed by one experienced neurosurgeon (Levy et al 1992), no deaths occurred, and only three haemorrhages occurred in 14 patients with PCNSL, with the haemorrhage confined to the tumour beds. In one patient, a permanent hemiparesis and aphasia developed following the biopsy. A similar rate of haemorrhage was noted by Chappell et al (1992): one haemorrhage with somnolence after biopsy in 25 biopsies. In other series, the morbidity and mortality rates have been higher. Four of 18 patients with assorted intracranial mass lesions had a significant complication from biopsy (Marks et al 1989). The diagnostic yield from stereotactic brain biopsy also varies among institutions and may depend on the number of tissue samples obtained by aspiration. In the Levy series, only two of 50 biopsies were non-diagnostic, and

Table 12.4   Indications for brain biopsy in AIDS

Failed empirical anti-toxoplasmosis therapy
Accessible lesion, no coagulopathy
Karnovsky function scale >70, i.e. independent
No immediate life-threatening systemic disease
Radiation therapy acceptable to patient

the diagnostic yield was 96%. Of 16 enhancing lesions biopsied in the Chappell series, nine were PCNSL, two toxoplasmosis and only two non-diagnostic. In the Marks series, all 11 PCNSL patients had a definitive biopsy. Thus, at least for PCNSL, stereotactic brain biopsy is a reliable diagnostic technique. Before committing to biopsy for what is suspected to be PCNSL, the patient should be agreeable to radiotherapy and should not have active life-threatening systemic opportunistic infections. We would also recommend not biopsying patients with severe dementia or functional impairment from neurological disease (Table 12.4).

Epstein et al (1986) reported primary cerebral lymphomas in three children with AIDS. This represented an incidence of 4% in their autopsy group and 3% of their clinical population. The children were 2, 5 and 10 years old. The clinical presentations included hemiparesis, dystonia, seizures and encephalopathy. All had multicentric tumours. Two were of large cell type, one a small cell non-cleaved tumour.

Treatment

To date, there have been no controlled trials comparing different radiotherapy (RT) regimens or chemotherapy. Even with aggressive early RT, survival is limited in most patients to a few months. PCNSL is radiosensitive, however, and in most cases, neurological improvement or stability can be achieved with RT. Because our current approach to the diagnosis of PCNSL requires brain biopsy, with its associated costs and morbidity, certain criteria may be helpful in deciding when to recommend biopsy and RT or RT/chemotherapy. These criteria are empirical and arbitrary and may not apply to all patients. Nonetheless, some patients with PCNSL present so late, with such advanced neurological disease, or have such a limited prognosis from their

systemic disease, that aggressive management with biopsy may not be justified (see Table 12.4 for suggested criteria). Partial response to radiation was seen in one of Epstein's paediatric cases (Epstein et al 1986).

The use of steroids in the management of a contrast-enhancing lesion is discussed in Chapter 11. Steroids should be avoided during an empirical anti-toxoplasmosis trial because of their non-specific effect. In biopsy-proven PCNSL, or with rapidly expanding lesions, dexamethasone 4–6 mg q.i.d. can be used to control oedema. Unlike non-AIDS PCNSL, steroids do not seem to have a tumorolytic effect.

In the largest published series, Baumgartner et al (1990) noted that 76% of 29 patients treated with 4000 cGY of whole brain RT showed clinical improvement and 69% complete or partial radiographic response. The mean survival was 134 days vs. 42 days for those who did not receive RT (Table 12.5). Most patients who received RT did not die of tumour regression, but rather from the subsequent development of systemic and CNS opportunistic infections (Table 12.6). In fact, of the eight RT patients who underwent autopsy, only one had uncontrolled CNS lymphoma, and their lymphoma had progressed outside the radiation portal. In another series of 10 patients receiving cranial RT, only two died with recurrent lymphoma and a half succumbed to opportunistic infections (Formenti et al 1989). The issues of chemotherapy for primary CNS lymphoma, as for the treatment of systemic lymphoma, revolve around the severity of the underlying immunodeficiency and poor bone marrow reserve with a high risk of opportunistic infections. DeAngelis et al (1992) showed a benefit for combined RT and chemotherapy for non-AIDS PCNSL using

Table 12.5   Survival data in 46 patients with primary CNS lymphoma

Radiation	Survival (days)		
	Mean	Median	Range
None ($n = 17$)	42	27	8–127
40 Gy ($n = 29$)	134	119	332–380

(Reproduced from Baumgartner et al 1990 with permission of Journal of Neurosurgery)

Table 12.6 Cause of death established at autopsy in 21 patients with primary CNS lymphoma

Radiation	Lymphoma	Other[a]
None ($n = 130$)	10	3
40 Gy ($n = 8$)	1[b]	7

[a] In those receiving RT, two had residual multifocal PCNSL, but died with other opportunistic infections, two died with PCP.
[b] Had a complete response to RT, but died of an inramedullary high-grade lymphoma of cervical cord outside radiation portal.
(Reproduced from Baumgartner et al 1990 with permission of Journal of Neurosurgery)

Table 12.7 Therapy for primary CNS lymphoma: CHOD + G-CSF regimen for ACTG/ECOG Trial

Cyclophosphamide	750 mg/m² i.v. day 1
Doxorubicin	50 mg/m² i.v. day 1
Vincristine	1.4 mg/m² i.v. day 1 (to a maximum dose of 2.0 mg)
Dexamethasone	12 mg/day
G-CSF	5 μg/kg s.c. beginning day 2 for a minimum of 10 days and until granulocytes are greater than 5000 for 2 days

CHOP (cyclophosphamide, doxorubicin, vincristine, prednisone) in combination with RT. This regimen is now used for non-AIDS primary CNS lymphoma before initiating RT, and preliminary data from the ECOG/NCCTG PCNSL study have shown a 75% objective response rate to CHOP chemotherapy before initiating RT. In AIDS PCNSL, a recently initiated regimen is under study within the ACTG and ECOG. A single cycle of CHOD (cyclophosphamide, doxorubicin, vincristine, dexamethasone) with a haematopoietic growth factor, G-CSF, is used in the doses listed in Table 12.7. Following chemotherapy, RT includes 12 daily 2.5 Gy fractions to the entire brain and four daily 2.5 Gy fractions to the identifiable lesions with a margin. This is equivalent to 40 Gy to the whole brain with an additional boost to the tumour.

HODGKINS' DISEASE

Although less common than NHL, there appears to be an increased incidence of Hodgkin's disease with HIV infection. The incidence is not higher, however, in immunosuppressed transplant recipients. Compared with Hodgkin's disease occurring separately from AIDS, with HIV infection, Hodgkin's disease is more likely to have mixed cellularity and to present with advanced disease (Kaplan et al 1987). As with NHL, treatment responses have been poor, with frequent relapses or development of opportunistic infections and a median survival of 1 year compared with 12 years in a comparison group of Hodgkin's patients. Hodgkin's disease has not yet been reported in the CNS.

OTHER CNS TUMOURS

Cerebral gliomas (Fig. 12.12), meningiomas, pituitary adenomas and arachnoid cysts have all been encountered in HIV-infected individuals, but there is no evidence of an increased incidence of any of these conditions.

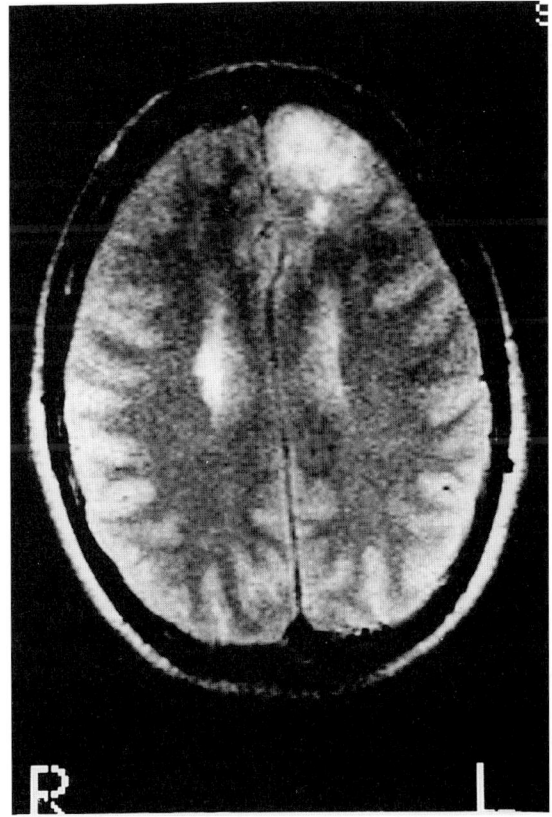

Fig. 12.12 Probably coincidental frontal glioma in an AIDS patient.

MANAGEMENT PLAN

Severely immunodeficient patients with seizures, focal cerebral deficit or mental changes will require neuroimaging. If a large periventricular mass of irregular enhancement is seen, lymphoma becomes the likely diagnosis, but biopsy is needed for confirmation. Distinction from *Toxoplasma* abscess may also be achieved by the response to anti-*Toxoplasma* therapy, and perhaps by thallium scanning. If the patient's general state permits aggressive treatment, the lymphoma may respond to radiotherapy and limited chemotherapy.

REFERENCES

Anders K H, Latta H, Change B S, et al. Lymphomatoid granulomatosis and malignant lymphoma of the central nervous system in the acquired immunodeficiency syndrome. Hum Pathol 1989; 20: 326–334

Baumgartner J E, Rachlin, J R, Beckstead J H, et al. Primary central nervous system lymphomas: natural history and response to radiation therapy in 55 patients with acquired immunodeficiency syndrome. J Neurosurg 1990; 73: 206–211

Beral V, Peterman T, Berkelman R, Jaffe H. AIDS associated non-Hodgkin lymphoma. Lancet 1991; 337: 805–809

Biggar R J, Rabkin C S. The epidemiology of acquired immunodeficiency syndrome related lymphomas. Curr Opin Oncol 1992; 4: 883–893

Broder S. Factors in the development of AIDS-related lymphomas. Leukemia 1992; 6 (supply 3): 6S–9S

Casey E B, Jellife A M, Le Quesne P M, Millett Y L. Vincristine neuropathy. Clinical and electrophysiological observations. Brain 1973; 96: 69–86

Centers for Disease Control. Revision of the CDC surveillance case definition for acquired immunodeficiency syndrome. MMWR 1987; 36 (suppl 1S): 3S–15S

Chappell E T, Guthrie B L, Orenstein J. The role of stereotactic biopsy in the management of HIV-related focal brain lesions. Neurosurgery 1992; 30: 825–829

DeAngelis L M. Cerebral lymphoma presenting as a non-enhancing lesion on computed tomographic/magnetic resonance scan. Ann Neurol 1993; 33: 308–311

DeAngelis L M, Yahalom J, Thaler H T, Kher U. Combined modality therapy for primary CNS lymphoma. J Clin Oncol 1992; 10: 635–643

Dina T S. Primary central nervous system lymphoma versus toxoplasmosis in AIDS. Radiology 1991; 179: 823–828

Eby N L, Grufferman S, Flannelly C M, et al. Increasing incidence of primary brain lymphoma in the US. Cancer 1988; 62: 2461–2465

Epstein L G, Sharer L R, Oleske J M, et al. Neurologic manifestations of human immunodeficiency virus infection in children. Pediatrics 1986; 78: 678–687

Formenti S C, Gill P S, Lean E, et al. Primary central nervous system lymphoma in AIDS. Results of radiation therapy. Cancer 1989; 63: 1101–1107

Gaidano G, Dalla-Favera R. Biologic aspects of human immunodeficiency virus-related lymphoma. Curr Opin Oncol 1992; 4: 900–906

Goldstein J D, Dickson D W, Moser F G, et al. Primary central nervous system lymphoma in acquired immune deficiency syndrome – a clinical and pathological study with results of treatment with radiation. Cancer 1991; 67: 2756–2765

Gorin F A, Bale J F Jr, Halks-Miller M, Schwartz R A. Kaposi's sarcoma metastatic to the CNS. Arch Neurol 1985; 42: 162–165

Hamilton-Dutoit S J, Pallesen G, Franzmann M B, et al. AIDS-related lymphoma. Histopathology, immunophenotype, and association with Epstein-Barr virus as demonstrated by in situ nucleic acid hybridization. Am J Pathol 1991; 138: 149–163

Heimans J J, DeVisser M, Polman C H, et al. Accuracy and inter-observer variation in the interpretation of computed tomography in solitary brain lesions. Arch Neurol 1990; 47: 520–523

Hill D R. The role of radiotherapy for epidemic Kaposi's sarcoma. Semin Oncol 1987; 14 (suppl 3): 19–22

Hoffman J M, Waskin H A, Schifter T, et al. FDG-PET in differentiating lymphoma from nonmalignant central nervous system lesions in patients with AIDS. J Nucl Med 1993; 34: 567–575

Ioachim H L, Dorsett B, Cronin W, et al. Acquired immunodeficiency syndrome-associated lymphomas. Hum Pathol 1991; 22: 659–673

Jacobson L P, Munoz A, Fox R, et al. Incidence of Kaposi's sarcoma in a cohort of homosexual men infected with the human immunodeficiency virus type 1. The Multicenter AIDS Cohort Study Group. J AIDS 1990; 3 (suppl 1): S24–S31

Kaplan L D, McGrath M S. AIDS-associated non-Hodgkin's lymphoma. AIDS Update 1991; 2: 1–11

Kaplan L D, Abrams D I, Feigal E, et al. AIDS-associated non-Hodgkin's lymphoma in San Francisco. JAMA 1989; 261: 719–724

Kaplan L D, Abrams D I, Volberding P A. Clinical course and epidemiology of Hodgkin's disease in homosexual men in San Francisco (abstract). III International Conference on AIDS, Washington, DC 1987.

Kaplan L D, Kahn J O, Crowe S, et al. Clinical and virologic effects of recombinant human granulocyte-macrophage colony-stimulating factor in patients receiving chemotherapy for human immunodeficiency virus-associated non-Hodgkin's lymphoma: results of a randomized trial. J Clin Oncol 1991; 9: 929–940

Knowles D M, Chamulak G A, Subar M, et al. Lymphoid neoplasia associated with the acquired immunodeficiency syndrome (AIDS). The New York University Medical Center experience with 105 patients (1981–1986). Ann Intern Med 1988; 108: 744–753

Koppel B S, Wormser G P, Tuchman A J, et al. Central nervous system involvement in patients with acquired immune deficiency syndrome (AIDS). Acta Neurol Scand 1985; 71: 337–353

Leger J M, Bouche P, Bolgert F, et al. The spectrum of

polyneuropathies in patients infected with HIV. J Neurol Neurosurg Psychiatr 1989; 52: 1369–1374

Levine A M, Meyer P R, Begandy M K, et al. Development of B-cell lymphoma in homosexual men. Clinical and immunologic findings. Ann Intern Med 1984; 100: 7–13

Levine A M, Shibata D, Sullivan-Halley J, et al. Case control study of HIV+ and HIV− lymphoma (NHL) in Los Angeles County (abstract). Proceedings of the Annual Meeting of the American Society for Clinical Oncology 1992; 11: A1140

Levine A M, Wernz J C, Kaplan L, et al. Low-dose chemotherapy with central nervous system prophylaxis and zidovudine maintenance in AIDS-related lymphoma. A prospective multi-institutional trial. JAMA 1991; 266: 84–88

Levy R M, Bredesen D E, Rosenblum M L. Neurological manifestations of the acquired immunodeficiency syndrome (AIDS): experience at UCSF and review of the literature. J Neurosurg 1985; 62: 475–495

Levy R M, Russell E, Yungbluth M, et al. The efficacy of image-guided stereotactic brain biopsy in neurologically symptomatic acquired immunodeficiency syndrome patients. Neurosurgery 1992; 30: 186–190

Lowenthal D A, Straus D J, Campbell S W, et al. AIDS-related lymphoid neoplasia. The Memorial Hospital experience. Cancer 1988; 61: 2325–2337

Macapinlac H A, Scott A M, Zhang J, et al. Comparison of TL-201 SPECT and F-18 FDG PET images with MRI in the evaluation of primary CNS lymphoma in non-AIDS patients. J Nucl Med 1993; 34: 56P (abstr)

MacMahon E, Glass J D, Hayward S D, et al. Epstein-Barr virus in AIDS-related primary central nervous system lymphoma. Lancet 1991; 338: 969–973

Marks W J, Jr, McArthur J C, Royal W R, et al. Intracranial mass lesions in AIDS: diagnosis and response to therapy. Neurology 1989; 39 (suppl): 380 (abstr)

McArthur J C. Neurologic manifestations of AIDS. Medicine (Baltimore) 1987; 66: 407–437

McLeod J G, Penny R. Vincristine neuropathy: an electrophysiological and histological study. J Neurol Neurosurg Psychiatr 1969; 32: 297–304

Mitsuyasu R T, Taylor J M, Glaspy J, Fahey J L. Heterogeneity of epidemic Kaposi's sarcoma. Implications for therapy. Cancer 1986; 57 (suppl 8): 1657–1661

Moore R D, Kessler H, Richman D D, et al. Non-Hodgkin's lymphoma in patients with advanced HIV infection treated with zidovudine. JAMA 1991; 265: 2208–2211

Munoz A, Schrager L K, Bacellar H, et al. Trends in the incidence of outcomes defining acquired immunodeficiency syndrome (AIDS) in the Multicenter AIDS Cohort Study: 1985–1991. Am J Epidemiol 1993; 137: 423–438

Odajnyk C, Muggia F M. Treatment of Kaposi's sarcoma: overview and analyses of clinical setting. J Clin Oncol 1985; 3: 1277–1285

Pluda J M, Yarchoan R, Jaffe E S, et al. Development of non-Hodgkin lymphoma in a cohort of patients with severe human immunodeficiency virus (HIV) on long-term antiretroviral therapy. Ann Intern Med 1990; 113: 276–282

Poon T, Matoso I, Tchertkoff V, et al. CT features of primary cerebral lymphoma in AIDS and non-AIDS patients. J Comput Assist Tomogr 1989 13: 6–9

Qunibi W, Akhtar M, Sheth K, et al. Kaposi's sarcoma: the commmonest tumour after renal transplantation in Saudi Arabia. Am J Med 1988; 84: 225–232

Rabkin C S, Biggar J, Horm J W. Increasing incidence of cancers associated with the human immunodeficiency virus epidemic. Int J Cancer 1991; 47: 692–696

Remick S C, Diamond C C, Migliozzi J A, et al. Primary central nervous system lymphoma in patients with and without acquired immunodeficiency syndrome. A retrospective analysis and review of the literature. Medicine (Baltimore) 1990; 69: 345–360

Ries L A G, Hankey B F, Miller B A, et al. Cancer statistics review 1973–88. Bethesda: National Cancer Institute, 1991: 2789

Rosenblum M L, Levy R M, Bredesen D E, et al. Primary central nervous system lymphomas in patients with AIDS. Ann Neurol 1988; 23; S13–S16

Rutherford G W, Schwarcz S K, Lemp G F, et al. The epidemiology of AIDS-related Kaposi's sarcoma in San Francisco. J Infect Dis 1989; 159: 569–572

Schaumburg H H, Spencer P S, Thomas P K. Disorders of peripheral nerves. Philadelphia: F A Davis, 1983

Sherman M E, Erozan Y S, Mann R B, et al. Stereotactic brain biopsy in the diagnosis of malignant lymphoma. Am J Clin Pathol 1991; 95: 878–883

Snider W D, Simpson D M, Nielsen S, et al. Neurological complications of acquired immune deficiency syndrome: analysis of 50 patients. Ann Neurol 1983; 14: 403–418

So Y T, Beckstead J H, Davis R L. Primary central nervous system lymphoma in acquired immune deficiency syndrome: a clinical and pathological study. Ann Neurol 1986; 20: 566–572

Urba W, Duffey P, Longo D. Treatment of patients with aggressive lymphomas: an overview. Nat Cancer Inst Monogr 1990; 10: 29–37

Vadhan-Raj S, Wong G, Gnecco C, et al. Immunological variables as predictors of prognosis in patients with Kaposi's sarcoma and the acquired immunodeficiency syndrome. Cancer Res 1986; 46: 417–425

Vinters H V, Anders K H. Lymphomatoid granulomatosis and the acquired immunodeficiency syndrome (AIDS) [letter]. Ann Intern Med 1987; 107: 945

Volberding P A. The role of chemotherapy for epidemic Kaposi's sarcoma. Semin Oncol 1987; 2 (suppl 3): 23–26

Welch K, Finkbeiner W, Alpers C E, et al. Autopsy findings in the acquired immune deficiency syndrome. JAMA 1984; 252: 1152–1159

Ziegler J L, Beckstead J A, Volberding P A, et al. Non-Hodgkin's lymphoma in 90 homosexual men. Relation to generalized lymphoadenopathy and the acquired immunodeficiency syndrome. New Engl J Med 1984; 311: 565–570

13. Cerebrovascular disease

Surveys of large numbers of patients with AIDS have suggested that cerebrovascular disease is sufficiently frequent to imply that it is in some way a complication of HIV infection or of the immunosuppression and its sequelae (Engstrom et al 1989). The registry at the University of California in San Francisco contained 1600 patients when searched by Engstrom and colleagues and yielded 12 cases of cerebral infarction. This prevalence (0.7%) was higher than expected for the age group. Autopsy studies also reveal a high prevalence of infarction or haemorrhage. Mizusawa et al (1988) found such lesions in 28 of 83 cases. A case control study of autopsies suggests that it may be wrong to conclude that there is always a causal connection with AIDS, however. Berger et al (1990) compared the prevalence of cerebral vascular disease at autopsy in a group dying of AIDS and in age-matched controls dying of unrelated conditions such as cancer. There was no excess of vascular lesions in the brains of those with AIDS, and there was no difference in the nature of the lesions, except that vasculitis was seen in two of the AIDS cases but in none of the non-AIDS cases. Of 154 adult AIDS cases coming to autopsy 13 had acute or recent cerebrovascular lesions. Four of these stroke cases had evidence of cardiac embolism, and 40% of the AIDS cases had evidence at autopsy of cardiac disease. Their control group of young people mostly dying of malignancy had a comparable incidence of heart disease and embolism. Their conclusion was that cerebrovascular lesions were a common terminal event in young patients with serious systemic illnesses. This suggests that HIV infection, per se, does not cause cerebrovascular disease or a propensity to stroke, but that stroke occurs in HIV-seropositive individuals as a secondary complication of systemic illness or of drug use.

AETIOLOGY

The nature of the vascular lesions seen in AIDS is revealed by autopsy studies. For example Mizusawa et al (1988) found four cases of haemorrhage and 23 of infarction, and one patient had both types of pathology. Many infarcts are small and appear to have been asymptomatic, though subtle deficits may easily be missed in terminally ill patients.

The cause of the ischaemic cerebrovascular lesions in AIDS patients is of considerable interest and many potential causes have been identified. At this point, there is no evidence that HIV infection of the brain leads directly to cerebrovascular disease.

Cardiac embolism

Cardiac disease may be found in as many as 50% of AIDS patients (Rodan et al 1987), with cardiac embolism a possibility. The cardiac disease varies from a viral myocarditis to a congestive cardiomyopathy, which may in some instances be due to zidovudine toxicity. Rarely, *Toxoplasma* can cause a myocarditis. Intravenous drug users are liable to infective endocarditis, with the potential for embolism (Fig. 13.1) and mycotic aneurysm formation (Fig. 13.2). Some patients have unrelated cardiac problems such as atrial fibrillation, patent foramen ovale or a prolapsing mitral valve. The latter lesions are controversially linked

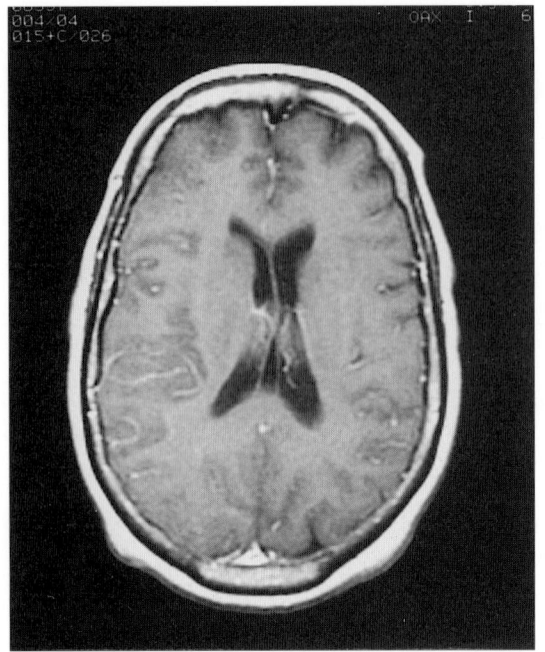

Fig. 13.1 Ischaemic stroke in an HIV-positive patient with vascular prominence ('luxury perfusion') in the territory of the left middle cerebral artery.

to the incidence of stroke in young subjects, regardless of HIV infection. Other patients have the type of terminal vascular event related to marantic endocarditis with embolism of non-bacterial vegetations, or cerebral venous thrombosis associated with cachexia and dehydration.

Atheroma

Most angiographic studies of young patients with strokes reveal a surprising prevalence of atheroma (Lisovoski & Rousseaux 1991), and thromboembolism from arterial plaques is a potential cause for stroke in AIDS. Arterial disease risk factors should be sought regardless of HIV status, and treated wherever possible. The dominant factor is hypertension, diabetes mellitus, tobacco use, hyperlipidaemia and fibrinogen levels having a weaker effect on incidence. Oral contraceptive use in females is a risk factor though the risk is small. Migraine probably accounts for some young strokes (Bousser et al 1985), but is a diagnosis of

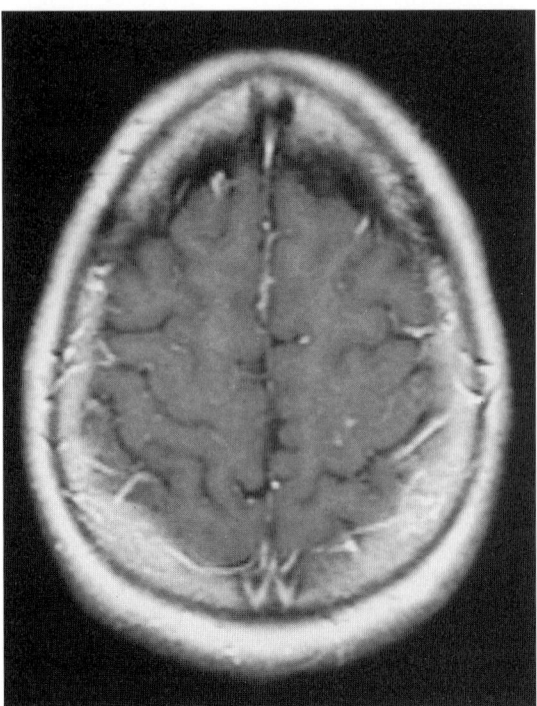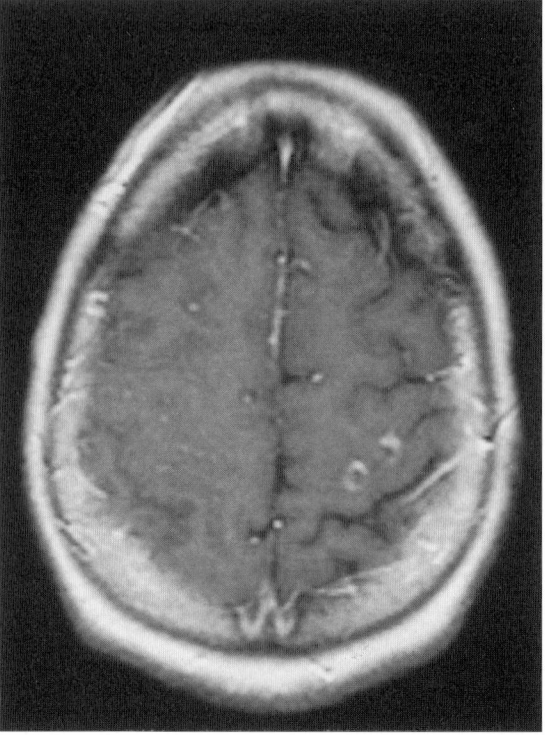

Fig. 13.2 Development of mycotic aneurysms/septic embolism in an HIV-positive patient with endocarditis seen on gadolinium-enhanced T1-weighted MRI (10 days between images).

exclusion in a migraineur with a history of classic attacks.

Haematological disorders

In non-HIV patients, antiphospholipid antibodies have been associated with a variety of neurological syndromes, including stroke and migraine. The antibodies may be IgG, IgM, IgA or mixed, which bind to negatively charged or neutral phospholipids and include anticardiolipin antibody and lupus anticoagulant (Brey et al 1990). These antibodies have also been associated with systemic thrombosis, fetal loss and thrombocytopenia. Brey et al (1990) found an excessive frequency of antiphospholipid antibodies in young patients with stroke or transient ischaemic attack (TIA). Levine et al (1990b) studied 48 patients with cerebral or visual dysfunction and circulating antiphospholipid antibodies and the majority of patients did not have systemic lupus erythematosus. Thrombocytopenia was present in almost one-third and a false positive VDRL in 23%. Cerebral angiography was either normal or showed large vessel occlusion or stenosis without vasculitic changes.

Anticardiolipin antibodies develop in a proportion of patients with HIV infection and may underlie some cases of ischaemic cerebral infarction. It is unknown how often strokes in HIV infection can be attributed to anticardiolipin antibodies. Cases have been described in which anticardiolipin antibodies develop or in which low levels of protein C or S are found (Brew & Miller 1993). One case control study of haemophiliacs showed that only those who had become HIV positive also had the procoagulant phospholipid antibodies (Naimi et al 1990). Some pathological series (Mizusawa et al 1988) have shown that many infarcts have been clinically silent and have been small and often located in the striatum and brainstem. A mural thickening of small vessels has been proposed as the cause for such 'lacunar' infarcts, though the common finding of calcification of small blood vessels did not appear to be closely linked to the presence or site of infarcts. Anticoagulants may be indicated if no other cause for cerebrovascular symptoms is found and if the titre of anticardiolipin antibodies is high. Levine et al (1990b) suggested the following clues to the presence of antiphospholipid antibodies: history of systemic lupus erythematosus, prolonged activated partial thromboplastin time (aPTT) or prothrombin time (PT) without explanation, miscarriages, thrombocytopenia, systemic thrombotic events, prior stroke of unknown cause, positive antinuclear antibody (ANA), prominent or recurrent visual disturbances, or a family history of premature stroke. False positive VDRL or low platelet count should also prompt screening for antiphospholipid antibodies. As a first step, anticardiolipin antibodies (ELISA) should be measured as well as an aPTT. If a circulating lupus anticoagulant is suspected, even with a normal aPTT, additional tests for a coagulopathy, such as Russell viper venom test, can be performed.

Vasculitis

AIDS patients are subject to vasculitic changes in intracerebral vessels. This can be due to opportunistic infections as diverse as *Candida albicans*, *Aspergillus fumigatus*, cryptococcus, cytomegalovirus (CMV), syphilis, herpes zoster and tuberculosis, or even to lymphoma (Kieburtz et al 1993). In some cases HIV itself appears to be the cause (Scaravilli et al 1989) and it is plausible that HIV might induce vasculitis in some instances. HIV antigens have been demonstrated in endothelial cells in some cases (Wiley et al 1986), or at least in the pericytes, and perivascular inflammation is a common neuropathological feature of HIV infection. How often a frank vasculitis develops is uncertain, and it is probably a rare event. Park et al (1990) in one paediatic case described an unusual dilated vasculopathy, which they tentatively attributed to HIV.

Herpes zoster

Zoster ophthalmicus can affect the middle cerebral artery through the trigeminal innervation of the dura, and a contralateral stroke (Fig. 13.3) can follow the skin lesions within days or weeks. This has sometimes been called the 'crossed zoster syndrome'. It was assumed that the cause was an arteritis of vessels supplied by the trigeminal nerve (Anastasopoulos et al 1958). In a careful autopsy

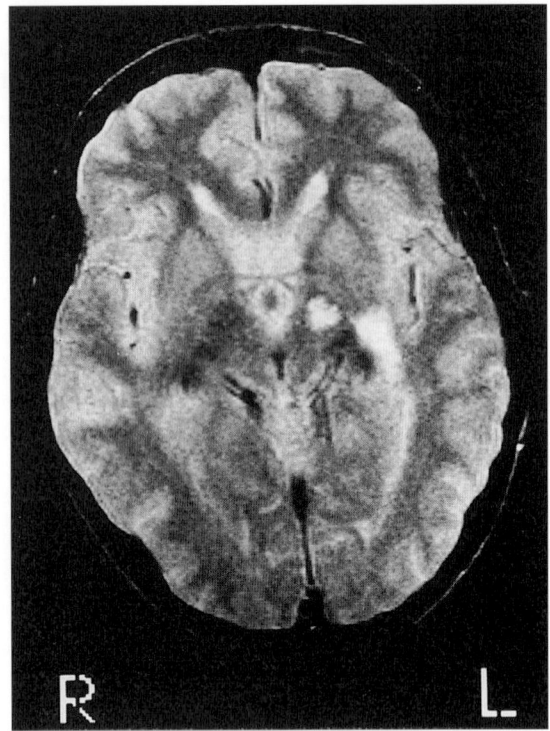

Fig. 13.3   Cerebral infarct on T2-weighted MRI due to zoster vasculitis.

ophthalmicus. The differential diagnosis includes the other causes of stroke and a zoster encephalitis. In the latter situation, focal deficit is unlikely, and the picture is dominated by a meningitic illness with confusion and disturbed consciousness and diffuse electroencephalographic (EEG) changes. Computed tomography (CT) or

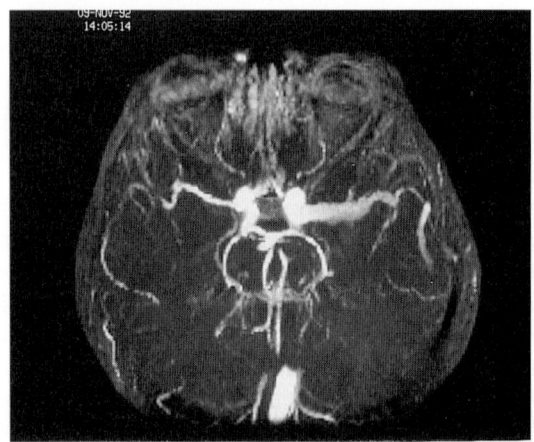

A

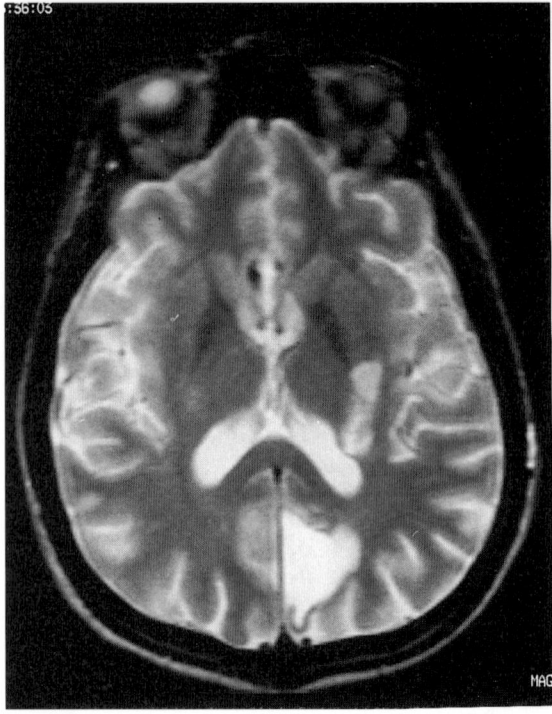

B

Fig. 13.4   Abnormal middle cerebral artery, possibly related to previous zoster infection. **A** MR angiography and **B** MRI (T2 weighted).

report, Eidelberg et al (1986) showed in three cases that there was a predominantly thrombotic process without striking arteritis. Varicella zoster viral antigens were detectable in the media of the walls of the thrombosed middle cerebral arteries, however, suggesting a spread from the trigeminal nerve. Rarely, there is aneurysm formation and sometimes the gross pathology shows haemorrhage. In some cases, the zoster infection has not been in the trigeminal territory (Eidelberg et al 1986). For example, Ross et al (1991) described a patient with pontine infarction after C2 herpes zoster. This was attributed to spread of virus through innervation of posterior fossa arteries from cervical roots (Saito & Moskowitz 1989). In the case of Rawlinson and Cunningham (1991), hemiplegia followed thoracic shingles suggesting the possibility of blood-borne spread of the virus.

The typical clinical picture is of the acute or subacute onset of contralateral hemiplegia weeks or perhaps up to 6 months after an attack of zoster magnetic resonance imaging (MRI) (Fig. 13.3) shows infarction.

Angiography (MacKenzie et al 1981) may be normal, but often shows areas of segmental constriction or vessel occlusion (Hilt et al 1983). In a personal case, dilatation of the middle cerebral artery (Fig. 13.4) followed zoster infection, but a causal relationship could not be confirmed in the absence of histology.

The cerebrospinal fluid (CSF) in non-AIDS cases shows a pleocytosis, but in AIDS this is less helpful because of the background changes related to HIV infection. Improvement may follow the use of antiviral therapy (Rawlinson & Cunningham 1991) so full doses of intravenous acyclovir should be prescribed even if there has been a long interval between the cutaneous eruption and the stroke.

Aspergillus infection

Invasive aspergillosis is relatively rare in AIDS and disseminated disease almost always results from primary lung infection. Central nervous system (CNS) aspergillosis is associated with multiple abscesses, which typically produce vascular invasion and haemorrhage. Haemorrhagic stroke or catastrophic subarachnoid haemorrhage may result from invasion of major blood vessel walls with subsequent thrombosis, occlusion or rupture (Fig. 13.5). Definitive diagnosis of aspergillosis is usually made from histopathological examination of tissue, and blood cultures are almost always negative, even with invasive disease. CSF in CNS aspergillosis may be haemorrhagic with either a neutrophilic or mononuclear pleocytosis, but positive cultures are unusual. Antigen tests are under development. Amphotericin B remains the first line of treatment for invasive aspergillosis in daily doses of up to 0.7 mg/kg to a total dose of at least 30 mg/kg. Itraconazole also has activity against *Aspergillus* species (Meyer et al 1973).

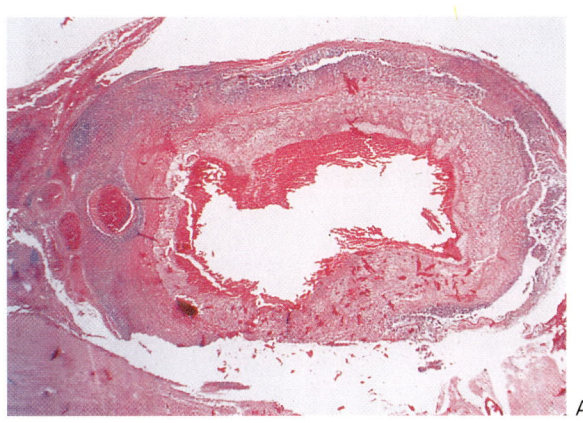

A

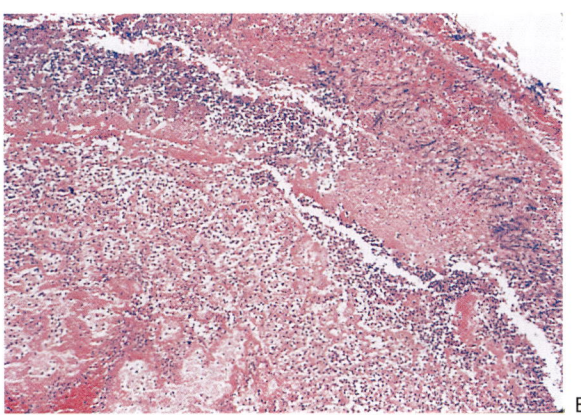

B

Fig. 13.5 *Aspergillus* invasion of the basilar artery. **A** Low power; **B** high power.

Meningovascular syphilis

Meningovascular syphilis (Chapter 10) can cause an endarteritis of small vessels up to the size of the middle cerebral artery with resultant infarction (Fig. 13.6). It has been suggested that AIDS patients progress to the stage of meningovascular disease more rapidly than was usual in the pre-AIDS era when an interval of 5–10 years commonly separated the primary spirochaetal infection and the stroke. Musher et al (1990) reported 11 cases of AIDS-related meningovascular syphilis, with CT evidence of infarction in 10. Berger (1992) reported a case of syphilitic spinal cord infarction with improvement after penicillin treatment. Katz and Berger (1989) also described CT evidence of silent cerebral infarction attributed to meningovascular syphilis. Syphilis serology in blood and CSF should be sought in the aftermath of a stroke in an HIV-infected person, and an appropriate treatment for neurosyphilis prescribed with intravenous penicillin if evidence of untreated neurosyphilis is suspected.

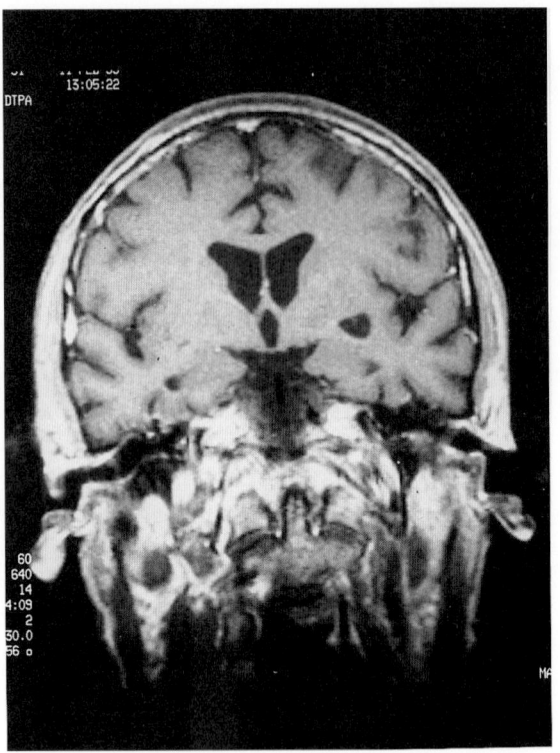

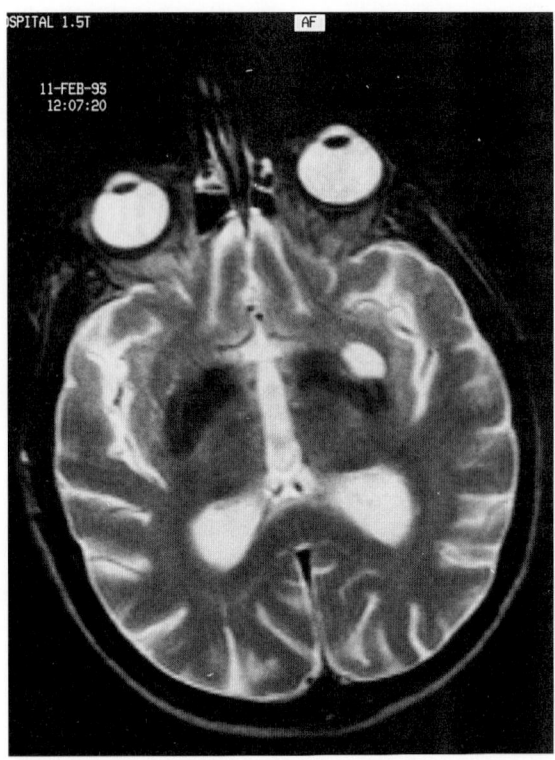

A

B

Fig. 13.6   Old cerebral infarct due to meningovascular syphilis in an AIDS patient. **A** T1 and **B** T2-weighted MR images.

Tuberculosis

Mycobacterium tuberculosis infection may cause a basal meningitis with associated arteritis of vessels as they penetrate the dura and at the base of the brain. The changes affect small- and medium-sized arteries and veins. The vessel walls show cellular infiltration with or without caseation. In some cases, the appearances suggest a delayed hypersensitivity reaction rather than direct infection. Superadded thrombosis is seen in both arteries and veins. The clinical picture of tuberculous meningitis (TBM) with a febrile ill patient with cranial nerve palsies and meningism may be complicated by the development of focal deficits due to infarction. The differential diagnosis includes a Todd's paresis after a focal seizure due to TBM, and other causes of stroke. Middle cerebral artery territory infarction is most frequent, but quadriplegia and involuntary movements have been reported, albeit in non-AIDS cases (Molavi & Le Frock 1985). There appear to be no differences in the presence of HIV infection.

Substance abuse

Patients whose HIV infection occurs in the context of drug abuse may also develop cerebrovascular problems due to amphetamine, cocaine, heroin, LSD, phencyclidine and proprietary sympathomimetics (Sloan et al 1991). Strokes due to amphetamine are well recognized and are thought to be due to a vasculitis that mimicks polyarteritis nodosa clinically and pathologically, with fever, leucocytosis, raised erythrocyte sedimentation rate (ESR), etc. (Citron et al 1970). A similar vasculitis with segmental narrowing of intracranial vessels and aneurysm formation on angiography has been described for other sympatheticomimetics such as phentermine (Kokkinos & Levine 1993). Cocaine-related strokes are being increasingly reported and a typical presentation would be the occurrence of a stroke a few hours after use. Cocaine produces vasospasm experimentally (Wang et al 1990) and a biopsy-proven vasculitis (Krendel et al 1990), which may be associated with multiple vessel occlusions and a clinical picture of focal deficit and diffuse cerebral dysfunction. It remains uncertain whether the vessel wall thickening and lymphocytic infiltration is a response to spasm or reflects a hypersensitivity reaction (Fredericks et al 1991). The route of administration does not appear to affect risk, and infarction may occur in any cerebrovascular territory. Daras et al (1991) reviewing 18 cases noted a hemisphere lesion in 13, brainstem infarction in two, spinal cord ischaemia in two and multiple infarctions in one. All cases may not be due to vasculitis as cocaine can cause a cardiomyopathy (Sauer 1991) or myocardial infarction (Sloan & Mattioni 1992), and the stroke may be due to cardiac embolism (Petty et al 1990). Cerebral haemorrhage due to cocaine (or amphetamine) use may relate to a surge of hypertension with consequent bleeding from coincident 'Berry' aneurysms or arteriovenous malformation (Levine et al 1990a). Sometimes there is no arterial lesion despite multiple haemorrhages (Green et al 1990).

Intravenous drug users also run the risk of injection of particulate matter, e.g. talc, which can rarely cause cerebral infarction, perhaps dependent on the presence of a patent foramen ovale. Bitar and Gomez (1993) recently described a patient with occipital infarction after injection of a melted opiate suppository.

Some pathological series (Mizusawa et al 1988) have shown that many infarcts in AIDS cases have been clinically silent and have been small and often located in the striatum and brainstem. A mural thickening of small vessels has been proposed as the cause for such 'lacunar' infarcts, though the common finding of calcification of small blood vessels did not appear to be closely linked to the presence or site of infarcts. The cause for such a microvascular change is as yet unknown, though immune complex deposition can cause a necrotizing arteritis in mice exposed to proteins of the murine leukaemia virus (Yoshika et al 1979). It is also not clear whether such small vessel changes underlie those cases of stroke in which no aetiology is discovered after investigation (Engstrom et al 1989).

Septic arteritis

Patients with bacterial endocarditis are prone to septic embolism, especially from the friable vegetations caused by virulent organisms (Pruitt et al 1978). Intravenous drug users may have a slightly smaller incidence of cerebral embolism as it is often the tricuspid valve that is infected. They do, however, develop patchy septic damage to the walls of intracerebral vasculature. It has been thought that these follow damage to the arterial wall after microembolism of the vasa vasorum. Some patients have a clear-cut episode of macroembolism to the intracerebral vessel before the aneurysm develops, however, so the septic arteritis may develop from the lumen. They are usually asymptomatic until they rupture, often fatally (Brust et al 1990). The aneurysms are usually single and small, and often are located on branches of the middle cerebral artery (Fig. 13.2). They can 'disappear' during antibiotic therapy. Some patients have cranial nerve signs or focal deficit before rupture and others have a picture more like a meningitis. Some authors advocate an aggressive policy of angiography and early craniotomy or endovascular embolization (Khayata et al 1993) in an attempt to reduce the morbidity and mortality. However, Kanter and Hart (1990, 1991) reviewed 133 consecutive cases of infective endocarditis. Nine had cerebral haemorrhage, but only one had a proven aneurysm. Three had negative angiography, and five had autopsy evidence of pyogenic arteritis without aneurysm formation. Histopathological analysis of autopsy specimens shows that many cases of haemorrhage are in fact due to haemorrhagic transformation of infarcts due to septic embolism, and some aneurysms are occluded by septic material without rupture (Masuda et al 1992). The low yield of aneurysms suggests that routine angiography is not appropriate (Van der Meulen et al 1992). It is our policy to consider angiography and intervention only if subarachnoid haemorrhage has occurred, or scanning suggests the presence of a large aneurysm especially in a patient with focal deficit or severe headache, not explained by embolism or meningitis. The differential diagnosis of CNS complications of infective endocarditis includes a diffuse encephalopathy attributed to microembolism, which is most likely in the presence of virulent organisms, and meningitis. Any focal deficit is assumed to represent the effect of septic embolism, but imaging must be carried out to exclude the unlikely possibility of an abscess.

Arterial dissection

In a survey of the causes of young stroke (Lisovoski & Rousseaux 1991) dissection of major cervical or cerebral arteries was found in 10% of cases. These may be predisposed by disorders of the vascular media such as fibromuscular dysplasia, but can be due to external trauma, for example that potentially inflicted on the cervical carotid or vertebral artery in some sexual 'games'. The practice of asphyxiation during intercourse with a noose or cord can damage the arteries in the neck. The diagnosis is suggested by ipsilateral face, eye or head pain and a Horner syndrome, followed by a TIA or stroke in the ipsilateral carotid territory. The diagnosis can be made by Doppler, magnetic resonance angiography, CT, or angiography. Short-term (6–8 weeks) anticoagulation is recommended to limit the risk of further mural thromboembolism.

Paediatric stroke

In children cerebrovascular disease rivals lymphoma as the cause of focal neurological deficit or of focal lesions on CT or MRI. Some have haemorrhages due to thrombocytopenia, others have infarcts related to cardiac embolism or small vessel disease. Park et al (1990) recorded that four of 68 children followed over 4.5 years had clinical or radiological evidence of stroke. At autopsy the incidence was much higher (24%). Four patients had intracerebral haemorrhages, six non-haemorrhagic infarcts and three had both. An unusual arteriopathy with aneurysmal dilatation of vessels of the circle of Willis was found in one case. In the absence of evidence of zoster vasculitis, a direct role for HIV was tentatively proposed. Antiviral therapy would be appropriate.

DIAGNOSIS

The differential diagnosis of transient focal neurological deficits includes non-vascular causes. Episodic dysfunction clinically indistinguishable from TIAs can accompany gliomas and other mass lesions (Loeb 1979), and rarer causes of a transient deficit include hypoglycaemia, hypercalcaemia, hyponatraemia and hepatic and renal failure (Harrison 1982). Engstrom et al (1989) found examples of 'pseudo-TIAs' due to *Toxoplasma* abscesses, lymphoma and cryptococcal

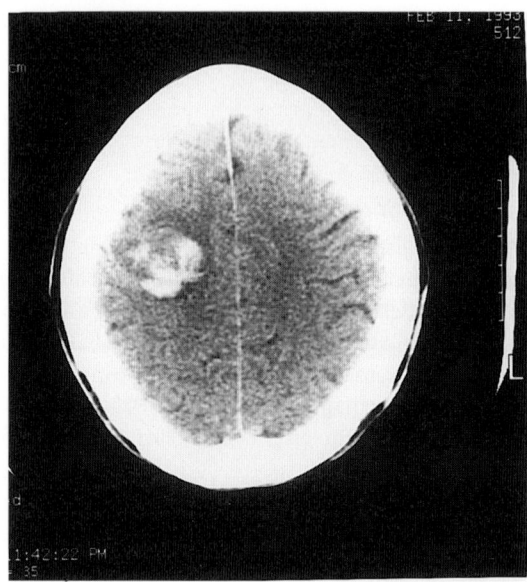

A

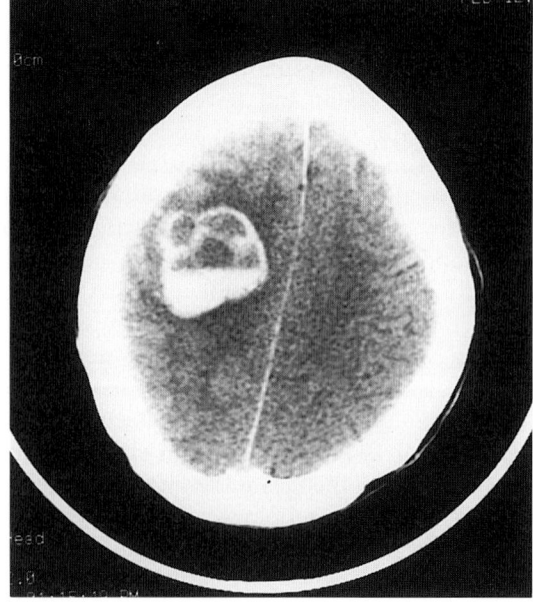

B

Fig. 13.7 (**A, B**) Evolving intraparenchymal haemorrhage from ruptured mycotic aneurysm in an HIV-positive patient with *Staphylococcus aureus* endocarditis.

infection. Brew and Miller (1993) have pointed out that patients with HIV-associated dementia complex may have frequent 'transient ischaemic attacks'. Although some of these may be associated with anticardiolipin antibodies and/or low platelet counts, their aetiology is uncertain and infarction rarely follows. Whether these 'attacks' are truly ischaemic is unknown.

CEREBRAL HAEMORRHAGE

Cerebral haemorrhage is not as common as infarction even in the autopsy series (Mizusawa et al 1988). Subarachnoid haemorrhage, subdural haematomas and parenchymal haemorrhages (Fig. 13.7) have all been described. Most, but by no means all, related to the presence of thrombocytopenia (Mizusawa et al 1988, Engstrom et al 1989, Berger et al 1990). The latter is a major factor in deciding whether to consider surgical evacuation of clots. Rarely, haemorrhage is due to the presence of Kaposi's sarcoma in the brain.

MANAGEMENT PLAN

In practice, mass lesions, infections and cardiac and haematological abnormalities should be sought. This will require CT or MRI of the brain, examination of the CSF, and cardiac screening, including echocardiography. If there is no such pathology a vasculitis should be considered and treatable causes pursued. This involves a search for evidence of *M. tuberculosis* and meningovascular syphilis with appropriate serological studies in the CSF, as this is a treatable option with a full course of intravenous penicillin (Labange et al 1991). Intravenous acyclovir should be prescribed in the presence of recent cranial zoster infection in an attempt to limit any associated angiitis.

Anticoagulants would be potentially hazardous in the presence of thrombocytopenia, and the prognosis does not seem to warrant their use except for dissection and some high-risk cardiac embolic sources (e.g. atrial fibrillation). In the absence of evidence of vascular disease, cardiac abnormality or coagulopathy, it is probably reasonable to prescribe aspirin in small dose, as long as the platelet count is normal. Attacks often continue unabated, raising doubts that the patient's TIAs are due to thromboembolism (Brew et al 1993).

REFERENCES

Anastasopoulos G, Routsonis K, Ierodiakonov C S. Ophthalmic herpes zoster with contralateral hemiplegia. J Neurol Neurosurg Psychiat 1958; 21: 210–212

Berger J R. Spinal cord syphilis associated with human immunodeficiency virus infection: a treatable myelopathy. Am J Med 1992; 92: 101–103

Berger J R, Harris J O, Gregorius J, Norenberg M. Cerebrovascular disease in AIDS: a case-control study. AIDS 1990; 4: 239–244

Bitar S, Gomez C R. Stroke following injection of a melted suppository. Stroke 1993; 24: 741–743

Bousser M G, Baron J C, Chiras J. Ischaemic strokes and migraine. Neuroradiology 1985; 27: 583–587

Brew B J, Miller J. Transient ischaemic attacks (TIAs) in HIV infection. Clin Neuropath 1993; 12 (suppl 1): S15

Brey R L, Hart R G, Sherman D G, Tegeler C H. Antiphospholipid antibodies and cerebral ischemia in young people. Neurology 1990; 40: 1190–1196

Brust J C, Taylor Dickinson P C, Hughes J E O, Holtzman N N. The diagnosis and treatment of cerebral mycotic aneurysms. Ann Neurol 1990; 27: 238–246

Citron B P, Halpern M, McCarron M, et al. Necrotizing angiitis associated with drug abuse. N Engl J Med 1970; 283: 1003–1011

Daras M, Tuchman A J, Marks S. Central nervous system infarction related to cocaine abuse. Stroke 1991; 22: 1320–1325

Eidelberg D, Sotrel A, Horoupian D S, et al. Thrombotic cerebral vasculopathy associated with herpes zoster. Ann Neurol 1986; 19: 7–14

Engstrom J W, Lowenstein D H, Bredesen D E. Cerebral infarctions and transient neurological deficits associated with acquired immunodeficiency syndrome. Am J Med 1989; 86: 528–532

Fredericks R K, Lefkowitz D S, Challa V R, Troost B T. Cerebral vasculitis associated with cocaine abuse. Stroke 1991; 22: 1437–1439

Green R M, Kelly K M, Gabrielsen T, et al. Multiple intracerebral haemorrhages after smoking 'crack' cocaine. Stroke 1990; 21: 957–962

Harrison M J G. Pathogenesis. In: Warlow C, Morris P, editors. Transient ischaemic attacks. Decker: New York, 1982: 21–46

Hilt D C, Buckholz D, Krumholz A, et al. Herpes zoster ophthalmicus and delayed contralateral hemiparesis caused by cerebral angiitis: diagnosis and management approaches. Ann Neurol 1983; 14: 543–553

Kanter M C, Hart R G. Cerebral mycotic aneurysms are rare in infective endocarditis. Ann Neurol 1990; 28: 590

Kanter M C, Hart R G. Neurological complications of infective endocarditis. Neurology 1991; 41: 1015–1020

Katz D A, Berger J R. Neurosyphilis in acquired immunodeficiency syndrome. Arch Neurol 1989; 46: 895–898

Khayata M H, Aymard A, Casasco A, et al. Selective endovascular techniques in the treatment of cerebral mycotic aneurysms. J Neurosurg 1993; 78: 661–665

Kieburtz K D, Eskin T A, Ketonen L, Tuite M J. Opportunistic cerebral vasculopathy and stroke in patients with the acquired immunodeficiency syndrome. Arch Neurol 1993; 50: 430–432

Kokkinos J, Levine S R. Possible association of ischaemic stroke with Phentermine. Stroke 1993; 24: 310–313

Krendel D A, Ditter S M, Frankel M R, Ross W K. Biopsy-proven cerebral vasculitis associated with cocaine abuse. Neurology 1990; 40: 1092–1094

Labange R, Tourniaire D, Bland J M. Infarction of the pons, neurosyphilis and HIV infection. Rev Neurol 1991; 147: 406–408

Levine S R, Brust J C M, Futrell N, et al. Cerebrovascular complications of the use of the 'crack' form of alkaloid cocaine. N Engl J Med 1990a; 323: 699–704

Levine S R, Deegan M J, Futrell N, Welch K M A. Cerebrovascular and neurologic disease associated with antiphospholipid antibodies: 48 cases. Neurology 1990b; 40: 1181–1189

Lisovoski F, Rousseaux P. Cerebral infarction in young people. A study of 148 patients with early cerebral angiography. J Neurol Neurosurg Psychiatr 1991; 54: 576–579

Loeb C. Clinical evaluation of patients with transient ischaemic attacks. Adv Neurol 1979; 25: 141–148

MacKenzie R A, Forbes G S, Karnes W E. Angiographic findings in herpes zoster arteritis. Ann Neurol 1981; 10: 458–464

Masuda J, Yutani C, Waki R, et al. Histopathological analysis of the mechanism of intracranial haemorrhagic complications of infective endocarditis. Stroke 1992; 23: 843–850

Meyer R D, Young L S, Armstrong D, Yu B. Aspergillosis complicating neoplastic disease. Am J Med 1973; 54: 6

Mizusawa H, Hirano A, Llena J F, Shintaku M. Cerebrovascular lesions in acquired immune deficiency syndrome (AIDS). Acta Neuropathol 1988; 76: 451–457

Molavi A, Le Frock J L. Tuberculous meningitis. Med Clin North Am 1985; 69: 315–344

Musher D M, Hamill R J, Baughn R D. Effect of human immunodeficiency virus (HIV) infection on the cause of syphilis and on the response to treatment. Ann Intern Med 1990; 113: 872–881

Naimi N, Plancherel C, Bosser C, et al. Anticardiolipin antibodies in HIV-negative and HIV-positive haemophiliacs. Blood Coag Fibrinolysis 1990; 1: 5–8

Park Y D, Belman A L, Kim T-S, et al. Stroke in pediatric acquired immunodeficiency syndrome. Ann Neurol 1990; 28: 303–311

Petty G W, Brust J C, Tatemichi T K, Barr M L. Embolic stroke after smoking 'crack' cocaine. Stroke 1990; 21: 1632–1635

Pruitt A A, Rubin R H, Karchmer A W, et al. Neurological complications of bacterial endocarditis. Medicine 1978; 57: 329–343

Rawlinson W D, Cunningham A L. Contralateral hemiplegia following thoracic herpes zoster. Med J Aust 1991; 155: 344–346

Rodan E O, Moskowitz L, Hensley G T. Pathology of the heart in AIDS. Arch Pathol Lab Med 1987; 111: 943–946

Ross M H, Abend W K, Schwartz R B, Samuels M A. A case of C2 herpes zoster with delayed bilateral pontine infarction. Neurology 1991; 41: 1685–1686

Saito K, Moskwitz M A. Contribution from upper cervical dorsal roots and ligamental ganglia to the feline circle of Willis. Stroke 1989; 20: 2524–2526

Sauer C M. Recurrent embolic stroke and cocaine-related cardiomyopathy. Stroke 1991; 22: 1203–1205

Scaravilli F, Daniel S E, Harcourt-Webster N, Guiloff R J. Chronic basal meningitis and vasculitis in acquired immunodeficiency syndrome: a possible role for human immunodeficiency virus. Arch Pathol Lab Med 1989; 113: 192–195

Sloan M A, Mattioni T A. Concurrent myocardial and cerebral infarctions after intranasal cocaine use. Stroke 1992; 23: 427–430

Sloan M A, Kittner S J, Rigamonti D, Price T R. Occurrence of stroke associated with use/abuse of drugs. Neurology 1991; 41: 1358–1364

Van der Meulen J H P, Weststrate W, Van Gijn J, Habbema J D F. Is cerebral angiography indicated in infective endocarditis. Stroke 1992; 23: 1662–1667

Wang A-M, Suojanen J N, Colucci V M, et al. Cocaine and methamphetamine induced acute cerebral vasospasm: an angiographic study in rabbits. AJNR 1990; 11: 1141–1146

Wiley C A, Schrier R D, Nelson J A, et al. Cellular localization of human immunodeficiency virus infection within the brains of acquired immune deficiency syndrome patients. Proc Natl Acad Sci USA 1986; 83: 7089–7093

14. Common neurological symptoms in HIV infection

MENTAL STATUS CHANGES

Because of the frequency of central nervous system (CNS) involvement with HIV or opportunistic infections, mental status changes and encephalopathies are common, particularly late in HIV infection. The development of encephalopathy with delirium, confusion and disorientation should initially prompt consideration of an opportunistic process. However, most opportunistic infections develop only after the CD4 count has dropped below 200. In an HIV-seropositive individual with a CD4 count above 200, the causes of encephalopathy include illicit drug use, Wernicke's encephalopathy, tuberculous (TB) meningitis, neurosyphilis, subarachnoid haemorrhage and primary HIV infection with seroconversion illness. After immune deficiency has developed with a CD4 count less than 200, common causes of altered mentation include cytomegalovirus (CMV) encephalitis, cryptococcal meningitis, primary CNS lymphoma and toxoplasmosis. Neuroimaging is essential in these cases, and may cause surprises as in a confused patient whose MRI revealed bilateral subdural haematomas (Fig. 14.1). Altered awareness is uncommon in progressive multifocal leucoencephalopathy (PML), except in the terminal phases. Similarly, in HIV dementia, delirium may be superimposed on the underlying features of dementia: 'decompensated dementia'. Usually, delirium in HIV dementia is triggered by inappropriate use of hypnotics, sedatives or antidepressants, or by systemic infection, hypoxia or metabolic derangement. There have been reports in individuals with HIV dementia of abrupt encephalopathy triggered by discontinua-tion of antiretroviral therapy. Although the mechanisms have not been completely worked out, it is possible that with the cessation of antiretroviral therapy, there is a sudden increase in viral replication in the brain, producing the encephalopathy (Pinching et al 1989).

With the polypharmacy common in the patient with advanced HIV disease, drug interactions or adverse effects are very common causes of encephalopathy. Particular culprits include phosphonoformate (foscarnet), amphotericin B, tricyclic antidepressants and opiates including

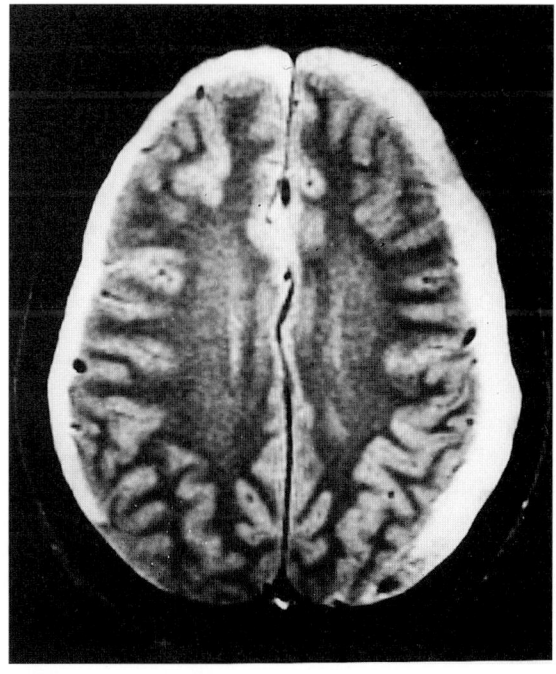

Fig. 14.1 T2-weighted MRI showing bright crescentic signal from bilateral subdural haematomas in a HIV-infected patient presenting with confusion.

Table 14.1   Clues to diagnosis of altered mentation in AIDS

Cause	Symptoms
Cryptococcal meningitis	Fever, headache, meningismus
CMV encephalitis	Progression over 1–4 weeks, electrolyte abnormalities
Toxoplasmosis ⎫ Primary CNS lymphoma ⎬	Focal neurological deficits Mass lesions on imaging
Wernicke's encephalopathy	Gait ataxia, ophthalmoparesis, nystagmus
TB meningitis	Pulmonary/extrapulmonary TB CSF: low glucose, high protein

Table 14.2   Common psychiatric disorders associated with HIV disease (Treisman, personal communication)

Disorder	Comments
Depression	Up to 50% life-time prevalence in homosexual and IVDU populations prior to serology testing Major depression commonly with insomnia, low energy and motivation, decreased appetite, decreased libido, guilt, suicidal ideation, decreased concentration Overlap with common constitutional symptoms of HIV infection Often chronic after initial 'adjustment reaction', especially in patients with prior history of depression
Substance abuse	Excluding IVDUs, 20–40% have history of non-opioid substance abuse
Anxiety disorders	Generalized chronic anxiety often develops as an outgrowth of acute adjustment reactions triggered by life stresses or losses Panic attacks are frequent, often associated with night sweats
Adjustment reactions	Usually remit, especially in those with no prior psychiatric history Part of initial adjustment to the diagnosis, or to change in disease status
Mania	New onset mania (with no personal or family history) may herald the onset of HIV dementia

IVDU, intravenous drug user.

codeine. Table 14.1 indicates some of the features helpful in the diagnosis of altered mentation in AIDS. Management of delirium depends on treatment of the underlying condition with reversal of the responsible hypoxia or electrolyte disturbance, for example, nursing in a quiet environment and cautious use of sedation. Neuroleptics should be avoided if possible, though they will be needed in mania or frank psychosis. Although there is some controversy over whether psychoses are truly more common in AIDS, there are some cases in whom such presentations herald an organic illness, or prove to be due to an opportunistic infection.

PSYCHIATRIC AND PSYCHOLOGICAL SYMPTOMS

A full discussion of the range of psychiatric disorders associated with HIV disease is beyond the scope of this book and several reviews are available (Holland & Tross 1985, Ostrow 1987, 1990). Since some of these disorders will be encountered by the hospital physician, infectious disease specialist or neurologist, and may cause confusion with organic disorders such as HIV dementia, they will be reviewed briefly (Table 14.2). Anxiety disorders and adjustment reactions are relatively common among individuals learning of their HIV serostatus, showing evidence of disease progression, e.g. first AIDS-defining illness, or experiencing loss of friends or partners. These acute psychological syndromes are frequently short-lived; however, they may become chronic, leading to symptoms of depression if appropriate interventions are delayed and social supports are absent. Sadness and depressive symptoms can develop because of multiple losses, as Atkinson et al (1988) describe, 'of health, income, independence, and relationships due to illness itself or social ostracism or self-imposed isolation because of fear of contagion'. In a systematic survey of 56 ambulatory homosexual men ranging from men with AIDS to HIV-seronegative individuals, Atkinson and colleagues found that homosexual men had a relatively high life-time prevalence of major psychiatric disorders, including generalized anxiety disorder (39%) and major depression (30%), and of alcohol or non-opiate drug abuse (39%). These disorders often preceded knowledge of HIV serostatus or other medical illnesses. Most psychiatric syndromes developed with the identification of seropositivity or the development of an HIV-related illness. Generalized anxiety was the most common condition and, overall, psychiatric disorders were not related to cognitive impairment.

Among patients attending the Johns Hopkins Hospital HIV Outpatient Clinic, which has a high proportion of injection drug users, in contrast to the Atkinson study, Treisman (personal communication) found a similarly high prevalence of psychiatric disease. The implications from these kinds of studies are that the patient's life-time history of psychiatric disorders is important both in interpreting current active symptoms and potentially in predicting future problems related to changes in physical health. Psychiatric or psychological consultation plays an important part in the management of patients with HIV infection at all stages of disease, and aggressive evaluation and management of psychiatric symptoms can improve the quality of life for the patient, facilitate compliance and reduce risky behaviours such as unprotected sex or continued substance abuse.

Treatment

Acute anxiety disorders can be treated with benzodiazepines. These are best for short-term treatment and have both anxiolytic as well as sedative effects. Tolerance develops quickly and there is a tendency for dose escalation. Lorazepam 0.5 mg t.i.d. increasing to 1–2 mg t.i.d. is useful because it has an intermediate half-life and no active metabolites. Alprazolam may have antidepressant properties, but has disadvantages of being very short-acting with a high risk of addiction. Buspirone is probably best for long-term treatment of anxiety disorders; it has a low abuse potential, and thus is useful for patients with a history of substance abuse. The usual dose is 5–10 mg t.i.d. with a slow onset of action (2–4 weeks). The non-tricyclic antidepressants, the serotonergic reuptake inhibitors sertraline, fluoxetine and paroxetine, are all equal in efficacy to tricyclic antidepressants for treatment of depression. They have virtually no anti-cholinergic, orthostatic or sedating effects. Insomnia, headache, nausea and diarrhoea are the most common side-effects. Paroxetine is associated with less insomnia. Extrapyramidal symptoms, including tremor and myoclonus, can occur in HIV infection with these agents. Drug treatment for depression is tabled in Appendix 6.

Drugs that cause psychiatric symptoms

Many drugs in common use can cause serious psychiatric symptoms, including delirium, depression, anxiety, and even psychotic reactions. Details are set out in Appendix 6.

VISUAL CHANGES

Several discrete causes of visual disturbance can occur in AIDS. These include visual field deficits, diplopia from oculomotor pareses, optic nerve involvement, retinal damage and uveitis. Each site of involvement may be associated with different visual complaints, and Table 14.3 indicates the common organisms or causes of the specific symptoms.

Visual field deficits

These usually occur late in HIV infection and are produced by opportunistic processes involving either the visual cortex, optic tracts or optic radiations. Depending on the specific entity, the onset of visual field deficits may be slow and unnoticed by the patient. This contrasts with ocular or oculomotor dysfunction. For example, PML commonly produces visual field dysfunction with a slow progression of deficits over several weeks to months.

Table 14.3 Causes of visual symptoms

Problem		Cause
Field defect	Optic tract radiation	Toxoplasmosis Lymphoma
	Visual cortex	PML Infarct/haemorrhage
Diplopia	Cranial nerve	Lymphomatous meningitis Neurosyphilis Cryptococcal meningitis Raised ICP
	Brainstem	PML, lymphoma, toxoplasmosis, infarct, Wernicke's encephalopathy Intoxication
Visual loss	Retina	CMV retinitis, Toxoplasma, Histoplasma
	Optic nerve	Syphilis, cryptococcosis, optic neuritis, raised ICP

ICP, intracranial pressure.

Oculomotor palsies

These include direct involvement of the IIIrd, IVth, or VIth cranial nerves with development of diplopia or the false localizing sign of bilateral VIth nerve palsies from elevated intracranial pressure. Common causes (Keane 1991) of direct cranial nerve involvement include lymphomatous meningitis with infiltration of the cranial nerves as they traverse the subarachnoid space or within the cavernous sinus. Cryptococcal infiltration of the cranial nerves can cause optic nerve or oculomotor nerve dysfunction and usually portends poor response to treatment. Cranial nerve involvement with neurosyphilis has been recognized frequently in HIV-seropositive individuals. In one series of 40 HIV-seropositive individuals with neurosyphilis, nine had syphilitic meningitis and 13 developed cranial nerve dysfunction. Involvement of the IInd cranial nerve was most frequent, followed by the VIIIth (Musher et al 1990). Cranial nerve lesions are also seen in TB meningitis and CMV ventriculoencephalitis.

Change in visual acuity

Visual blurring, the development of scotoma, or blindness are frequent manifestations of CMV retinitis (see Chapter 9). While peripheral retinal involvement may be visually silent, when CMV retinitis affects central vision, patients describe painless onset of visual blurring with black spots or field deficits. The fundoscopic appearance of CMV retinitis is characteristic with haemorrhagic exudates involving blood vessels. Many patients, particularly when at high risk for CMV infection (CD4 count less than 200), perform regular checks of vision using an Amsler grid (Fig. 14.2). Less common causes of visual loss include toxoplasmic or histoplasmic retinitis, papilloedema from elevated intracranial pressure associated with cryptococcal meningitis, or syphilitic optic neuritis (Winward et al 1989). The latter is often accompanied by recognizable inflammation of the anterior chamber with uveitis and iritis. A reversible optic neuritis with focal enhancement in the optic nerve (Fig. 14.3) on MRI has been described in a patient

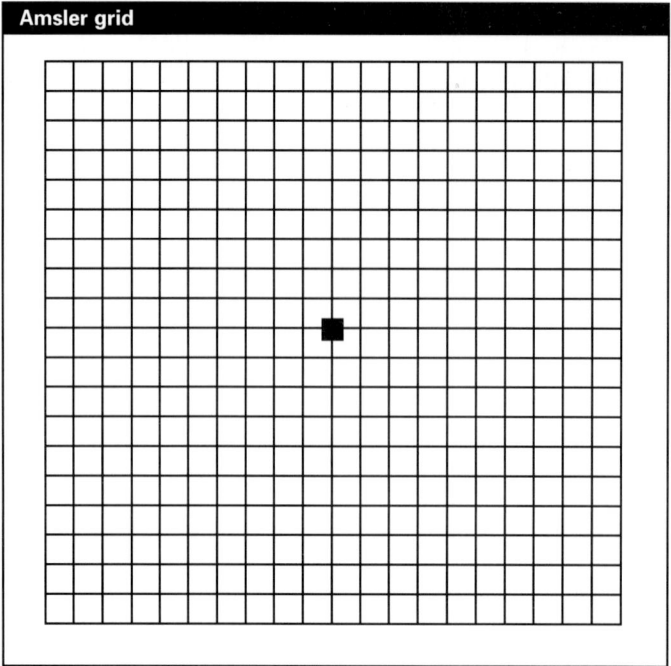

Fig. 14.2   Visual field grid for self-assessment of field defects. (Courtesy of Syntex Laboratories, Inc.) (See footnote p. 216.)

Table 14.4 Causes of headache

Immunocompetent	Tension headache
	Migraine
	Chronic HIV meningitis (CSF pleocytosis)
	Sinusitis
Immunodeficient	Cryptococcal meningitis
	Toxoplasmosis
	Lymphoma

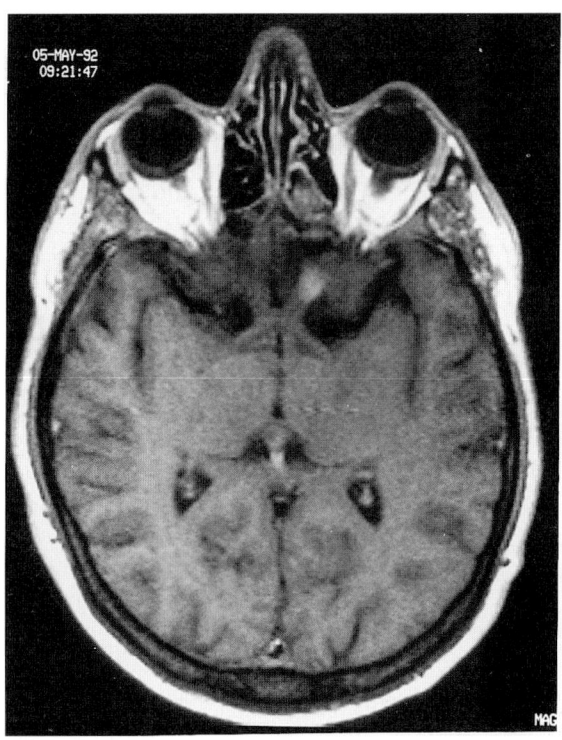

Fig. 14.3 Gadolinium-enhanced T1-weighted MRI showing a lesion in the right optic nerve. (Reproduced from Sweeney et al 1993 with permission of BMJ Publishing Group.)

who later developed lymphoma (Sweeney et al 1993).

HEADACHE

Headache is an extremely common symptom in HIV infection because of the frequency of intracranial infections and mass lesions, and of pyrexial systemic disorders related to immunosuppression. As with mentation change, the degree of immunodeficiency is a critical factor in the differential diagnosis. As Table 14.4 indicates, with a CD4 count in the normal range (e.g. above 500), opportunistic infections occur rarely, and other causes of headaches predominate. Below 500, the development of headache, particularly if new in onset and accompanied by fever, meningismus or neurological symptoms, should prompt an urgent search for intracranial infection.

Headache in the immunocompetent HIV-seropositive patient

As discussed above, during this phase of HIV infection, opportunistic processes are unlikely to develop. The most common causes of headaches are chronic 'tension' headaches, chronic HIV meningitis and sinusitis. Chronic tension headaches may be recognized by their chronicity and the descriptions of a band-like, vertex pressure occurring daily. Typically, the headaches worsen as the day progresses, are not accompanied by neurological symptoms or visual phenomena, and worsen during periods of anxiety or stress. As discussed later in this chapter, HIV is commonly associated with a cerebrospinal fluid (CSF) pleocytosis. In most individuals this is silent and not accompanied by meningism. In a small proportion of patients, usually very early in HIV infection, an acute aseptic meningitis develops. Far more common is a chronic low-grade meningitis from HIV. It is often difficult to separate the headache of chronic HIV meningitis from 'tension' headache, and indeed the two may overlap. A persistent CSF pleocytosis with greater than 20 white blood cells (WBC)/mm^3 favours an HIV chronic meningitis. The headache with chronic HIV meningitis may result from the intrathecal release of cytokines such as tumor necrosis factor-alpha (TNF-α). Sinus disease and sinusitis are a common cause of headache, usually frontal and aching in character and associated with nasal symptoms. MRI studies (Fig. 14.4) have shown a high frequency of sinus congestion and mucosal thickening in HIV-seropositive individuals (Chong et al 1993). Finally, migraine is an extremely common cause of headache and has been estimated to affect between 8 and 15% of the general population. Episodic headache with

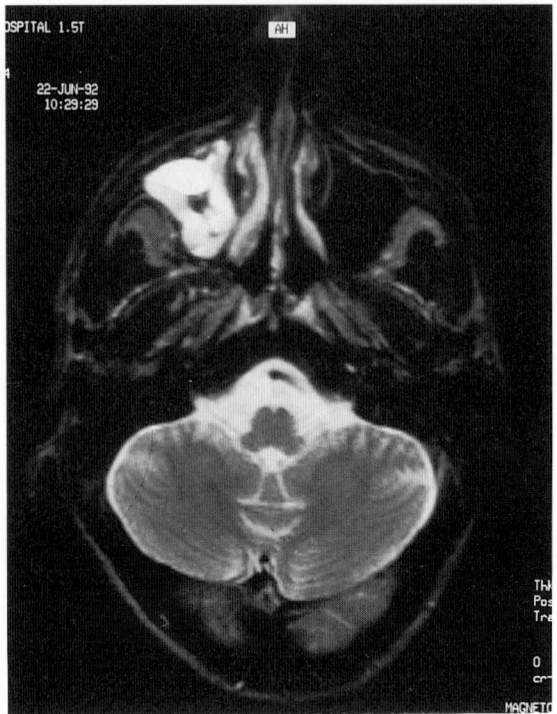

Fig. 14.4   T2-weighted MRI showing sinus disease.

nausea, vomiting and migrainous visual phenomena, such as scintillating scotoma or fortification spectra, are usually easily diagnosable as migrainous. It has been suggested that there is an increased frequency of migraine in HIV infection. This has not been confirmed by rigorous surveys. The initiation of zidovudine is frequently accompanied by temporary headaches lasting 2–4 weeks after drug initiation. In a migraineur, zidovudine can induce a flurry of migraine attacks. Usually these subside within a few weeks of initiation.

Headaches in the immunodeficient HIV-positive patient

In the setting of immunodeficiency with a CD4 count less than 500, the development of new headache has to be considered a marker of possible intracranial pathology, particularly if accompanied by meningism, localizing neurological symptoms and signs, or altered mentation. The exception is if the patient is obviously 'toxic' with a systemic infection such as pneumonia and

a pyrexial headache. The most common cause of new headache in an immunodeficient HIV-seropositive patient is cryptococcal meningitis. Forty-five per cent of patients developing cryptococcal meningitis have had no previous AIDS-defining illness (Chuck & Sande 1989), and in the USA it is not uncommon for an injecting drug user to present to medical attention for the first time with fulminant cryptococcal meningitis. The headache is usually severe, fronto-temporal and accompanied by fever, nausea and a stiff neck. Visual blurring from papilloedema occurs in about 10% of cases, but lateralizing neurological symptoms are rare. The average duration of headache before diagnosis is about 7 days. Because of the frequency of cryptococcal meningitis and the impracticality of performing lumbar puncture on every HIV-seropositive patient with a low CD4 count and headache, the measurement of serum cryptococcal antigen has come into widespread use. Chuck and Sande (1989) reviewed 106 cases of cryptococcal meningitis. Serum titres of cryptococcal antigen had been measured in 71; only one proved negative. Eight of 88 CSF samples were negative. Serum cryptococcal antigen is thus a reasonable screening test.

Other opportunistic processes, including cerebral toxoplasmosis and primary CNS lymphoma, are less common causes of head pain. Headache is described in about 60% of patients with toxoplasmosis (Navia et al 1986) and 40% of patients with lymphoma (Levy & Bredesen 1988). Headache is usually associated with nausea, vomiting, hemiparesis, language dysfunction, behavioural or personality change, or altered mentation. It may be frontal, nuchal, generalized or unilateral, and may be increased by head jolt, coughing, stooping and straining. A management scheme is shown in Fig. 14.5.

SEIZURES

Both focal and generalized seizures are common in HIV infection, affecting 5–10% of patients with AIDS. Seizures may be the initial presenting symptom indicating an underlying CNS opportunistic process, or may signal systemic illness, or the effects of drug or alcohol abuse. In two series studying the cause of seizures in HIV clinics in

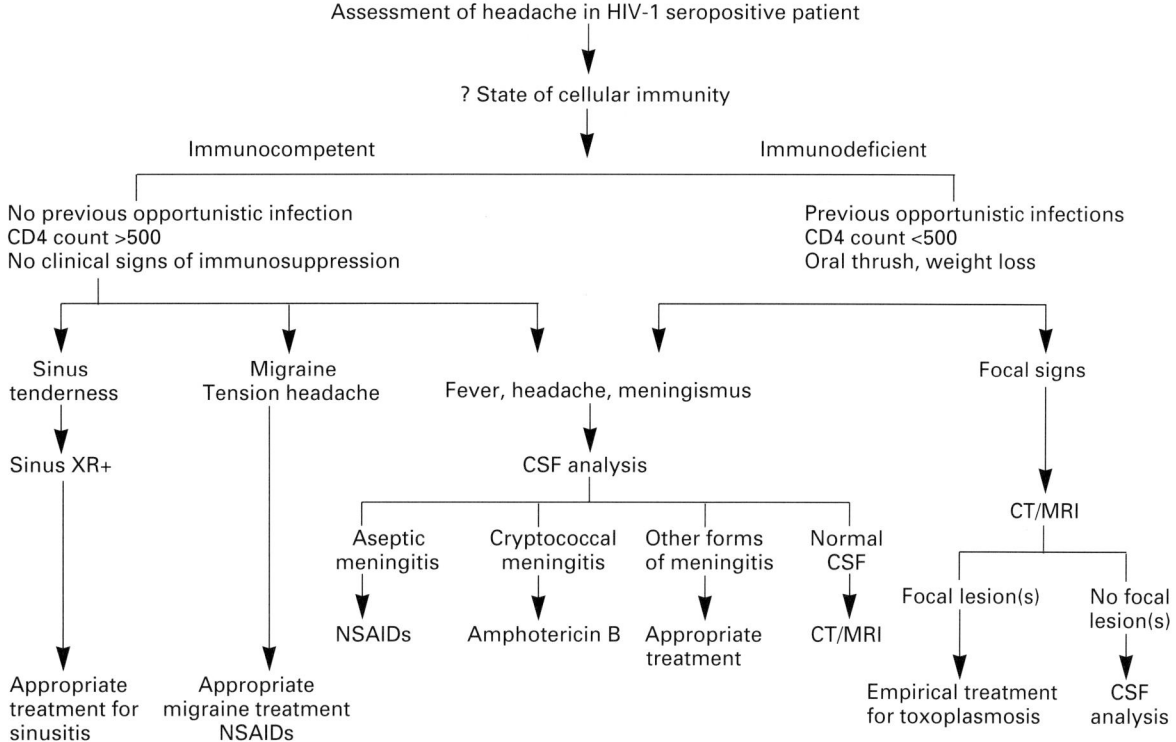

Fig. 14.5   Management protocol for headache.

New York and San Francisco (Holtzman et al 1989, Wong et al 1990), half had no obvious explanation in terms of structural deficits, metabolic causes or intoxication. The implication was that in these cases, seizures might result directly from brain infection with HIV. Long-term follow-up studies will reveal whether this interpretation is correct.

Amongst the more clearly defined causes for seizures in AIDS are focal intracranial lesions such as abscesses and lymphomas, meningitis, metabolic problems and strokes (Table 14.5). Rarer causes include viral encephalitides related to herpes simplex, herpes zoster, CMV and JC virus. In the immunocompetent HIV-infected patient, CNS opportunistic processes are unlikely and especially careful questioning for alcohol abuse or illicit drug use should be made with appropriate toxicological confirmation. The presence of neurological signs is predictive of an underlying structural cause. In Holtzman's study, 53 of 76 patients with neurological signs had a detectable cause, while only two of 24 patients with a normal neuro-

logical examination had a mass lesion or meningitis (Holtzman et al 1989). Focal seizures more frequently indicate underlying structural lesions.

The investigation of seizures in this setting should include contrast imaging for mass lesions and CSF examination for meningitis. Electroencephalography (EEG) recordings add little to the diagnostic work-up, except when the patient remains confused or encephalopathic. Here, EEG is useful to exclude frequent epileptiform dis-

Table 14.5   Causes of seizures

Cause	San Francisco (Wong et al 1990)	Cornell (Holtzman et al 1989)	Total
Toxoplasmosis	28	11	39 (23%)
Lymphoma	4	8	12 (7%)
Meningitis	16	7	23 (14%)
Cerebrovascular	3	4	7 (4%)
Metabolic	3	8	11 (6%)
Uncertain HIV encephalitis	46	32	78 (46%)
Total	100	70	170

charges or status, and to search for the characteristic periodic lateralizing epileptiform discharges of herpes simplex encephalitis. If neurodiagnostic studies and the neurological examination are normal, the patient can usually be reassured that the seizure has no sinister implications. Advice about driving should be given and secondary prophylaxis considered.

USE OF ANTICONVULSANTS

If the seizure can be linked to drug or alcohol use, prophylactic anticonvulsants are generally not advisable. If neuroimaging or CSF examination is abnormal, medication should possibly be started even after a single fit. However, anticonvulsant sensitivity is high and rashes and granulocytopenia are common both with phenytoin and carbamazepine. Phenobarbital can be used as a second-line agent, although its sedating properties pose a major disadvantage. For patients presenting with seizures who have identified mass lesions, there is an immediate risk of further seizures or status epilepticus and intravenous loading with phenytoin or valproate is appropriate.

Involuntary movements

The spectrum of abnormal involuntary movements is wide, including tremor, dystonia, akathisia and myoclonus. Symmetrical tremor may represent the exaggeration of physiological tremor or benign essential tremor in the setting of systemic infection or may be related to medication. Medications that commonly induce tremor include foscarnet, neuroleptics including phenothiazines and metaclopromide, and pyrimethamine. Tremor may be a part of a Parkinsonian syndrome from medications. Productive HIV infection has a predilection for the basal ganglia and brainstem and direct damage or the release of cytokines may trigger tremor and other movement disorders. Reyes et al (1991) demonstrated loss of neurones in the substantia nigra in AIDS patients, which may explain the higher risk of extrapyramidal symptoms in AIDS patients, especially those prescribed neuroleptics for agitation, delirium or frank psychosis (Hollander et al 1985, Hriso et al 1991). Hriso reported that the risk was

more than doubled. On less than the equivalent of 4 mg/kg day of chlorpromazine, 50% of the AIDS patients developed extrapyramidal problems. Over that dose, the rate rose to 78%. One personal case with writing tremor had a coincidental old focal lesion due to meningovascular syphilis that preceded his HIV infection.

In addition to tremor and Parkinsonism, a variety of involuntary movements have been described in patients with AIDS (Nath et al 1987). These have included hemidystonia (Nath et al 1987), hemichorea (Navia et al 1986), hemiballismus (Namer et al 1990) and unilateral akathisia (Carrazone et al 1989). Almost all have been related to *Toxoplasma* abscesses in the basal ganglia (see Fig. 11.1, p. 171). Rarer causes have included lymphoma, PML and zoster vasculitis (see Fig. 13.4, p. 200). The precise localization has varied between the head of the caudate, putamen, thalamus and subthalamic nucleus. Management of involuntary movement disorders depends on treatment of the underlying structural lesion, e.g. toxoplasmosis, or dose reduction of the provoking medication.

Gait disturbance

Many of the neurological disorders encountered during HIV infection can affect gait. Presentation for evaluation of gait disturbance is one of the more common reasons for neurological evaluation. Table 14.6 lists the most common causes of gait disturbance, their neurological syndromes and the symptoms that a patient may report. Additional details of clinical features, diagnostic evaluation and treatment are included in the appropriate chapters. Most of these conditions occur late in HIV infection. Patients' descriptions of their gait disturbance and associated symptoms often define the underlying cause. The examination should include observation of gait, evaluating cerebellar performance on tandem testing, and checking the ability to rise from a squat. Proximal weakness seen in difficulty rising from a low squat or chair, difficulty with brushing hair or working with the arms above the head will usually prove to be due to myopathy. Weakness of the feet on car pedals, and scuffing or tripping when walking, especially if combined with weakness of hand

Table 14.6 Causes of gait disturbance

Cause	Neurological syndrome	Gait	Symptoms
Intracranial mass lesion	Focal CNS signs	Hemiparetic	Weakness on one side: arm and leg
		Truncal ataxic	Drunken gait, wide-based, staggering
Myelopathy	Spastic paraparesis	Spastic	Legs stiff, toes scuff and catch, stumbling when walking or going up steps
CMV radiculitis	Lumbar radiculopathy	Asymmetrical weakness	Progressive asymmetrical leg weakness; variable sensory loss, bladder/bowel loss and back pain
Myopathy	Proximal weakness	Waddling	Difficulty rising from chair, knee bend, or climbing stairs. Difficulty brushing hair, shampooing. Muscle aching
Sensory neuropathy	Distal sensory loss; minimal weakness	Antalgic	Numb, 'frost-bitten' or painful feet

muscles, e.g. when opening jars, by contrast implies a peripheral neuropathy. A stiff-legged gait with dragging of both legs, associated with the findings of spasticity, hyperreflexia and extensor plantars, will suggest a myelopathy. Unsteadiness can be due to sensory loss (Romberg positive) or ataxia of stance and gait with a broad irregular base due to cerebellar deficit. Unilateral dragging of one leg can be due to a pyramidal lesion when the pattern of weakness (weakness of hip flexion, hamstrings and tibialis anterior) combined with an extensor plantar will prompt the search for a hemispheric lesion such as toxoplasmosis, lymphoma, PML or cerebrovascular disease. Weakness of one leg can also arise from a root lesion (perhaps restricted to L5/S1 with weak hip abduction, hamstrings and extensor hallucis longus with reduced hamstring and/or ankle jerk). Myelography or MRI and CSF examinations will be needed to exclude lymphoma, and to try to diagnose CMV or a coincidental disc prolapse. A foot drop due to a common peroneal nerve lesion when weakness is restricted to the anterior tibial compartment and peroneii with normal reflexes can also disturb the gait and will usually be due to a pressure palsy or to a mononeuritis perhaps related to CMV or a vasculitis.

DIZZINESS AND FAINTNESS

These are common symptoms, particularly in patients with advanced HIV infection. Probably the most common cause is orthostatic hypotension from anaemia or volume depletion. Because anaemia is so common in AIDS, resulting from advanced HIV infection, opportunistic processes such as *Mycobacteria avium complex* (MAC) and the effects of therapies, including zidovudine, many patients come to recognize a drop in haematocrit by the return of familiar symptoms of postural hypotension. This almost always responds to transfusion or growth factor therapy with erythropoietin. Adrenal insufficiency is another common feature of AIDS and frequently results from involvement of the adrenal glands with CMV (Tapper et al 1987). At autopsy, up to 75% of patients will have pathological evidence of CMV adrenalitis. HIV-associated cardiomyopathies may cause dizziness, faintness and syncope, as well as dyspnoea and arrhythmias. Cardiomyopathy can occur at all stages of HIV infection and clues to its occurrence include the typical features of congestive heart failure with paroxysmal nocturnal dyspnoea, exertional dyspnoea, peripheral oedema and cardiomegaly. Medications represent another common cause of dizziness. Particular culprits include foscarnet, tricyclic antidepressants, amphotericin and narcotics. Combinations are particularly prone to cause dizziness, even at normal dosages. Several studies have suggested that an autonomic neuropathy may develop in AIDS (Freeman et al 1990) and autonomic function tests, such as measurement of the R-R variation on EKG with the Valsalva manoeuvre, have been abnormal with a high frequency in AIDS. However, it seems more likely that these autonomic abnormalities are secondary to systemic disease, rather than representing primary neurological involvement of the autonomic nervous system.

REFERENCES

Atkinson J H, Grant I, Kennedy C J, et al. Prevalence of psychiatric disorders among men infected with human immunodeficiency virus. Arch Gen Psychiatr 1988; 45: 859–864

Carrazone E J, Rossitch E, Martinez J. Unilateral 'akathisia' in a patient with AIDS and a *Toxoplasma* subthalamic abscess. Neurology 1989; 39: 449–450

Chong W K, Hall-Craggs M A, Wilkinson I D, et al. The prevalence of paranasal sinus disease in HIV infection and AIDS on cranial MR imaging. Clin Radiol 1993; 47: 166–169

Chuck S L, Sande M A. Infections with *Cryptococcus neoformans* in acquired immunodeficiency syndrome. N Engl J Med 1989; 321: 794–799

Freeman R, Roberts M S, Friedman L S, Broadbridge C. Autonomic function and human immunodeficiency virus infection. Neurology 1990; 40: 575–580

Holland J C, Tross S. The psychosocial and neuropsychiatric sequelae of the acquired immunodeficiency syndrome and related disorders. Ann Intern Med 1985; 103: 760–764

Hollander H, Golden J, Mendelson T, Cortland D. Extrapyramidal symptoms in AIDS patients given low-dose metoclopramide or chlorpromazine [letter]. Lancet 1985; 2: 1186

Holtzman D M, Kaku D A, So Y T. New-onset seizures associated with human immunodeficiency virus infection: causation and clinical features in 100 cases. Am J Med 1989; 87: 173–177

Hriso E, Kuhn T, Masdeu J C, Grundman M. Extrapyramidal symptoms due to dopamine-blocking agents in patients with AIDS encephalopathy. Am J Psychiatr 1991; 148: 1558–1561

Keane J R. Neuro-ophthalmologic signs of AIDS: 50 patients. Neurology 1991; 41: 841–845

Levy R M, Bredesen D E. Central nervous system dysfunction in acquired immunodeficiency syndrome. In: Rosenblum M L et al, editors. AIDS and the nervous system. New York: Raven Press, 1988: 29–63

Musher D M, Hamill R J, Baughn R D. Effect of human immunodeficiency virus (HIV) infection on the course of syphilis and on the response to treatment. Ann Intern Med 1990; 113: 872–881

Namer I J, Tan E, Akalim E. Un cas d'hemiballisme au cours d'une meningite a cryptococque. Rev Neurol 1990; 146: 153–154

Nath A, Jankovic J, Pettigrew L C. Movement disorders and AIDS. Neurology 1987; 37: 37–41

Navia B A, Petito C K, Gold J W, et al. Cerebral toxoplasmosis complicating the acquired immune deficiency syndrome: clinical and neuropathological findings in 27 patients. Ann Neurol 1986; 19: 224–238

Ostrow D G. Psychiatric consequences of AIDS: an overview. Int J Neurosci 1987; 32: 669–676

Ostrow D G. Behavioral consequences of AIDS. New York: Plenum, 1990

Pinching A J, Helbert M, Peddle B, et al. Clinical experience with zidovudine for patients with acquired immune deficiency syndrome and acquired immune deficiency syndrome-related complex. J Infect 1989; 18 (suppl I): 33–40

Reyes M G, Faraldi F, Senseng C S, et al. Nigral degeneration in acquired immune deficiency syndrome (AIDS). Acta Neuropathol 1991; 82: 39–44

Sweeney B J, Manji H, Gilson R J C, Harrison M J G. Optic neuritis and HIV-1 infection. J Neurol Neurosurg Psychiatr 1993; 56: 705–707

Tapper M L, Rotterdam H Z, Lerner C W, et al. Adrenal necrosis in the acquired immunodeficiency syndrome. Ann Intern Med 1987; 100: 239–241

Winward K E, Hamad L M, Glaser J S. The spectrum of optic nerve disease in human immunodeficiency virus infection. Am J Ophthalmol 1989; 107: 373–380

Wong M C, Suite N D A, Labar D R. Seizures in human immunodeficiency virus infection. Arch Neurol 1990; 47: 640–642

NOTE (See Fig. 14.2)

The following patient advice regarding self-testing of vision is taken from an educational pamphlet by Syntex Laboratories Inc.

Here is a list of the important vision problems; they may occur in both eyes or in just one. Call your doctor right away if you notice *any* of the following:

1. Any sudden changes of vision
2. A significant increase in the number of 'floaters' (small, moving 'spots before the eyes' that are seen most easily when you look at the sky or at a plain background; many people without eye disease have a few floaters)
3. A sense that a curtain or veil is blocking vision
4. Distortion or blurring of an area of vision
5. An area of vision that is missing.

The type of vision problem depends on the part of the retina that is infected. Also, these problems can be caused by diseases other than CMV retinitis. A physician must make the diagnosis after careful examination, which includes using eye drops to dilate the eyes so that more of the retina can be seen.

Peripheral vision

If the edges of the retina are affected by CMV retinitis, you may have problems with side (peripheral) vision. You can check your peripheral vision while reading the newspaper:

1. If you use reading glasses, wear them when you check your vision
2. Close one eye
3. Focus on a word in the middle of an opened-out newspaper
4. Move the paper close enough so that print fills your field of vision (all you can see is print)
5. Notice if any area seems blurred, darkened or is missing
6. Repeat for the other eye

7. Call your doctor right away if you notice that an area seems blurred, darkened or is missing.

Central vision

If the infection is in the centre of the retina (the macula), the central part of your vision will be affected. The best way to check your central vision each day at home is by using the Amsler Grid. Here are the steps to follow:

1. Test yourself in good light. If you use reading glasses, wear them while you use the Amsler Grid
2. Make sure that you put the Amsler Grid at a comfortable reading distance
3. Cover one eye
4. Look directly at the black dot in the centre
5. Keeping your eye on the centre, notice whether all the lines are straight and all the squares are equal (like graph paper)
6. If any area of the Amsler Grid looks distorted, blurred, discoloured or is missing, call your doctor immediately
7. Repeat the steps for the other eye.

15. Investigations

ELECTROENCEPHALOGRAPHY

Although magnetic resonance imaging (MRI) and computed tomography (CT) are clearly the most reliable ways of identifying structural lesions in the brain, clinical electrophysiology offers ways of monitoring function that are complementary.

Abnormal electroencephalography (EEG) records in symptomatic subjects can help confirm the organic nature of the cause of symptoms, and for example help distinguish depressive pseudo-dementia from HIV-associated dementia complex (Fig. 15.1), and can identify seizure activity (Gabuzda et al 1988, Parisi et al 1989a). Gabuzda et al (1988) reported a high incidence of EEG abnormality in AIDS-related complex (ARC) and AIDS patients (27/47), and Tinuper et al (1990) reported an even higher yield of abnormal records

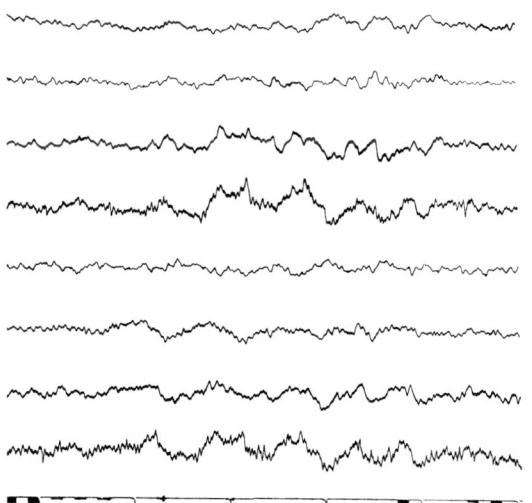

Fig. 15.1 EEG showing excessive slow activity in a case of HIV-associated dementia.

in patients with the AIDS dementia complex. Focal lesions can be suspected from EEG records (Tinuper et al 1990), but imaging is vastly superior and the EEG is non-discriminatory between the different pathologies. A high incidence of abnormality in patients with secondary central nervous system (CNS) disease (20/24) (Tinuper et al 1990) suggests that the EEG can have a role in screening for such complications. Diffuse abnormality correlated in Tinuper's study with meningitis and cytomegalovirus (CMV) encephalitis, whilst focal abnormalities proved to be associated with *Toxoplasma*, other abscesses and cerebral infarction. A focal EEG abnormality with a normal CT scan should raise the possibility of progressive multifocal leucoencephalopathy (PML) and prompt MRI.

Attempts to diagnose neurological involvement in HIV infection at an early stage have led to investigation of the sensitivity of the EEG in asymptomatic subjects. Parisi et al (1989a) examined a cohort of 185 asymptomatic patients in CDC stage A and found normal records in 73%. The most common 'abnormality' consisted of an excess of theta activity, particularly anteriorly ($n = 50$), though 16 subjects had frontal delta. There were no controls so the implications of these findings are difficult to estimate. Tinuper et al (1990) in their albeit smaller study found no abnormal records in 42 asymptomatic patients, though 14 were said to be borderline.

Quantitative studies began to be described in 1990 (Parisi et al 1989b, Itil et al 1990). Itil et al (1990) in asymptomatic ARC and AIDS patients found an increase in abundance of theta, delta and beta activity, with a reduction of alpha resembling a shift to the pattern seen in dementias of

Alzheimer type. Parisi et al (1989b) carried out a prospective study on asymptomatics. They found that 22 out of 40 patients with an EEG abnormality developed signs of CNS involvement. By contrast only two of 37 with normal records so progressed ($p<0.001$). The large prospective Multicenter AIDS Cohort Study (MACS), however, found no difference in the incidence of EEG abnormalities in asymptomatic HIV infection when compared with seronegatives (Nuwer et al 1992). The mean dominant frequency was 10.3 Hz for seropositives and 10.1 Hz for seronegatives. The relative abundance of theta activity was 14.1% in seropositive records and 13.8% in seronegatives.

There is thus at this juncture no proof that an abnormal EEG record in asymptomatic patients should change management policies except perhaps to intensify clinical monitoring of such an individual, and lower the threshold for further investigation of suspicious early symptoms. Later the EEG can have a role in screening patients with HIV-associated dementia or possible secondary CNS disease.

EVOKED POTENTIALS

Neurophysiological investigation of central sensory and motor pathways has been revolutionized by the development of simple evoked potential technology. Visual (VER), auditory (AER) and somatosensory evoked potentials (SSEP) are now routinely available in most laboratories and event-related or so-called 'cognitive' potentials are being increasingly used in the field of dementia research. At a more preliminary stage are techniques for pain, temperature and olfaction. Electrophysiological techniques for motor pathway assessment include electromagnetic stimulation of the cortex and spinal roots with recording from distal limb muscles, sometimes referred to as muscle evoked potentials or MEPs.

The clinical usefulness of evoked potentials lies in their ability to detect abnormalities when the clinical picture is unclear, to help define the site of lesions, for example in the brainstem (AER) or sensory pathway (SSEP). They also offer an objective way of monitoring the natural history or therapeutic response. Long latency potentials are in general less useful than those of shorter latency because the former are more variable in waveform and latency, and more sensitive to levels of attention and concentration. VERs, AERs and short latency SSEPs have been extensively studied in normals. Because of variability it is conventional to define a prolonged latency as one exceeding 2.5 SD over the normal mean for an age-matched population.

VERs (Fig. 15.2) are dependent on visual acuity and luminance and on the individual pattern stimulator so local control data are always necessary. Age affects latency and must be controlled. The dominant positive deflection at about 100 ms is routinely measured to whole- and half-field stimulation with a chequerboard pattern. Because of the sensitivity of the test it is claimed that if the VERs are entirely normal, there should be no signs of visual pathway lesions (Chiappa 1990). The converse is not true. Patients in CDC stage A have normal latencies (Farnarier & Somma-Mauvais 1990), but neurological symptomatic AIDS patients do show prolongation (Table 15.1).

Brainstem AERs (Fig. 15.3) in response to an auditory click signal are of complex waveform. Wave I is believed to be generated in the VIIIth nerve and is the first prominent negative deflection on scalp electrodes > 1.4 ms after the stimulus. Wave V is the largest wave after 5.5 ms and has a characteristic steep trough following its peak. Its generator is believed to be the lateral lemniscus. Wave III, also a negative deflection, is

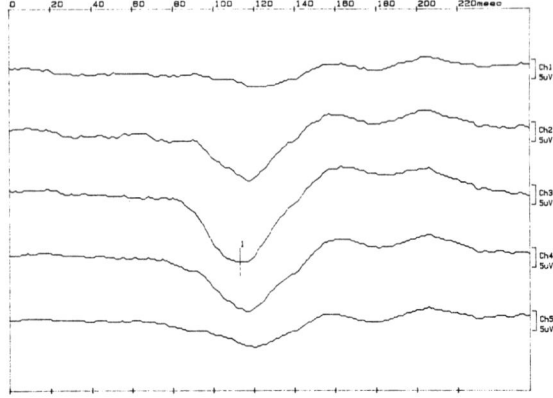

Fig. 15.2   Appearance of a normal visual evoked response.

Table 15.1 Evoked potentials in asymptomatic seropositives and AIDS

Latency	Normals (n = 40)	Asymp. seropos. (n = 30)	AIDS (n = 90)
VER P100 (ms)	110.7 (4.7)	113.4 (7.5)	117.3 (12)*
AER I–V (ms)	4.04 (0.09)	4.06 (0.19)	4.24 (0.2)*
SSEP N20 (ms)	19.4 (0.72)	19.7 (0.66)	20.7 (1.5)*

VER, visual evoked response; AER, auditory evoked response; SSEP, somatosensory evoked potential. *$p < 0.05$.
Results expressed as mean (SD).
(Middlesex Hospital data, SSEP; Farnarier & Somma-Mauvais 1990, VER/AER.)

halfway between I and V and is believed to emanate from the medullary olive. In practice the amplitude of waves is unreliable. Age again has to be considered in looking at latencies. If wave I is normal the later intervals can be used to impune abnormalities of the auditory pathway in the brainstem. Delay from I to III suggests a lower pontine lesion, and a prolonged III to V interval suggests the abnormality is between low pons and midbrain. Smith has claimed that HIV-infected patients have prolonged I–V latencies (Smith et al 1988), as have Farnarier and Somma-Mauvais (1990), though the latter only find significant abnormalities in patients with frank AIDS. Boccellari et al (1993) studied 55 HIV-seropositive and 37 seronegative homosexual men. HIV-seropositive individuals had increased wave III through five latencies and the majority with abnormalities had CD4 counts below 400/mm³. These findings conflict with those of Koralnik et

al (1990) who found no association between evoked potentials and immune status, but Koralnik's cases had higher CD4 counts (mean 635). The possibility that brainstem evoked potentials detect changes in asymptomatic individuals with early immune suppression is intriguing but still sub-judice.

SSEPs can be recorded from a wide area over the posterior hemispheres. They are height dependent, though this factor is not marked when looking at scalp responses to stimulation at Erb's point. They require cooperation from the subject as they depend on relaxation. It is essential that a peripheral response is monitored to exclude abnormalities due to delayed conduction in the peripheral nerve before the stimulus reaches the CNS. The diphasic positive–negative wave at Erb's point is used for this purpose in the upper limb whilst the median nerve is being stimulated. In the lower limb a response can be picked up from L1, which excludes peripheral sources of delay (or diagnoses them!). Waves from the dorsal column, dorsal horn, cuneate nucleus and medial lemniscus are discernible but are not robust clinical tools. Most laboratories concentrate on thalamic and cortical generated waves on scalp electrodes. These are at N18 and P22 from the upper limb and N30–34 and P40 for the leg (Fig. 15.4). Comparisons of intervals between the peripheral and these central waveforms allow an interpretation of possible abnormality in the roots, below the thalamus or in the cortex, or combinations of these options. SSEPs, whilst

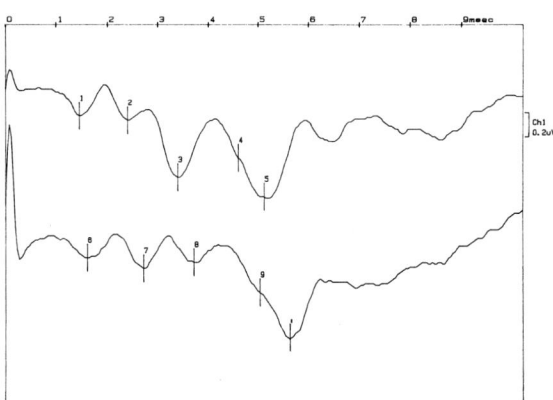

Fig. 15.3 Normal brainstem evoked response.

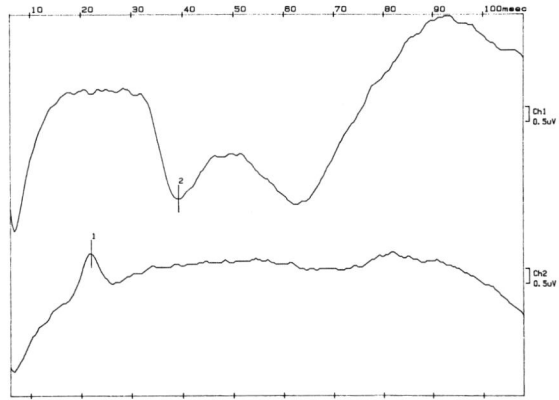

Fig. 15.4 Normal somatosensory evoked potential.

Table 15.2   Latency of posterior tibial somatosensory evoked potentials

	Seroneg. (n = 24)	Asymp. seropos. (n = 44)
Cortical latency (ms)	42.1	42.7
Spinal latency (ms)	24.1	24.3
Central latency (ms)	17.9	18.1

(Middlesex Hospital data)

testing the posterior columns, medial lemnisci, etc., cannot totally exclude a lesion of the sensory pathway and do not interrogate the spinothalamic tracts. Abnormalities have been described, however, in patients with AIDS, and HIV infection (Farnarier & Somma-Mauvais 1990). Several laboratories have tested all three main primary evoked potentials (VER, AER, SSEP) in patients with HIV infection and AIDS. There is general agreement that abnormalities are detectable in patients with symptomatic HIV infection or AIDS presumably reflecting the widespread brainstem and hemispheric pathology. Asymptomatic patients with AIDS may also show lesser prolongations of latency (Farnarier & Somma-Mauvais 1990). Patients in CDC stage A have given less clear-cut findings. Some studies with appropriate seronegative controls from the same backgrounds have, for example, found no abnormality of lower limb SSEPs in these groups (McAllister et al 1992) (Table 15.2). By contrast, others report delay in the latency from gluteal crease to D12 followed by a later central prolongation held to demonstrate an evolving subclinical myelopathy (Smith et al 1990). The discrepancies in these studies probably reflect different control and normal range criteria and different exclusion criteria or other strategies to deal with confounding factors such as alcohol and drugs. Neither Koralnik et al (1990) nor Boccellari et al (1993) found any association between immune deficiency and SSEPs in asymptomatic patients. The greatest practical usefulness of SSEPs is in the investigation of sensory symptoms. Peripheral nerve conduction tests need to be combined with SSEPs in order to locate the cause of any prolonged latencies. Long cortical latencies with normal conduction velocities in the limb and responses at L1 or C7 imply the presence of

myelopathy or encephalopathy. Prolonged intervals between Erb's point and C7, or to L1, without peripheral slowing suggest root lesions.

MEPs can be elicited from limb muscles such as the abductor digiti minimi, flexor pollicis brevis or the tibialis anterior, in response to electrical or magnetic stimulation of the cerebrum through the intact skull (Fig. 15.5). Magnetic stimulation is preferred as it is not painful. Responses are of higher amplitude and of shorter latency if the patient makes a small voluntary contraction of the target muscle. The clinical usefulness of MEPs follows from the fact that they represent the only way to demonstrate abnormal function in central motor pathways. Normal latencies between the

ROOT STIMULATION

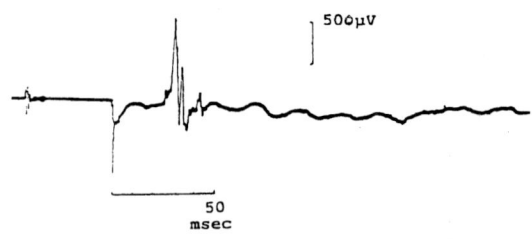

CORTICAL STIMULATION

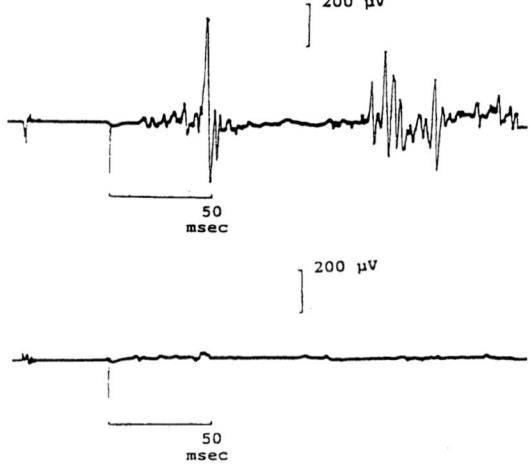

Fig. 15.5   Magnetic stimulation. Top trace, normal muscle response to root stimulation; middle trace, cortical stimulation with facilitation; and bottom trace, normal cortical stimulation without facilitation.

Table 15.3 Latency of muscle evoked responses in flexor pollicis brevis to magnetic stimulation

	Seroneg. (n = 24)	Asymp. seropos. (n = 44)
Cortical latency (ms)	44.1	45.4
Root latency (ms)	26.0	26.5
Central conduction time (ms)	17.9	18.9

(Middlesex Hospital data)

cortex and muscle are useful findings in patients with doubtful physical signs or weakness of non-organic origin. Our own experience in asymptomatic HIV-seropositive patients has been that MEP latencies are normal both from the scalp and from the lumbar region, providing no evidence of a subclinical leucoencephalopathic or myelopathic disturbance of pyramidal tracts (Table 15.3).

Long latency evoked potentials in response to cognitive tasks are gaining in popularity in the investigation of dementia. The usual paradigm requires the subject to identify rare signals in a train of more familiar ones. The response to the 'odd' (i.e. rare) stimulus (10% or 15% of presentations) has a maximal symmetrical positive wave called the P300 or P3 (Fig. 15.6), although its latency depends on various external factors and on degree of difficulty. This 'odd-ball' paradigm is easily set up with two different tones of different pitch presented through earphones. The subject must be awake and alert, which limits the usefulness of the test in severely impaired patients and those with toxic confusional states. Goodin et al (1978) have described prolonged P3 latencies in patients with presumed Alzheimer's disease. There is a relationship between the latency and the severity of dementia, and progressive dementias show increasing abnormalities on retesting. There has been much interest in their applicability to the early detection and monitoring of HIV-associated dementia (Arendt et al 1990, Goodin et al 1990, Goodwin et al 1990). Some have reported consistent abnormalities, for example in HIV-infected intravenous drug users. Goodwin et al (1990) studied 206 HIV-positive patients using a two-tone AER. Their results highlight the need for appropriate control groups. They found differences in latency and amplitude between the

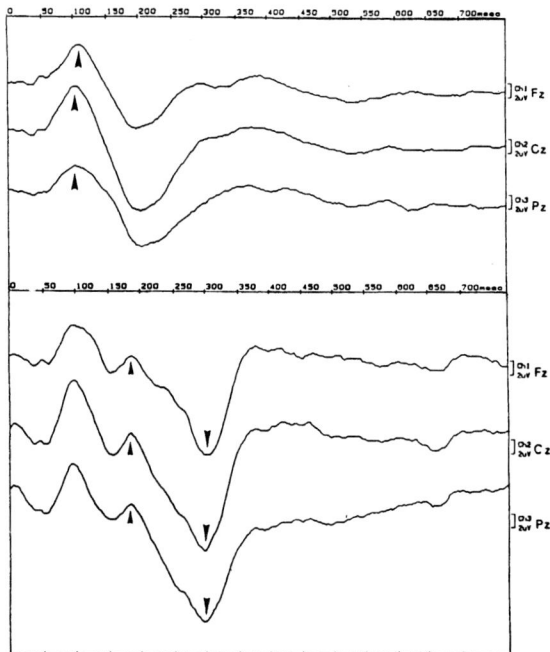

Fig. 15.6 Cognitive event-related P300.

HIV-positive and normal control subjects but not in comparison with seronegative intravenous drug users. Clear abnormalities were confined to the AIDS patients in whom P3 amplitude was lower, and over 1 year this group showed a lengthening of latency. Our own experience has been in agreement with this as we have found no differences between the results from patients in CDC stage A and seronegative at-risk controls (Table 15.4).

Table 15.4 P300 latencies (ms) in asymptomatic seropositives and AIDS

Electrode	Seroneg. (n = 23)	Asymp. seropos. (n = 45)	AIDS (n = 25)
Frontal	319 (29.5)	330 (34.1)	322 (22.8)
Central	321 (29.8)	333 (37.8)	330 (31.8)
Parietal	335 (38.1)	348 (38.1)	348 (28.0)

Results expressed as mean (SD).
(Middlesex Hospital data)

NEUROIMAGING

As discussed in Chapter 2, there is little evidence that neuroimaging detects subclinical pathology in the CNS. For example, Sonnerborg et al (1990) found abnormal-looking white matter on low field strength MRI in 64% of patients with lymphadenopathy, 50% of asymptomatic seropositives and 55% of seronegative at-risk controls. There is no evidence of any greater prevalence of visible changes in HIV-infected subjects than in seronegative at-risk controls, but both groups may show some subtle differences when compared with blood donors, for example. The implication is that there are factors common to groups with similar lifestyles and exposure to drugs and sexually transmitted disease that relate to a higher prevalence of mild abnormality. McAllister et al (1992) reported a similar finding for both atrophy and the presence of small white matter hyperintensities (Table 15.5). Alcohol intake may be a factor in the prevalence of atrophy (McAllister et al 1992). Thus patients with atrophy defined by the presence of enlarged sulci, or ventricles, or both, and as assessed by radiologists, drank more alcohol (median 50.1 units/week) than those without (median 30.8 units/week; Mann-Whitney $U=133.5$, $p < 0.001$). There was no correlation between the use of recreational drugs and the finding of atrophy, and none between soft neurological signs and imaging abnormalities.

Quantitative image-analytic techniques were used in a similar study of 67 asymptomatic seropositives with two groups of seronegative controls (39 high risk, 26 low risk) (Jernigan et al 1993). Volumes of ventricles, sulcal CSF space, white matter and deep grey matter were calculated. No differences were found (Table 15.6). Ongoing studies of relaxometry and proton spectroscopy also reveal no differences between asymptomatic groups (Chapter 2).

Table 15.5 Changes visible on MRI in asymptomatic subjects

	Seroneg.	Asymp. seropos.	AIDS	Significance
Atrophy	6/22	5/38	0/12	NS
Focal white matter lesions	7/22	2/38	1/12	NS
Follow-up: development or increase in atrophy	1/22	1/35	7/18	$p<0.005$

(Middlesex Hospital data)

Table 15.6 CSF and white matter volumes in asymptomatic individuals

	Asymp. seropos.	High-risk neg.	Low-risk neg.
Ventricles	0.2 (1.3)	0.2 (1.2)	0.0 (1.1)
Sulci	0.4 (1.3)	1.0 (1.1)	0.1 (1.2)
White matter	−0.2 (1.2)	0.0 (−1.0)	0.1 (1.0)
Caudate	−0.1 (1.1)	−0.6 (1.2)	0.2 (0.9)

Z-scores (SD) after estimation of subject's deviation from age and skull size predicted volumes.
(© 1993 American Medical Association Reproduced from Jernigan et al 1993 with permission of the American Medical Association)

In AIDS, imaging is more frequently abnormal, though the great sensitivity of MRI is not matched by high specificity, and many opportunistic infections and tumours can be very difficult to separate on imaging criteria alone. Biopsy (PML, lymphoma) or therapeutic trials of specific antimicrobials (toxoplasmosis) may be needed. What follows is a précis of the imaging characteristics of the major neurological infections and tumours (Fig. 15.7).

Cytomegalovirus (see Chapter 9)

Although CMV is a frequent finding in the CNS, with scattered microglial nodules in the cerebrum (Wiley et al 1986), these are not detected on CT or MRI. A florid ventriculitis with high signal in periventricular white matter on T2, occasionally with enhancement of ventricular walls, is relatively rare, but may be found in the context of sytemic CMV infection and a clinical picture of encephalitis with multiple cranial nerve lesions and nystagmus (Kalayjian et al 1993). Hydrocephalus can follow acqueductal involvement (Vinters 1989). Areas of necrosis/infarction associated with CMV were detected as foci of increased T2 signal at autopsy by Grafe et al (1990). CMV radiculopathy may be suspected from a nodular appearance of lumbar roots on myelography or MRI, but lymphomatous infiltration can cause the same appearances, to be distinguished by CSF cytology or biopsy.

Progressive multifocal leucoencephalopathy (see Chapter 9)

CT shows non-enhancing (except rarely) hypo-

MRI of brain in AIDS

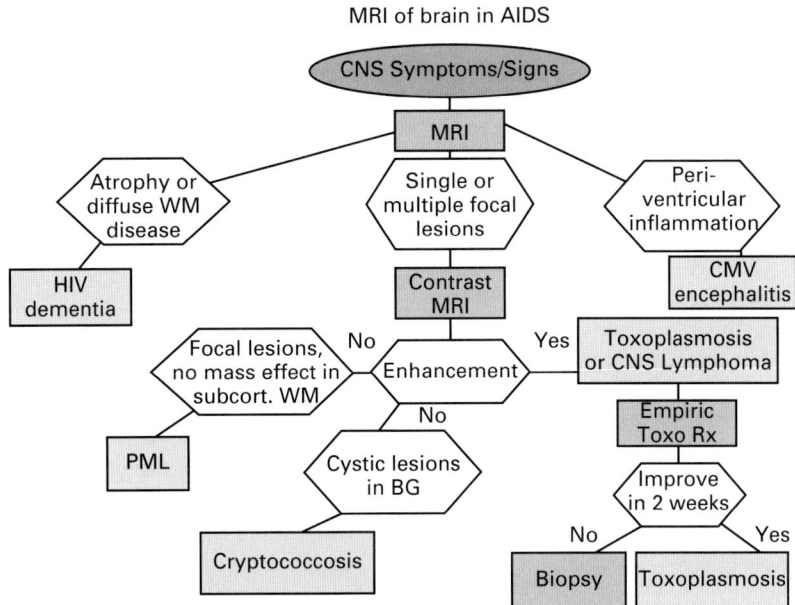

Fig. 15.7   Protocol for interpretation of MRI.

dense white matter lesions without mass effect. These are mostly sited in the periventricular, perioccipital and cerebellar regions. A normal CT scan in a patient with a striking slow wave focus on EEG or with a marked focal deficit is suspicious.

On MRI (T1), PML is seen as single or multiple white matter areas of low signal. On T2 these are of high signal with a scalloped but ill-defined edge. The abnormal area is homogeneous, and on sequential slices appears to map the motor or sensory tracts. For example, an area in the hemisphere may be contiguous with high signal all the way down through the brainstem into the medullary pyramid. Separate posterior fossa lesions are seen in some 10%. Whilst all affected patients have white matter lesions, only about half show grey matter involvement. Mass effect is rare; there is little or no oedema, and enhancement is the exception not the rule. The differential diagnosis includes toxoplasmosis and lymphoma, which usually have mass effect, multiple sclerosis and infarction, which is usually discernible from its site and shape, and HIV leucoencephalopathy, which is less visible on T1 images.

Herpes simplex encephalitis (see Chapter 9)

Because of the tendency for herpes simplex to produce infection and then necrosis of the temporal and inferior frontal lobes, it can be suspected if these areas show low density on CT, perhaps with some haemorrhage, or high T2 signal on MRI. The problem is that in AIDS the disease is milder and these imaging changes are less definite. It is said that sparing of the basal ganglia and a well-demarcated insula are additional imaging clues (Kendall 1993).

Toxoplasmosis (see Chapter 11)

CT shows single or multiple masses, 60% of which are sited in the deep grey matter. There is almost always enhancement and a nodular pattern may be seen. More characteristic is a thin wall ring enhancement. Smaller abscesses are more likely to show 'solid' enhancement, whilst larger abscesses are likely to have ring enhancement. Abscesses are characteristically spherical, unlike the more oblong lesions of lymphoma. Sometimes area(s) of vasogenic oedema are seen without revealing the causative focus of infection. This is often the case with small or cortical abscesses.

MRI is more sensitive, and may reveal multiple lesions in a patient whose CT scan showed only a single lesion. Abscesses are of low signal on T1. On T2 there is a high-signal centre and a low-signal capsule surrounded by high-signal oedema. Rare lesions are of high signal on T1 and T2 owing to haemorrhagic necrosis. Evidence of a haemorrhagic rim is a pointer in favour of *Toxoplasma* rather than lymphoma. Rare meningitis with enhancing meninges or diffuse encephalitis may be seen, but the imaging changes are non-specific. The differential diagnosis of abscesses with mass effect and enhancement is principally with lymphoma. Despite the imaging clues just described, the distinction ultimately depends on biopsy or response to treatment.

Cryptococcosis (see Chapter 8)

CT is usually normal, though occasionaly a low-density lesion(s), which may enhance, represents a cryptococcoma. MRI can be more revealing with small, usually non-enhancing nodules and dilated Virchow-Robin spaces. Some patients develop hydrocephalus, and others show meningeal enhancement.

Tuberculosis (see Chapter 10)

CT can be normal in tuberculous meningitis or show meningeal basal enhancement and hydrocephalus. Tuberculomas are solid homogeneously enhancing masses of high density. On MRI they are of high signal on T2 with oedema. They may ring enhance. If large and caseating they may show central calcification. It is easy for them to be mistaken for toxoplasmosis.

Lymphoma (see Chapter 12)

On CT, lymphomas are low-density ring- or irregular-enhancing masses with oedema (in non-AIDS patients the lesions are usually iso- or hyperdense with little oedema). On MRI the pattern of enhancement and oedema is often indistinguishable from that accompanying *Toxoplasma* abscesses. Solitary and very large lesions are more likely to be lymphomas. The lesions are more likely to be due to lymphoma

when periventricular or in the corpus callosum. Solid enhancement of large lesions suggests lymphoma. The best discriminating point may be the observation that the lymphoma, if adjacent to a ventricle, often seems to 'grow' along the ventricular wall.

HIV-associated dementia complex
(see Chapter 3)

The microscopic foci of encephalitis do not seem to be detectable by CT or MRI (Post et al 1988).

The blood–brain barrier disturbance associated with leucoencephalopathy can be seen (Post et al 1988). The white matter on CT is of low density and on MRI is of high signal on T2 weighting. The trigonal area appears the first affected. The changes consist of ill-defined patches with fluffy edges (unlike the stronger, better-defined appearance of PML). Such changes are symmetrical, and the matching T1 images are normal. There is no enhancement. This picture is often accompanied by atrophy. Some neurologically normal but medically symptomatic patients with AIDS show these changes, and their white matter shows abnormal relaxometry and proton spectroscopy (Menon et al 1990).

Spinal cord (see Chapter 5)

Imaging of the spinal cord is primarily carried out to detect compressive masses either due to lymphoma, which may be contiguous with paraspinal masses, or an epidural abscess. Myelitis may be seen as an area of high T2 signal, but the distinction between inflammation and lymphoma is difficult, even when the meninges enhance. Vacuolar myelopathy is not routinely detectable.

SINGLE-PHOTON EMISSION COMPUTED TOMOGRAPHY

All forms of cerebral imaging have been employed in the search for objective criteria for the diagnosis of organic mental syndromes in HIV-infected individuals. EEG changes are non-specific and CT and MRI can be normal in patients with cognitive impairment. Positron emission tomography (PET), though more sensitive, is less available, as is magnetic resonance spectroscopy.

There has therefore been much interest in the use of single-photon emission computed tomography (SPECT) scanning in AIDS, particularly with ^{99m}Tc-HMPAO as a marker of regional cerebral blood flow (Ell et al 1987). It is assumed that, in the absence of infarcts or mass lesions, cerebral blood flow and metabolism are still metabolically coupled together. If so, regional depressed blood flow is held to reflect an area of impaired metabolism indicative of functional damage or structural damage that may be below the threshold of X-ray imaging or MRI.

'Blind' reading of scans in one published series revealed a heterogeneous pattern of cortical uptake with or without focal abnormalities in cortex and grey matter. There was good agreement between the degree of scan abnormality and a crude clinical rating of cognitive impairment (Masdeu et al 1991). Pohl et al (1988) also recorded a high yield of abnormal scans in patients diagnosed as having the AIDS dementia complex. Clinically normal patients also had abnormal scans (LaFrance et al 1988, Masdeu et al 1991). These findings need replication in a prospective study using formal psychometry to define dementia, appropriate at-risk seronegative controls, and blind assessments. Only then will it be clear whether the technique can help define the clinical picture.

Thallium scanning (see Fig. 12.11, p. 191) may prove useful in the differentiation of lymphoma (high uptake) and other mass lesions.

NEUROPSYCHOLOGICAL TESTING

Because of the frequency of cognitive impairment, particularly with advanced HIV infection, neuropsychological testing has become an important component of the routine evaluation of patients with AIDS. While there is still some debate about the frequency and clinical relevance of cognitive abnormalities appearing early in HIV infection during the asymptomatic phase, there is now clear evidence that 20–30% of patients develop HIV dementia after AIDS and probably a further 20–30% will develop minor degrees of cognitive impairment. Neuropsychological testing is an important adjunct to the neurological examination. However, because of its relative lack of specificity in distinguishing the effects of HIV infection within the brain from those of opportunistic infections, or other confounding medical conditions, it should not be relied on solely for diagnostic purposes. The design and use of a neuropsychological test battery for use in HIV infection depends on the specific question to be addressed. Thus, designing neuropsychological tests to screen for the earliest signs of cognitive impairment in healthy asymptomatic HIV seropositive individuals involves a different strategy from a battery used to monitor treatment effects in patients with established HIV dementia. Similarly, any battery of neuropsychological tests must consider educational and cultural differences in patient populations because of the powerful impact of these factors on test performance. As an example, in the WHO multicultural study in which neuropsychological testing was performed at six centres across the world, novel test instruments had to be devised to replace existing 'Western' instruments, which were culture-specific.

Selnes and Miller (1993) have outlined a number of factors important in planning a neuropsychological test battery for the longitudinal assessment of cognitive impairment in HIV infection:

1. The neuropsychological tests should be sensitive to a wide range of impairments
2. Tests should be robust to the effects of serial repetition or 'practice'
3. The test battery should include tests proven to be sensitive to HIV-associated cognitive change
4. Normative data appropriate to age and education for the population under study should be used
5. The overall testing period should be relatively short, particularly for patients with advanced HIV infection.

Selnes and Miller used factor analysis to identify major areas of cognitive functioning or 'domains' using the 24 separate neuropsychological tests used in the MACS. Subjects with symptomatic HIV infection had impairment in motor performance, speed of processing and abstraction, with some minor impairment of both verbal and non-verbal memory. These findings agree with other studies in this area (Perry et al 1989, Van Gorp et al 1989). Factor analysis of the test battery confirmed that it measured at least seven major functional domains: brief attention (Digit Span), verbal memory (Rey Auditory Verbal Learning Test), motor speed (Grooved Pegboard Test), visuoconstructional skills (Rey Ostereich Complex Figure, Wais-R Block Design), simple reaction time, choice reaction time, and affect (CES Depression Scale, Beck Depression Scale). This factor analysis permitted Selnes, Miller and the MACS Neuropsychology Group to reduce the number of neuropsychological tests in the battery so that it could be substantially shortened and yet still probe all of the relevant functional cognitive domains. The brief test battery developed for longitudinal evaluation of cognitive function in the MACS includes all of the neuropsychological tests that discriminate between the performance of patients with AIDS and that of seronegative controls. It incorporates measures of verbal (Rey Auditory Verbal Learning Test) and non-verbal memory (Rey Ostereich Complex Figure Recall), attention (Rey Auditory Verbal Learning Test, Digit-Symbol), visuoconstructional skills (Rey Ostereich Complex Figure), motor speed (Trails A, Digit-Symbol, Grooved Pegboard), executive functions (Trails B, Digit-Symbol), simple and choice reaction time (California Computerized Assessment Package), and mood (CES-Depression). The battery (see Fig. 3.5, p. 37) takes approximately 45 minutes and is sensitive to the earliest signs of HIV-associated cognitive impairment. This battery would be useful, for example, in the initial assessment of a patient with suspected HIV dementia. For screening large numbers of patients in the earlier stages of HIV infection, an even more abbreviated battery consisting simply of Trailmaking A and B and Digit-Symbol may be used.

For monitoring treatment effects in patients with established dementia, a shorter battery has been developed by Sidtis, Price and the AIDS Clinical Trial Neurology Group, which measures treatment response well, is robust, and resistant to practice effects. The 'micro' battery includes four tests: Timed Gait, Grooved Pegboard dominant hand, Digit-Symbol, and Finger Tapping non-dominant. The 'macro' battery consists of 10 measures: WAIS-R Vocabulary (administered only at baseline), Timed Gait, Grooved Pegboard dominant, Grooved Pegboard non-dominant, Trailmaking A and B, Digit-Symbol, Finger Tapping dominant and non-dominant, Rey Auditory Verbal Learning Test, and Profile of Mood State. Price and Sidtis have evaluated the test–retest stability of these neuropsychological tests and found a variability ranging from less than 1% for tests of psychomotor speed to around 9% for the Digit-Symbol. The summary score was even more stable with an average difference of less than 1% with little evidence of practice effect.

Conversion of raw scores with age- and education-specific norms to units of standard deviation or 'z-scores' is recommended and allows for the easy comparison of scores between individuals. In trials of HIV dementia, a composite score representing the average of the sum of z-scores from all completed neuropsychological tests has provided a simple single measure of neuropsychological function. The neuropsychological summary score correlates well with the clinical severity of HIV dementia as judged by the MSK stage (Price and Sidtis, personal communication).

The National Institute of Mental Health has published specific recommendations for neuropsychological assessment of HIV-associated cognitive changes (Butters et al 1990), including a suggested battery that includes 25 different neuropsychological tests covering 10 separate domains (and requiring 7–9 hours for administration!) (see Table 3.11, p. 40). While this type of extensive battery might be feasible in a healthy HIV-positive patient, it is unlikely to be tolerated by an individual with more advanced HIV infection or with established dementia. Ingraham et al (1990) have stressed the importance of considering the number of neuropsychological tests performed. As the number of neuropsychological tests in a battery increases, so the likelihood of a type II error, i.e. appearing to find a significant difference when in fact one does not exist, increases. This is another argument for keeping neuropsychological test batteries short.

NERVE CONDUCTION STUDIES

Nerve conduction studies can be very valuable in a number of situations. The diagnosis of peripheral neuropathy is confirmed by finding generalized abnormalities of motor and/or sensory conduction. Normal studies make it more likely that limb weakness or sensory symptoms are due to root or more central lesions when evoked potential studies (vide supra) may be more revealing. The pathological substrate for peripheral neuropathy can be inferred from the results of nerve conduction studies. Thus axonal loss, as in the toxic neuropathies and in the common sensory neuropathy of advanced AIDS, is accompanied by small or absent sensory action potentials, small muscle compound action potentials and little if any reduction in maximum motor conduction velocity. By contrast the acute and chronic varieties of inflammatory demyelinating neuropathies show marked slowing of conduction velocities and evidence of conduction block. Thus the amplitude of the muscle action potential recorded by surface electrodes may be smaller from a proximal site of nerve stimulation than from a site close to the muscle. The comparison gives a measure of the number of intact axons whose myelin sheath is damaged between the points of stimulation. F waves, which represent the effect of retrograde stimulation of anterior horn cells after distal nerve stimulation, are particularly likely to show abnormalities in Guillain-Barré and chronic inflammatory demyelinating polyneuropathy (CIDP) cases as they represent a measure of conduction 'to-and-fro' from the periphery through the roots and back again. The sheer length of the tested segment of nerve increases sensitivity, and the demyelinating neuropathies (acute inflammatory demyelinating polyneuropathy (AIDP) and CIDP) often show a concentration of pathology in the roots, not revealed by conduction studies in the periphery.

In the case of single nerve lesions, nerve conduction tests are able to locate the site of damage usually by comparing the results of stimulation either side of an abnormal area, but also by employing electromyography to support the findings on clinical examination of the precise distribution of affected muscles. An important adjunct in such cases is to demonstrate whether the patient has instead a generalized neuropathy not clinically obvious or whether the symptomatic isolated nerve lesion is on the background of a mild diffuse neuropathy predisposing the patient to the effects of even modest trauma or compression. Localization by nerve conduction tests to part of a nerve not liable to pressure immediately raises suspicions of a vasculitic lesion or the effects of something like CMV. This is particularly true when the clinical picture and/or the electrical tests show evidence of multiple nerve lesions rather than a diffuse generalized conduction abnormality. Such a mononeuritis multiplex may only be revealed by nerve conduction tests, being clinically unsuspected, the symptoms and signs appearing diffuse.

The tests can also give some prognostic information. Electromyographic evidence of denervation with extensive fibrillation potentials and rapid firing of a much diminished number of motor units implies a worse prognosis especially in a Guillain-Barré style neuropathy, for example. A local conduction block in a single nerve exposed to trauma carries a good prognosis as recovery only awaits remyelination of the short area of damage for power to return, rather than the lengthy interval required for axon regrowth.

It should be recalled that nerve conduction tests interrogate only the largest motor and sensory fibres. Small fibres, which are involved in the later stages of AIDS-related painful axonal sensory neuropathy and in autonomic neuropathy, are more difficult to test. Quantitative testing of temperature thresholds in the periphery may be one way of filling this gap.

The main role of electromyography is in distinguishing neurogenic from myopathic weakness. Neurogenic weakness is recognized by the presence of fibrillation potentials and fasciculation at rest and by rapid firing of large prolonged polyphasic potentials. The latter develop as collateral axonal sprouts from surviving neurones reconnect to muscle fibres formerly innervated by a now-degenerated axon. In acute cases, fibrillation takes

2–3 weeks to develop and only rapid firing of surviving units may be seen, or the muscle may be silent. By contrast muscle disease is characterized by a full interference pattern at weak effort comprising small polyphasic potentials, which reveal their loss of constituent muscle fibres. Some fibrillation may be seen, especially in inflammatory polymyositis. Quantitative measures of size and duration of potentials and of their number of component phases sharpen the electromyographer's ability to distinguish such changes.

Clinical neurophysiological testing has been extensively employed in asymptomatic seropositive individuals in the search for evidence of subclinical neuropathy. In patients with AIDS, defined for example by non-neurological events such as *Pneumocystis carinii* pneumonia (PCP), nerve conduction tests do show abnormalities. For example, Fuller et al (1991) found the amplitude of compound action potentials from distal muscles and sural nerve sensory action potentials to be reduced by about a third when compared with healthy controls. Conduction velocities and F wave latencies were reduced but only by 5–10%. The picture thus suggests a mild axonal damage, and nerve biopsies in five asymptomatic volunteers showed loss of larger axons without inflammation or demyelination. The interpretation of such results is not straightforward. First, there was no HIV-seronegative group from a comparable background and no formal attempt was made to allow for the effects of alcohol and drugs. Second, the findings are entirely non-specific and mimic those seen in patients with malignancies and critical illness neuropathy. A similar study of nerve conduction in a prospective cohort (Harrison M J G, unpublished data) revealed clinical and/or neurophysiological evidence of neuropathy in 17 of 119 (14%) patients, but this number was reduced to nine of 119 (7.5%) when iatrogenic and unrelated causes were eliminated. None of 28 seronegative subjects had signs of neuropathy, whilst five of 61 (8%) asymptomatic seropositive individuals did, compared with four of 22 (18%) with AIDS. The difference is not significant, however. Patients with neuropathy so detected tended to have lower CD4 counts and higher serum β_2-microglobulin levels, though this trend also failed to reach conventional levels of significance. There remains a suspicion that a small number of patients, as they develop AIDS, begin to show nerve conduction abnormalities, presumably reflecting the subclinical form of axonal sensory neuropathy destined to develop in 20–30% of long-term survivors.

CEREBROSPINAL FLUID

The study of CSF in HIV infection has proved to be both useful diagnostically and to advance our understanding of the neurobiology of HIV. CSF abnormalities are found early in HIV infection and, in addition, most of the CNS opportunistic infections also influence CSF constituents. The combined effect of multiple infectious processes on the CSF profile is sometimes difficult to interpret, for example, in the setting of neurosyphilis in the HIV-positive patient. The use of CSF for prediction of neurological disease has been studied through the measurement of immune activation markers and measures of viral load. In this section, we will review the CSF abnormalities found during HIV infection and with some of the opportunistic processes that develop with AIDS. For the latter, the useful diagnostic abnormalities are summarized in Table 15.7.

CSF abnormalities during HIV infection

As we have discussed in earlier chapters (Chapters 1 and 2), the nervous system is invaded early in HIV infection. While only about 1–2% of individuals develop an acute aseptic meningitis with HIV seroconversion, CSF abnormalities reflecting a chronic 'silent' meningitis can be detected in about 60% of asymptomatic seropositive individuals. Numerous studies of the frequency of CSF abnormalities during this phase of HIV infection have been completed and recently been reviewed by Nogales-Gaete and colleagues (1992). The results of studies may vary depending on the exact level of immunodeficiency in study subjects. The frequency of CSF pleocytosis in HIV-seropositive patients (white blood cells (WBC) >5 cells/mm^3) ranges from 15 to 100%, averaging 30%. When pleocytosis is present, it is predominantly lymphocytic and the

Table 15.7 Typical CSF findings in the different neurological disorders associated with HIV infection.

Condition	WBC count	Protein	Glucose	Other
Acute aseptic meningitis	Up to 100 lymphocytes/mm^3, rarely >200/mm^3	Elevated, usually < 100 g/dl	Normal	HIV isolated frequently
Chronic 'silent' meningitis	Usually <25/mm^3	May be elevated, usually <100 g/dl	Normal	HIV isolated in 30%
HIV dementia	Usually acellular; >20/mm^3 in 5% of cases	Up to 100 g/dl in one-third of cases; normal in remainder of cases	Normal	Elevated neopterin, quinolinic acid, β_2-microglobulin Non-specific increase in IgG
CMV polyradiculitis	Polymorphonuclear pleocytosis	Elevated in majority of cases	Low	CMV culture positive in 50% of cases
CMV encephalitis	Lymphocytic pleocytosis or normal	Elevated	Normal	CMV usually not isolated from CSF; PCR positive in 33%
Cryptococcal meningitis	Lymphocytic pleocytosis >20 WBC/mm^3 in 35%	Elevated in 70%	Low in 25%	Cryptococcal antigen present in CSF in most cases Fungal cultures positive in most cases
Neurosyphilis	Usually elevated	Usually elevated	Normal	CSF VDRL positive in 20–70% of cases
Tuberculous meningitis	Mononuclear pleocytosis	May be markedly elevated (>100 mg/dl)	Usually <40 mg/dl	Acid-fast bacillus cultures or smears positive in many cases
Guillain-Barré syndrome	Up to 50/mm^3	Up to 200 g/dl	Normal	
Toxoplasmosis	Lymphocytic pleocytosis in 75%	Elevated	Normal	Intrathecal synthesis of *Toxoplasma* antibody in 60%
Primary CNS lymphoma	Lymphocytic pleocytosis in 60%	Elevated	Normal	Cytology positive in 5%
Progressive multifocal leucoencephalopathy	Normal in most	Normal	Normal	JC virus PCR positive in 30–50%

(After Dal Pan & McArthur 1993)

distribution of CSF lymphocyte subtypes parallels the blood (Margolick et al 1988, McArthur et al 1989). The CSF pleocytosis is, in general, mild with values ranging up to 40 WBC/mm^3. To date, the presence of this 'viral' meningitis early in HIV infection has not been shown to predict subsequent neurological disease and is probably silent in most patients. In some patients there appears to be an association between pleocytosis and chronic complaints of headache and other neurological symptoms (Hollander & Levy 1987). As HIV infection progresses, the frequency of CSF pleocytosis decreases, and after AIDS, pleocytosis is unusual unless certain CNS opportunistic infections are present. As previously discussed, some of the CNS opportunistic infections such as CMV encephalitis and PML do not typically induce a pleocytosis. Similarly, with the primary HIV-related neurological diseases, dementia, myelopathy and sensory neuropathy, the CSF is generally acellular.

The temporal profile of CSF pleocytosis has been elucidated by serial CSF sampling performed in the Multicenter AIDS Cohort Study. In these studies, lumbar punctures have been performed annually on a group of HIV-positive homosexual men followed prospectively since 1986. These longitudinal studies in men with documented dates of HIV seroconversion have permitted the exploration of the relationship between CSF pleocytosis and other abnormalities, the degree of immunodeficiency and the duration of HIV infection. Figure 15.8 illustrates these findings. From these longitudinal studies in homosexual men with known dates of HIV seroconversion, the CSF WBC count peaks at about 27 months after seroconversion and declines thereafter. These findings in HIV infection are analogous to the situation with SIV infection in experimentally infected macaques. Meningitis develops early within the first few weeks of infection and subsequently clears (Mori et al 1993).

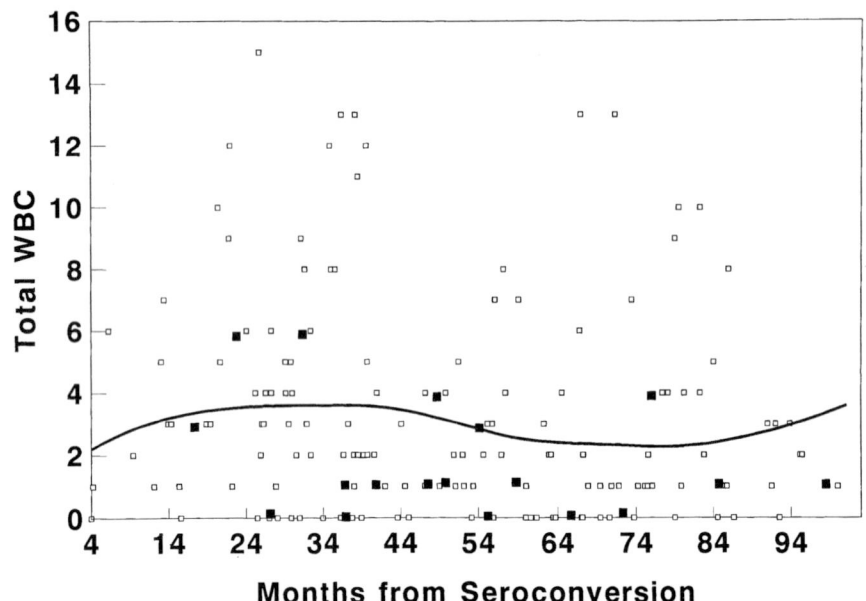

Fig. 15.8 Change in level of pleocytosis with duration of HIV infection. The pleocytosis is relatively mild, and tends to peak at 27 months after seroconversion, falling subsequently. There are no discernible differences between neurologically normal individuals (open squares) and those developing HIV dementia (closed squares). (Reproduced from Nance-Sproson et al 1993.)

Elevations in total protein, albumin and in the CSF serum/albumin ratio (a measure of breakdown in the blood–brain barrier (Tibbling et al 1977)) are frequent in all stages of HIV infection. While patients with HIV dementia tend to have higher levels of CSF protein and more evidence of blood–brain barrier disruption than non-demented individuals, the differences are rarely dramatic enough to be useful clinically (Fig. 15.9). CSF glucose levels are usually within the normal range, although patients with AIDS may have slightly lower levels than asymptomatic seropositive patients (Marshall et al 1988). Increased concentrations of IgG are often found and tend to increase with duration of infection. Only a small fraction of the CSF IgG component represents HIV-specific antibodies. Initially, it was thought that the detection of intrathecal synthesis of HIV-specific IgG was a good marker for neurological disease (Resnick et al 1985). However, it now seems that an intrathecal synthesis tends to increase with duration of infection, rather than providing a specific marker of neurological disease (Van Wielink et al 1990).

Oligoclonal bands are often found both in patients with and without neurological symptoms (McArthur et al 1988, Resnick et al 1988, Sonnerborg et al 1989) and their measurement is not particularly useful.

HIV identification in CSF

The identification of HIV infection within the CSF is possible with a number of different techniques, including HIV isolation from cell-free and unprocessed CSF (Sonnerborg et al 1988), detection of HIV antigens and, recently, through the use of polymerase chain reaction (PCR) techniques to detect HIV DNA or RNA. It remains unclear, however, whether the level of virus in CSF is reflective of HIV in lymphocytes trafficking through the CSF, or represents the state of productive HIV transcription in the brain. Combining results from a number of studies, HIV can be isolated by lymphocyte co-cultivation techniques from 23% of asymptomatic seropositive patients and 46% of those with frank AIDS (Nogales-Gaete et al 1992). There seems to be no

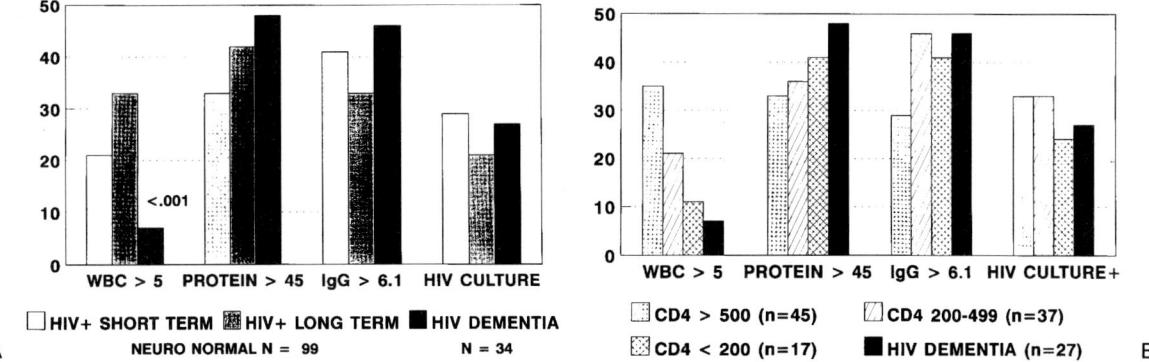

Fig. 15.9 Frequency of CSF abnormalities in HIV dementia related to duration of HIV infection (short term c. 18 months; long term c. 36 months) (**A**) and CD4 count (**B**).

correlation between the frequency of HIV isolation and duration of infection or the presence of dementia (Fig. 15.9). Aside from technical differences in isolation techniques, the biggest factor determining culture positivity is CSF WBC count. The higher the CSF WBC count, the more likely the HIV culture will be positive. This association explains why HIV isolation frequency may be quite low in patients with advanced AIDS, because during this phase of infection, CSF pleocytosis is uncommon. Concomitant antiretroviral therapy does not influence the rate of HIV recovery substantially (Tartaglione et al 1991). The detection of p24 antigen is a much simpler and cheaper method of HIV detection than virus isolation; however, its relative insensitivity has limited its usefulness in CSF. To maximize sensitivity, p24 antigen assay is now performed with acid pretreatment to dissociate immune complexes (Nishanian et al 1990). Even with this additional step, the majority of HIV-infected patients have no detectable CSF p24. Royal and colleagues (1994) performed assays for HIV p24 antigen from 83 CSF samples using acid dissociation. HIV p24 was detected in 19 of 40 dementia samples, one of 26 neurologically normal and one of 17 individuals with minor cognitive motor disorder. The sensitivity of the antigen capture assay in CSF was 48%, specificity 95% and the positive predictive value 72%. Two-thirds of subjects with moderate or severe dementia were positive for p24 antigen, which suggests that measurement of CSF p24 antigen after acid dissociation can estimate CNS HIV load and may correlate with

the severity of cognitive symptoms. The limitation, of course, is that the sensitivity is low, and particularly in mild dementia, CSF p24 is frequently negative. A direct correlation between CSF β_2-microglobulin and p24 antigen was found. Whether CSF p24 is truly reflective of *brain* viral burden remains questionable. Achim and colleagues (1993) found no specific association between brain tissue levels of p24 and postmortem CSF p24; however, these results need to be confirmed using CSF obtained ante-mortem. Several other studies have associated detectable p24 with HIV dementia (D'Agaro et al 1990) or from children with progressive encephalopathy (Epstein et al 1987). CSF p24 has been shown to decline with zidovudine therapy (de Gans et al 1988). At this point, because of the relative insensitivity of currently available antigen detection methods, the measurement of CSF p24 seems to add little in most clinical settings.

PCR techniques have been used to detect HIV proviral sequences (DNA) from CSF. Shaunak et al (1990) found no correlation between systemic stage and proviral detection. Steuler et al (1992) found a strong association between detection of proviral sequences in CSF and neurological findings. Currently, the role of PCR in the clinical setting remains uncertain, but as PCR techniques develop, it may be possible to use reverse transcriptase PCR to detect HIV transcripts in CSF as a measure of HIV load. This could be used as a tool to monitor changes with treatment, or, perhaps, to identify individuals at high risk of dementia.

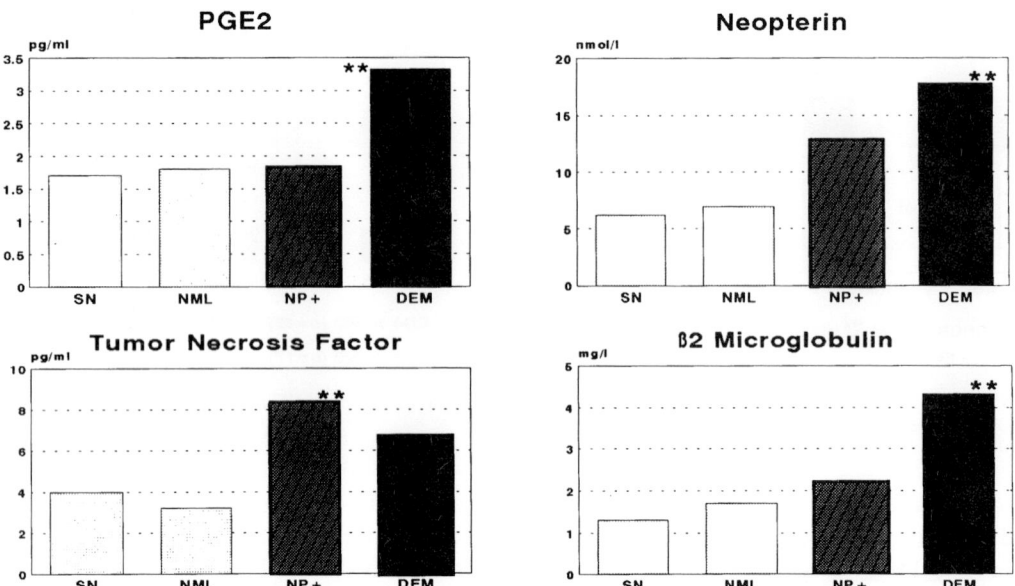

Fig. 15.10   Increased levels of PGE_2, β_2-microglobulin and neopterin in HIV dementia (DEM), compared with HIV seronegative controls (SN), HIV seropositive neurologically normal (NML) and HIV seropositive with minor neurological signs (NP+).

Lymphokines and monokines in CSF

A wide range of soluble products of lymphocytes and monocytes have been measured in CSF. It is difficult to compare directly the combined data from a number of published studies because of differences in the descriptions of neurological impairment and variability in the levels of immune dysfunction among subjects. During the early phases of HIV infection when CSF pleocytosis is common, there is a predominance of CD8+ lymphocytes in the CSF (McArthur et al 1989) and soluble CD8 is increased correspondingly (Griffin et al 1990). Levels of soluble CD8 decline later with increasing duration of infection. A number of these products reflect T cell activation (interferon γ, interleukin (IL)-2) while others reflect macrophage activation (neopterin, quinolinic acid, β_2-microglobulin). Pathological studies of brain and spinal cord have documented that macrophage infiltration and activation is an almost universal event in AIDS, with expression of class I and II major histocompatibility complex (MHC) molecules and the production of various cytokines within the nervous system (Tyor et al 1992). It remains uncertain, however, exactly how

well CSF levels reflect the production of cytokines within the brain (Achim et al 1993). These surrogate markers of immune activation have been widely studied and are highly intercorrelated (Peter et al 1991). Several groups have now confirmed that increases in CSF β_2-microglobulin, neopterin and quinolinic acid are consistently correlated with the presence of HIV dementia (Fig. 15.10).

β_2-microglobulin, probably the most stable and easily measured, has been extensively evaluated as a potential diagnostic marker for disease progression and HIV dementia (Table 15.8). β_2-microglobulin is a low-molecular-weight protein in the immunoglobulin super-family that is expressed on the surface of most nucleated cells and forms part of the class I MHC molecule. Elevated serum levels of β_2-microglobulin are associated with activated T lymphocytes and macrophages and appear to predict accelerated progression to AIDS independently of the CD4 count. Elevated CSF β_2-microglobulin has been found in CNS lymphoma and with HIV-related neurological disease. In demented individuals, CSF β_2-microglobulin is elevated independently of serum levels, suggesting that it is produced within the brain in HIV dementia. In one study

Table 15.8 Sensitivity of various CSF markers for HIV dementia

	Sensitivity	Specificity	Efficiency	Positive predictive value
β_2-microglobulin >3.8 mg/l	44%	90%	61%	88%
β_2-microglobulin >2.2 mg/l	85%	55%	74%	76%
p24 antigen	48%	95%	72%	90%
PGE$_2$	72%	54%	61%	48%
Neopterin >16.0 nmol/l	89%	NA	NA	NA

PGE$_2$, prostaglandin E$_2$; NA, not available.

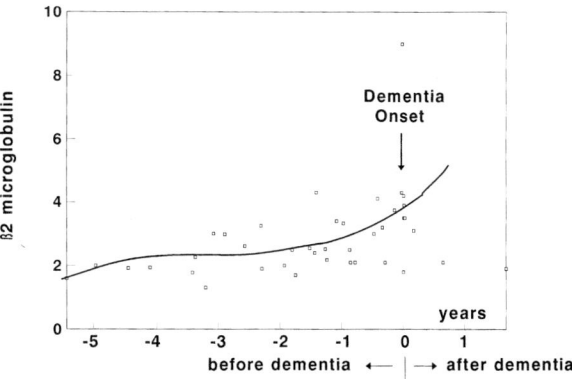

Fig. 15.11 CSF β_2-microglobulin before and after development of HIV dementia. Note the gradual rise in the 18 months before diagnosis. (Reproduced from Nance-Sproson et al 1993.)

(McArthur et al 1992), using a cut-off of 2.2 mg/l, determination of CSF β_2-microglobulin had a sensitivity of 85%, specificity of 55% and a positive predictive value of 76% for diagnosis of HIV dementia compared with non-demented subjects with CD4 counts less than 200. The specificity was improved to 90% by using a higher cut-off of 3.8 mg/l, suggesting that β_2-microglobulin may be useful in the differentiation of HIV dementia from other causes of cognitive symptoms. In general, CSF β_2-microglobulin levels remain stable in individuals who remain neurologically normal, even with declining CD4 counts. Those who develop dementia show rising levels over time (Fig. 15.11). Unfortunately, this rise is not dramatic enough for serial measurements of CSF β_2-microglobulin to become a clinically useful predictor of dementia.

Neopterin (dihydro-neopterin) is a pteridine compound considered to be a marker of cell-mediated immune reactions and thought to be another surrogate marker of immune activation. Activated macrophages and T lymphocytes produce neopterin under the influence of interferon γ (Peter et al 1991). Like β_2-microglobulin and quinolinic acid, neopterin is elevated in a variety of diseases and has been found to be increased in CSF of patients with HIV dementia (Fuchs et al 1989, Sonnerborg et al 1989, Brew et al 1990).

CSF levels of tumor necrosis factor (TNF) are, in general, higher in patients with HIV dementia; however, the correlation is less precise, perhaps

because of tissue binding of TNF-α. Increased levels of TNF-α mRNA have been measured in the brains of patients with HIV dementia (Wesselingh et al 1993) and Grimaldi et al (1991) have shown elevated levels of TNF-α in CSF. This was not confirmed in a paediatric group (Mintz et al 1989), although serum levels were higher in children with progressive encephalopathy.

Interferon γ is a product of activated CD8 T cells and CSF levels are, in general, higher in HIV-seropositive individuals than controls. Interferon γ stimulates macrophages to produce neopterin. Interferon α is increased in CSF in HIV dementia (Rho M, personal communication). IL-1β, IL-6, and granulocyte-macrophage colony stimulating factor (GM-CSF) are not increased in HIV dementia.

Arachidonic acid metabolites in brain and CSF have been examined because activated macrophages and microglia produce either prostaglandin E$_2$ (PGE$_2$) and other eicosanoids via the cyclo-oxygenase pathway or the leukotrienes LTC$_4$, LTD$_4$ and LTE$_4$ via the lipo-oxygenase pathways. Astrocytes may also produce PGE$_2$, as well as other prostaglandins. Platelet-activating factor (PAF) may also be produced in excess, although its measurement in CSF is difficult because of insta-bility (Gendelman H, personal communication). The increase in eicosanoid synthesis may be mediated through cytokines such as TNF and possibly by HIV gp/120 cell binding. Griffin et al

(1993) found that at least three different products of the cyclo-oxygenase pathway, PGE_2, PGF_{2a} and thromboxane B_2 (TXB_2) are increased in the CSF of patients with HIV dementia. Products of the lipo-oxygenase pathway were not elevated. The levels of PGE_2 increased in parallel with the severity of dementia and correlated with elevations in other immune activation markers – neopterin and β_2-microglobulin. Other groups have detected elevations in PAF in CSF from demented subjects (Swindell S, Gendelman H, unpublished observation).

Quinolinic acid is another measurable immune activation marker, a metabolite of L-tryptophan whose production is induced through the actions of interferon γ on indoleamine-2,3-dioxygenase, an enzyme that shunts L-tryptophan into the kynurenine pathway. Studies in experimental animals had established that quinolinic acid was an excitotoxic metabolite and an agonist of N-methyl-D-aspartate (NMDA) receptors. Subsequent observations (Heyes et al 1989) that levels were elevated in CSF from patients with AIDS raised the issue as to whether quinolinic acid might be directly involved in the pathogenetic mechanisms. In addition to HIV dementia, quinolinic acid levels are elevated with aseptic meningitis, opportunistic infections and neoplasms, consistent with the well-documented relationship between immune activation and increased quinolinic acid levels. Using reaction time as a measure of neurocognitive impairment, Martin et al (1992) showed that progressive slowing of reaction time was highly correlated with increasing levels of CSF quinolinic acid. Similar observations from the MACS have shown that CSF quinolinic acid levels rise before the development of clinically defined HIV dementia (Nance-Sproson et al 1993). A similar correlation between elevations in CSF quinolinic acid has been seen in SIV-infected macaques with neurological signs and rapidly progressive systemic disease (Heyes et al 1992). The significance of these elevations in quinolinic acid remains uncertain. The presence of elevated levels in CSF may simply serve as another marker of immune activation. Alternatively, because quinolinic acid is an NMDA receptor agonist, greatly increased tissue levels could directly mediate neuronal dysfunc-

tion. A third possibility is that induction of indoleamine-2,3-dioxygenase could deplete intracellular tryptophan by metabolic shunting with subsequent impairment of synthesis of serotonin. This might in turn lead to neurobehavioural consequences from deficiency of serotonin.

In conclusion, the study of CSF has provided important clues to the natural history of HIV infection in the nervous system. Pleocytosis appears to be a relatively early event and is accompanied by a degree of immune activation. During the asymptomatic phase of infection, when neurological disease is rare, the CSF profile remains stable, apart from a rising frequency of specific HIV antibodies. In individuals who develop dementia (and perhaps myelopathy), the levels of surrogate markers of immune activation rise with, and sometimes before, the development of neurological disease. Measures of virus load in CSF are higher in patients with neurological disease, and like the soluble markers, may decrease with antiretroviral treatment. The usefulness of measurement of these markers is becoming clearer. For example, the measurement of CSF β_2-microglobulin or acid-dissociated p24 in a patient with evolving cognitive symptoms may help differentiate mild HIV dementia from other causes. Hopefully, the continued study of the markers will contribute to our understanding of the pathogenesis of HIV dementia and to the management of the neurological complications of AIDS.

BIOPSIES

Given the diagnostic difficulties and the lack of specificity of imaging and clinical neurophysiological findings, it is not surprising that the issue of obtaining a tissue diagnosis often arises.

Brain biopsy is frequently needed to diagnose lymphoma and PML, and to exclude other treatable infections when abscesses fail to respond to anti-*Toxoplasma* treatment. Many units have a policy of biopsying mass lesions that do not respond to anti-*Toxoplasma* therapy within about 2 weeks. Lymphoma is the usual finding, though all reported series include some examples of toxoplasmosis that has been slow to respond, or for which treatment has failed. The distinction has important therapeutic implications. The need to confirm a radiological diagnosis of lymphoma is influenced by the patient's general state and whether it would be appropriate to arrange radiotherapy. Before committing to biopsy for what is suspected to be primary CNS lymphoma (PCNSL), the patient should be agreeable to radiotherapy and should not have active life-threatening systemic opportunistic infections. We would also recommend not biopsying patients with severe dementia or functional impairment from neurological disease (see Table 12.4, p. 192).

The need to confirm PML depends on a decision to use experimental treatment protocols involving toxic materials such as cytosine arabinoside.

Open biopsy is not without hazard, including a risk of haemorrhage. Stereotactically CT or MR guided biopsy is preferred (Fig. 15.12). Two types of stereotactic frames are in widespread use: the Brown-Roberts-Wells system or the Leksell frame. The neurosurgical techniques have been described elsewhere (Levy et al 1992); the CT or MR coordinates of the lesion are used to guide the needle approach to the lesion and the aspiration of tissue for microhistological and cytopathological examination. Tissue specimens should be examined using the algorithm devised by Levy and colleagues. In addition to routine haematoxylin and eosin (H&E) staining, material from brain biopsies should be submitted for bacterial and fungal cultures, immunostaining for herpes simplex and SV40 (which cross reacts with JC virus) and Giemsa-stained for *Toxoplasma gondii*. For lymphoma diagnosis, a panel of monoclonal antibodies including common leucocyte antigen (LCA), pan-T cell antibody (UCHL-1) and pan B antibody (L26) are used in addition to H&E staining. Recently, a dioxigenin-labelled probe for Epstein-Barr virus RNA transcripts has been developed for research applications which is highly sensitive for PCNSL (MacMahon et al 1991).

The haemorrhagic complications of stereotactic biopsy can be minimized by avoiding aspirin or aspirin-containing compounds for 7 days preoperatively, and by excluding thrombocytopenia and coagulopathies. In the largest series to date, with 50 biopsies performed by one experienced neuro-

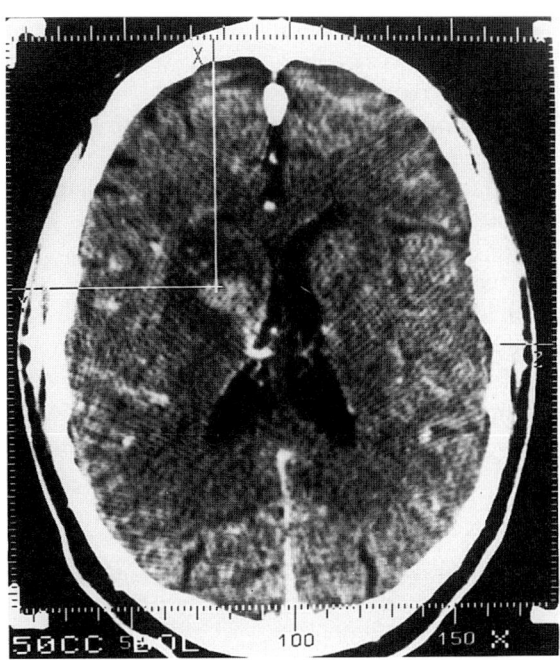

Fig. 15.12 Stereotactic coordinates for guided biopsy of cerebral lymphoma.

surgeon (Levy et al 1992), no deaths occurred and three haemorrhages occurred in 14 with PCNSL, with the haemorrhage confined to the tumour beds. In one patient, a permanent hemiparesis and aphasia developed following the biopsy. A similar rate of haemorrhage was noted by Chappell et al (1992) – one haemorrhage with somnolence after biopsy in 25 biopsies. In other series, the morbidity and mortality rates have been higher. Four of 18 patients with assorted intracranial mass lesions had a significant complication from biopsy (Marks et al 1989). The diagnostic yield from stereotactic brain biopsy also varies among institutions and may depend on the number of tissue samples obtained by aspiration. In the Levy series, only two of 50 biopsies were non-diagnostic, and the diagnostic yield was 96%. Of 16 enhancing lesions biopsied in the Chappell series, nine were PCNSL, two toxoplasmosis and only two non-diagnostic. In the Marks series, all 11 PCNSL patients had a definitive biopsy. Thus, at least for PCNSL, stereotactic brain biopsy is a reliable diagnostic technique.

Nerve biopsy is occasionally indicated to detect vasculitis and CMV, and to distinguish demyelinating from axonal neuropathy, although nerve conduction tests can point strongly one way or the other. The picture in cases of acute or chronic inflammatory demyelinating neuropathy is the familiar one of demyelination with variable axonal loss. Macrophage stripping of myelin lamellae and variable degrees of T cell infiltration are seen (Cornblath et al 1987). In situ hybridization for HIV has been universally negative and HIV only cultured once (Ho et al 1985). The changes in the more common axonal neuropathy consist of bland loss of myelinated fibres with axonal thinning and some oedema. Cellular infiltration is sparse (Fuller et al 1989). In patients with mono-neuritis multiplex, vasculitis with fascicular necrosis is the usual biopsy finding. Other cases may show CMV inclusions or infiltration with lymphoma.

Muscle biopsy can be important in distin-guishing an inflammatory polymyositis with T cell infiltration and fibre necrosis from non-specific type II fibre atrophy associated with weight loss and cachexia. Some believe zidovudine-related myopathy is characterized by ragged red fibres and electronmicroscopic evidence of abnormal mitochondria with paracrystalline inclusions. These findings are described in more detail in Chapter 11.

REFERENCES

Achim C L, Heyes M P, Wiley C A. Quantitation of human immunodeficiency virus, immune activation factors, and quinolinic acid in AIDS brains. J Clin Invest 1993; 91: 2769–2775

Arendt G, Hefter H, Hoemberg V, et al. Early abnormalities of cognitive event-related potentials in HIV-infected patients without clinically evident CNS deficits. EEG Clin Neurophysiol 1990; suppl 41: 370–380

Boccellari A A, Dilley J W, Yingling C D, et al. Relationship of CD4 counts to neurophysiological function in HIV-1 infected homosexual men. Arch Neurol 1993; 50: 517–521

Brew B J, Bhalla R B, Paul M, et al. Cerebrospinal fluid neopterin in human immunodeficiency virus type-I infection. Ann Neurol 1990; 28: 556–560

Butters N, Grant I, Judd L L, et al. Assessment of AIDS-related cognitive changes: recommendations of the NIMH workshop on neuropsychological assessment approaches. J Clin Exp Neuropsychol 1990; 12: 963–978

Chappell E T, Guthrie B L, Orenstein J. The role of stereotactic biopsy in the management of HIV-related focal brain lesions. Neurosurgery 1992; 30: 825–829

Chiappa K H. Evoked potentials in clinical medicine, 2nd edn. New York: Raven Press, 1990

Cornblath D R, McArthur J C, Kennedy P G E. Inflammatory demyelinating peripheral neuropathies associated with human T-cell lymphotropic virus type III infection. Ann Neurol 1987; 21: 32–40

D'Agaro P, Andrian P, Roscioli B, et al. HIV-1 isolation and p24 antigen detection in cerebrospinal fluid of subjects with neurological abnormalities related to AIDS. Acta Neurol (Napoli) 1990; 12: 49–52

Dal Pan G J, McArthur J C. Human immunodeficiency virus type 1 infection and its neurological complications. In: Hanley D F, Borel C, McPherson R, et al, editors. Principles and practices of neurocritical care. Baltimore: Williams & Wilkins, 1993

de Gans J, Lange J M, de Wolf F, et al. Decline of HIV antigen levels in cerebrospinal fluid during treatment with low-dose zidovudine. AIDS 1988; 2: 37–40

Ell P J, Costa D C, Harrison M J G. Imaging cerebral damage in HIV infection. Lancet 1987; 2: 569–570

Epstein L G, Goudsmit J, Paul D A, et al. Expression of human immunodeficiency virus in cerebrospinal fluid of children with progressive encephalopathy. Ann Neurol 1987; 21: 397–401

Farnarier G, Somma-Mauvais H. Multimodal evoked potentials in HIV infected patients. Electroencephalogr Clin Neurophysiol 1990; 41: 355–364

Fuchs D, Chiodi F, Albert J, et al. Neopterin concentrations in cerebrospinal fluid and serum of individuals infected with HIV-1. AIDS 1989; 3: 285–288

Fuller G N, Jacobs J M, Guiloff R J. Association of painful peripheral neuropathy in AIDS with cytomegalovirus infection. Lancet 1989; 2: 937–941

Fuller G N, Jacobs J M, Guiloff R J. Subclinical peripheral nerve involvement in AIDS: an electrophysiological and pathological study. J Neurol Neurosurg Psychiatr 1991; 54: 318–324

Gabuzda D H, Levy S R, Chiappa K H. Electroencephalography in AIDS and AIDS-related complex. Clin Electroencephalogr 1988; 19: 1–6

Goodin D S, Squires K C, Starr A. Long latency event-related components of the auditory evoked potential in dementia. Brain 1978; 101: 635–648

Goodin D S, Aminoff M J, Chernoff D N, Hollander H. Long latency event-related potentials in patients infected with human immunodeficiency virus. Ann Neurol 1990; 27: 414–419

Goodwin G M, Chiswick A, Egan V, et al. The Edinburgh cohort of HIV-positive drug users: auditory event-related potentials show progressive slowing in patients with Centers for Disease Control stage IV disease. AIDS 1990; 4: 1243–1250

Grafe M A, Press G A, Berthoty D P, et al. Abnormalities of the brain in AIDS patients: correlation of postmortem MR findings with neuropathology. AJNR 1990; 11: 905–911

Griffiin D E, McArthur J C, Cornblath D R. Soluble interleukin-2 receptor and soluble CD8 in serum and cerebrospinal fluid during human immunodeficiency virus-associated neurologic disease. J Neuroimmunol 1990; 28: 97–109

Griffin D E, Wesselingh S L, McArthur J C. Elevated central nervous system prostaglandins in HIV-associated dementia. Ann Neurol 1993; in press

Grimaldi L M E, Martino G V, Franciotta D M, et al. Elevated alpha-tumor necrosis factor levels in spinal fluid from HIV-1-infected patients with central nervous system involvement. Ann Neurol 1991; 29: 21–25

Heyes M P, Jordan E K, Lee K, et al. Relationship of neurologic status in macaques infected with the simian immunodeficiency virus to cerebrospinal fluid quinolinic acid and kynurenic acid. Brain Research 1992; 570: 237–250

Heyes M P, Rubinow D, Lane C, Markey S P. Cerebrospinal fluid quinolinic acid concentrations are increased in acquired immune deficiency syndrome. Ann Neurol 1989; 26: 275–277

Ho D D, Rota T R, Schooley R T, et al. Isolation of HTLV-III from cerebrospinal fluid and neural tissue of patients with neurological syndromes related to the acquired immunedeficiency syndrome. N Engl J Med 1985; 313: 1493–1498

Hollander H, Levy J A. Neurologic abnormalities and recovery of human immunodeficiency virus from cerebrospinal fluid. Ann Intern Med 1987; 106: 692–695

Ingraham L J, Bridge T P, Janssen R, et al. Neuropsychological effects of early HIV-1 infection: assessment and methodology. J Neuropsychiatr Clin Neurosci 1990; 2: 174–182

Itil T M, Ferracuti S, Freedman A M, et al. Computer-analysed EEG (CEEG) and dynamic brain mapping in AIDS and HIV related syndrome: a pilot study. Clin Electroencephalogr 1990; 21: 140–144

Jernigan et al. In: Hanley D F, Borel C, McPherson R, et al (editors). Principles and practices of neurocritical care. Baltimore: Williams & Wilkins, 1993

Jernigan T L, Archibald S, Hesselink J R, et al. Magnetic resonance imaging morphometric analysis of cerebral volume loss. Arch Neurol 1993; 50: 250–255

Kendall B E. Neuroradiological imaging. In: Scaravilli F, editor. The neuropathology of HIV infection. London: Springer-Verlag, 1993: 35–52

Koralnik I J, Beaumanoir A, Hausler R, et al. A controlled study of early neurologic abnormalities in men with asymptomatic human immunodeficiency virus infection. N Engl J Med 1990; 323: 864–870

LaFrance N D, Pearlson G, Schaerf F, et al. SPECT imaging with I-123-isopropyl amphetamine in asymptomatic HIV seropositive persons. J Nucl Med 1988; 29: 42

Levy R M, Russell E, Yungbluth M, et al. The efficacy of image guided stereotactic brain biopsy in neurologically symptomatic acquired immunodeficiency syndrome patients. Neurosurgery 1992; 30: 186–190

Margolick J B, McArthur J C, Scott E R, et al. Flow cytometric quantitation of T cell phenotypes in cerebrospinal fluid and peripheral blood of homosexual men with and without antibodies to human immunodeficiency virus type I. J Neuroimmunol 1988; 20: 73–81

Marks W J, McArthur J C, Royal W R, et al. Intracranial mass lesions in AIDS: diagnosis and response to therapy. Neurology 1989; 39 (suppl): 380 (abstr)

Marshall D W, Brey R L, Cahill W T, et al. Spectrum of cerebrospinal fluid findings in various stages of human immunodeficiency virus infection. Arch Neurol 1988; 45: 954–958

Martin A, Heyes M P, Salazar A M, et al. Progressive slowing of reaction time and increasing cerebrospinal fluid concentrations of quinolinic acid in HIV-infected individuals. J Neuropsychiatr Clin Neurosci 1992; 4: 270–279

Masdeu J C, Yudd A, Van Heertum R L, et al. Single-photon emission computed tomography in human immunodeficiency virus encephalopathy: a preliminary report. J Nucl Med 1991; 32: 1471–1475

McAllister R, Herns M V, Harrison M J G, et al. Neurological and neurophysiological performance in HIV seropositive men without symptoms. J Neurol Neurosurg Psychiatr 1992; 55: 143–148

McArthur J C, Cohen B A, Farzedegan H, et al. Cerebrospinal fluid abnormalities in homosexual men with and without neuropsychiatric findings. Ann Neurol 1988; 23: S34–S37

McArthur J C, Nance-Sproson T E, Griffin D E, et al. The diagnostic utility of elevation in cerebrospinal fluid β_2-microglobulin in HIV-1 dementia. Neurology 1992; 42: 1707–1712

McArthur J C, Sipos E, Cornblath D R, et al. Identification of mononuclear cells in CSF of patients with HIV infection. Neurology 1989; 39: 66–70

MacMahon E, Glass J D, Hayward S D, et al. Epstein–Barr virus in AIDS-related primary central nervous system lymphoma. Lancet 1991; 338: 969–973

Menon D K, Baudouin C J, Tomlinson D, et al. Proton MR spectroscopy and imaging of the brain in AIDS: evidence of neuronal loss in regions that appear normal. J Comput Assist Tomogr 1990; 14: 882–885

Mintz M, Rapaport R, Oleske J M, et al. Elevated serum levels of tumor necrosis factor are associated with progressive encephalopathy in children with acquired immunodeficiency syndrome. Am J Dis Child 1989; 143: 771–774

Mori K, Ringler D J, Derosiers R C. Restricted replication of simian immunodeficiency virus strain-239 in macrophages is determined by env but is not due to restricted entry. J Virol 1993; 67: 2807–2814

Nance-Sproson T, McArthur J C, Selnes O A, Griffin D E. Predictive value and temporal trends in cerebrospinal fluid abnormalities during HIV infection. Neurology 1993; A265 (abstr)

Nishanian P, Huskins K R, Stehn S, et al. A simple method for improved assay demonstrates that HIV p24 antigen is present as immune complexes in most sera from HIV-infected individuals. J Infect Dis 1990; 162: 21–28

Nogales-Gaete J, Syndulko K, Tourtellotte W W. Cerebrospinal fluid (CSF) analyses in HIV-1 primary neurological disease. Ital J Neurol Sci 1992; 13: 667–683

Nuwer M R, Miller E N, Visscher B R, et al. Asymptomatic HIV infection does not cause EEG abnormalities. Neurology 1992; 42: 1214–1219

Parisi A, Di Perri G, Strosselli M, et al. Usefulness of computerized electroencephalography in diagnosing, staging and monitoring AIDS-dementia complex. AIDS 1989a; 3: 209–213

Parisi A, Strosselli M, Di Perri G, et al. Electroencephalography in the early diagnosis of HIV-related subacute encephalitis: analysis of 185 patients. Clin Electroencephalogr 1989b; 20: 1–5

Perry S, Belsky-Barr D, Barr W B, Jacobsberg L. Neuropsychological function in physically asymptomatic, HIV-seropositive men. J Neuropsychiatr 1989; 1: 296–302

Peter J B, McKeown K L, Barka N E, et al. Neopterin and beta-2-microglobulin and the assessment of intra-blood–brain-barrier synthesis of HIV-specific and total IgG. J Clin Lab Analysis 1991; 5: 317–320

Pohl P, Vogl G, Fill H, et al. Single photon emission

computed tomography in AIDS dementia complex. J Nucl Med 1988; 29: 1382–1386

Post M J D, Tate L G, Quencer R M, et al. CT, MR and pathology in HIV encephalitis and meningitis. AJR 1988; 151: 373–380

Resnick L, Berger J R, Shapshak P, Tourtellotte W W. Early penetration of the blood–brain barrier by HIV. Neurology 1988; 38: 9–14

Resnick L, diMarzo-Veronese F, Schupbach J, et al. Intra-blood–brain-barrier synthesis of HTLV-III-specific IgG in patients with neurologic symptoms associated with AIDS or AIDS-related complex. N Engl J Med 1985; 313: 1498–1504

Royal W, Selnes O A, Concha M, et al. Cerebrospinal fluid HIV-1 p24 antigen levels in HIV-1-related dementia. Ann Neurol 1994; in press

Selnes O A, Miller E N. Development of a screening battery for HIV related cognitive impairment: the MACS experience. In: Grant I, Martin A, editors. Neuropsychology of HIV infection: current research and directions. New York: Oxford University Press, 1993

Shaunak S, Albright R E, Klotman M E, et al. Amplification of HIV-1 provirus from cerebrospinal fluid and its correlation with neurologic disease. J Infect Dis 1990; 161: 1068–1072

Smith T, Jacobsen J, Gaub J, et al. Clinical and electrophysiological studies of human immunodeficiency virus-seropositive men without AIDS. Ann Neurol 1988; 23: 295–297

Smith T, Jacobsen J, Trojaborg W. Myelopathy and HIV infection. AIDS 1990; 4: 589–591

Sonnerborg A B, Ehrnst A C, Bergdahl S K, et al. HIV isolation from cerebrospinal fluid in relation to immunological deficiency and neurological symptoms. AIDS 1988; 2: 89–93

Sonnerborg A, Saaf J, Alexius B, et al. Quantitative detection of brain alterations in human immunodeficiency virus type 1-infected individuals by magnetic resonance imaging. J Infect Dis 1990; 162: 1245–1251

Sonnerborg A B, von Stedingk L-V, Hansson L-O, Strannegard O O. Elevated neopterin and beta-2-microglobulin levels in blood and cerebrospinal fluid occur early in HIV-1 infection. AIDS 1989; 3: 277–283

Steuler H, Munzinger S, Wildemann B, Storch-Hagenlocher B. Quantitation of HIV-1 proviral DNA in cells from cerebrospinal fluid. J Acquired Immunodeficiency Syndromes 1992; 5: 405–408

Tartaglione T A, Collier A C, Coombs R W, et al. Acquired immunodeficiency syndrome: cerebrospinal fluid findings in patients before and during long-term oral zidovudine therapy. Arch Neurol 1991; 48: 695–699

Tibbling G, Link H, Ohman S. Principles of albumin and IgG analyses in neurological disorders. I. Establishment of reference values. Scand J Clin Invest 1977; 37: 385–390

Tinuper P, de Carolis P, Galeotti M, et al. Electroencephalogram and HIV infection: a prospective study in 100 patients. Clin Electroencephalogr 1990; 21: 145–150

Tyor W R, Glass J D, Griffin J W, et al. Cytokine expression in the brain during AIDS. Ann Neurol 1992; 31: 349–360

Van Gorp W G, Satz P, Hinkin C, et al. The neuropsychological aspects of HIV-1 spectrum disease. Psychiatr Med 1989; 7: 59–78

Van Wielink G, McArthur J C, Moench T, et al. Intrathecal synthesis of anti-HIV-IgG: correlation with increasing duration of HIV-1 infection. Neurology 1990; 40: 816–819

Vinters H V. AIDS, cytomegalovirus, and the brain stem. Ann Neurol 1989; 25: 311–312

Wesselingh S L, Power C, Glass J, et al. Intracerebral cytokine messenger RNA expression in acquired immunodeficiency syndrome dementia. Ann Neurol 1993; 33: 576–582

Wiley C A, Schrier R D, Denaro F J, et al. Localisation of cytomegalovirus proteins and genome during fulminant central nervous system infection in an AIDS patient. J Neuropath Exp Neurol 1986; 45: 127–139

16. Appendices

APPENDIX 1

CDC CLASSIFICATION SYSTEM FOR
HIV-1 INFECTION AND EXPANDED
AIDS SURVEILLANCE CASE
DEFINITION FOR ADOLESCENTS AND
ADULTS

The joint CDC/WHO classification system for
HIV disease in adolescents and adults is tabulated
below and incorporates both clinical conditions
and CD4 count. It is similar in some respects to
the Walter Reed staging system, which is less
commonly used (Redfield et al 1986). The WHO
criteria were published in *Weekly Epidemiological
Record* 1990; 65: 221–224 and are reproduced
with permission of WHO.

Category A

Asymptomatic HIV-1 infection
Persistent generalized lymphadenopathy
(PGL)
Acute (primary) HIV-1 infection with
accompanying illness or history of acute HIV-1
infection

Category B

Symptomatic conditions occurring in an
HIV-1 infected adolescent or adult, excluding
those in Category C, include, but are not limited
to:

CD4 + cell categories	Clinical categories*		
	(A) Asymptomatic or PGL	(B) Symptomatic not (A) or (C) conditions	(C) AIDS-indicator conditions
(1) $\geq 500/mm^3$	A1	B1	C1**
(2) $200-499/mm^3$	A2	B2	C2**
(3) $< 200/mm^3$ AIDS-indicator cell count	A3**	B3**	C3**

PGL, persistent generalized lymphadenopathy.
* See below for definition of clinical categories.
**AIDS-defining category:
    Lymphoma, immunoblastic (or equivalent term)
    Lymphoma primary in brain
    Mycobacterium avium complex or *M. Kansasii*, disseminated or extrapulmonary
    Mycobacterium tuberculosis, disseminated extrapulmonary or pulmonary
    Mycobacterium, other species or unidentified species, disseminated or extrapulmonary
    Pneumocystis carinii pneumonia
    Progressive multifocal leucoencephalopathy
    Salmonella septicaemia, recurrent
    Toxoplasmosis of brain
    Wasting syndrome due to HIV-1

Bacterial endocarditis, meningitis, pneumonia, or
  sepsis
Candidiasis, vulvovaginal: persisting
  (>1 month duration) or poorly responsive to
  therapy
Candidiasis, oropharyngeal (thrush)
Cervical dysplasia
Constitutional symptoms, such as fever
  (>38.5°C) or diarrhoea lasting > 1 month
Hairy leukoplakia, oral
Herpes zoster (shingles), involving at least two
  distinct episodes or more than one
  dermatome
Idiopathic thrombocytopenic purpura
Listeriosis
Nocardiosis
Pelvic inflammatory disease
Peripheral neuropathy

Category C

Bacterial pneumonia, recurrent
Candidiasis of bronchi, trachea or lungs
Candidiasis, oesophageal
Cervical cancer, invasive
Coccidioidomycosis, disseminated or
  extrapulmonary
Cryptococcosis extrapulmonary
Cryptosporidiosis, chronic intestinal (>1 month
  duration)
Cytomegalovirus disease (other than liver, spleen
  or nodes)
Cytomegalovirus retinitis (with loss of vision)
HIV-1 encephalopathy
Herpes simplex: chronic ulcer(s) (>1 month
  duration) or bronchitis, pneumonitis or
  oesophagitis
Histoplasmosis, disseminated or
  extrapulmonary
Isosporiasis, chronic intestinal (>1 month
  duration)
Kaposi's sarcoma
Lymphoma, Burkitt's (or equivalent term)

REFERENCE

Redfield R R, Wright D C, Tramont E C. The Walter Reed
  staging classification for HTLV-III/LAV infection. N Engl J
  Med 1986; 314: 131–132

APPENDIX 2

CRITERIA FOR CLINICAL DIAGNOSIS OF CENTRAL NERVOUS SYSTEM DISORDERS IN ADULTS AND ADOLESCENTS

All of the following diagnoses require laboratory evidence for systemic HIV-1 infection (ELISA test confirmed by Western blot, polymerase chain reaction or culture).

I. Sufficient for diagnosis of AIDS

*(A) HIV-1 associated dementia complex**

Probable (must have each of the following):

1. Acquired abnormality in at least two of the following cognitive abilities (present for at least 1 month): attention/concentration, speed of processing of information, abstraction/reasoning, visuospatial skills, memory/learning and speech/language. The decline should be verified by reliable history and mental status examinations. In all cases, when possible, history should be obtained from an informant and examination should be supplemented by neuropsychological testing. Cognitive dysfunction causing impairment of work or activities of daily living[†] (objectively verifiable or by report of a key informant). This impairment should not be attributable solely to severe systemic illness.
2. At least one of the following:
   (a) Acquired abnormality in motor function or performance verified by clinical examination (e.g. slowed rapid movements, abnormal gait, limb incoordination, hyperreflexia, hypertonia or weakness), neuropsychological tests (e.g. fine motor speed, manual dexterity, perceptual motor skills), or both.
   (b) Decline in motivation or emotional control or change in social behaviour. This may be characterized by any of the following: change in personality with apathy, inertia, irritability, emotional lability, or new onset of impaired judgement characterized by socially inappropriate behaviour or disinhibition.
3. Absence of clouding of consciousness during a period long enough to establish the presence of # 1.

4. Evidence of another aetiology, including active CNS opportunistic infection or malignancy, psychiatric disorders (e.g. depressive disorder), active alcohol or substance use, or acute or chronic substance withdrawal, must be sought from history, physical and psychiatric examination and appropriate laboratory and radiological investigation (e.g. lumbar puncture, neuroimaging). If another potential aetiology (e.g. major depression) is present, it is not the cause of the above cognitive, motor or behavioural symptoms and signs.

Possible (must have one of the following):

1. Other potential aetiology present (must have each of the following):
   (a) As above (see Probable) # 1, 2 and 3
   (b) Other potential aetiology is present but the cause of # 1 above is uncertain.
2. Incomplete clinical evaluation (must have each of the following):
   (a) As above (see Probable) # 1, 2 and 3
   (b) Aetiology cannot be determined (appropriate laboratory or radiological investigations not performed).

(B) HIV-1-associated myelopathy

Probable (must have each of the following):

1. Acquired abnormality in lower-extremity neurological function disproportionate to upper-extremity abnormality verified by reliable history (lower-extremity weakness, incoordination and/or urinary incontinence) and neurological examination (paraparesis, lower extremity spasticity, hyperreflexia, or the presence of Babinski signs with or without sensory loss).
2. Myelopathic disturbance (see # 1) is severe enough[††] to require constant unilateral support for walking.
3. Although mild cognitive impairment may be present, criteria for HIV-1-associated dementia complex are not fulfilled.
4. Evidence of another aetiology, including neoplasm, compressive lesion or multiple sclerosis, must be sought from history,

physical examination, appropriate laboratory and radiological investigations (e.g. lumbar puncture, neuroimaging, myelography). If another potential aetiology is present, it is not the cause of the myelopathy. This diagnosis cannot be made in a patient infected with both HIV-1 and HTLV-I; such a patient should be classified as having possible HIV-1-associated myelopathy.

Possible (must have one of the following):

1. Other potential aetiology present (must have each of the following):
   (a) As above (see Probable) # 1, 2 and 3
   (b) Other potential aetiology is present but the cause of the myelopathy is uncertain.
2. Incomplete clinical evaluation (must have each of the following):
   (a) As above (see Probable) # 1, 2 and 3
   (b) Aetiology cannot be determined (appropriate laboratory or radiological investigations not performed).

II. Not sufficient for diagnosis of AIDS

HIV-1 associated minor cognitive/motor disorder

Probable (must have each of the following):

1. Cognitive/motor/behavioural abnormalities (must have each of the following):
   (a) At least two of the following acquired cognitive, motor or behavioural symptoms (present for at least 1 month) verified by reliable history (when possible, from an informant): impaired attention or concentration; mental slowing; impaired memory; slowed movements; incoordination; personality change, irritability or emotional lability.
   (b) Acquired cognitive/motor abnormality verified by clinical neurological examination or neuropsychological testing (e.g. fine motor speed, manual dexterity, perceptual motor skills, attention/concentration, speed of processing of information, abstraction/reasoning, visuospatial skills, memory/learning, or speech/language).
2. Disturbance from cognitive/motor/behavioural

abnormalities (see # 1) causes mild impairment of work or activities of daily living (objectively verifiable or by report of a key informant)**.

3. Does not meet criteria for HIV-1 associated dementia complex or HIV-1 associated myelopathy.
4. No evidence of another aetiology, including active CNS opportunistic infection or malignancy, or severe systemic illness determined by appropriate history, physical examination (e.g. lumbar puncture, neuroimaging). The above features should not be attributable solely to the effects of active alcohol or substance use, acute or chronic substance withdrawal, adjustment disorder, or other psychiatric disorders.

Possible (must have one of the following):

1. Other potential aetiology present (must have each of the following):
   (a) As above (see Probable) # 1, 2 and 3
   (b) Other potential aetiology is present and the cause of the cognitive/motor/behavioural abnormalities is uncertain.
2. Incomplete clinical evaluation (must have each of the following):
   (a) As above (see Probable) # 1, 2 and 3
   (b) Aetiology cannot be determined (appropriate laboratory or radiological investigations not performed).

Notes

* For research purposes, HIV-1-associated dementia complex can be coded to describe the major factors:

1. HIV-1-associated dementia complex requires criteria 1, 2a, 2b, 3 and 4
2. HIV-1-associated dementia complex (motor) requires criteria 1, 2a, 3 and 4
3. HIV-1-associated dementia complex (behaviour) requires criteria 1, 2b, 3 and 4.

† The level of impairment due to cognitive dysfunction should be assessed as follows:

Mild: Decline in performance at work including in the home, that is conspicuous to others. Unable to work at usual job, although may be able to work at a much less demanding job. Activities of daily living or social activities are impaired but not to a degree making the person completely dependent on others. More complicated daily tasks or recreational activities cannot be undertaken. Capable of basic self-care such as feeding, dressing and maintaining personal hygiene, but activities such as handling money, shopping, using public transportation, driving a car or keeping track of appointments or medications is impaired.

Moderate: Unable to work, including work in the home. Unable to function without some assistance of another in daily living, including dressing, maintaining personal hygiene, eating, shopping, handling money and walking, but able to communicate basic needs.

Severe: Unable to perform any activities of daily living wihout assistance. Requires continual supervision. Unable to maintain personal hygiene, nearly or absolutely mute.

†† The severity of HIV-1-associated myelopathy should be graded as follows:

Mild: Ambulatory, but requires constant unilateral support (e.g. cane) for walking
Moderate: Requires constant bilateral support (e.g. walker) for walking
Severe: Unable to walk even with assistance, confined to bed or wheelchair.

** Able to perform all but the most demanding aspects of work or activities of daily living. Performance at work is mildly impaired but also able to maintain usual job; social activities may be mildly impaired.

APPENDIX 3

NEUROPATHOLOGICAL DIAGNOSTIC CRITERIA (extracts from Budka et al 1991 with permission of International Society of Neuropathology)

HIV encephalitis (including HIV encephalomyelitis and HIV myelitis)

Morphological definition: Multiple disseminated foci are composed of microglia, macrophages and multinucleated giant cells. If multinucleated giant cells are not found, the presence of HIV antigen or nucleic acids as determined by immuno-cytochemistry or in situ hybridization is required.

Possible associated clinical syndromes: HIV-1 associated cognitive/motor complex, HIV-1 associated progressive encephalopathy of childhood.

HIV leucoencephalopathy

Morphological definition: Diffuse damage to white matter includes myelin loss, reactive astro-gliosis, macrophages and multinucleated giant cells but little or no inflammmatory infiltrates. If multinucleated giant cells are not found, the presence of HIV antigen or nuclei acids as deter-mined by immunocytochemistry or in situ hybridization is required.

Possible associated clinical syndromes: HIV-1 associated cognitive/motor complex, HIV-1 associated progressive encephalopathy of childhood.

Vacuolar myelopathy

Morphological definition: Multiple areas of the spinal cord, predominantly in the dorsolateral spinal tracts, exhibit numerous vacuolar myelin swellings (vacuolar myelinopathy) and macrophages; some macrophages typically reside within vacuoles.

Possible associated syndromes: HIV-1 associated myelopathy.

Vacuolar leucoencephalopathy

Morphological definition: Numerous vacuolar myelin swellings (vacuolar myelinopathy) and macrophages are prominent in cerebral white matter; some macrophages typically reside within vacuoles.

Possible associated clinical syndromes: HIV-1 associated cognitive/motor complex.

Lymphocytic meningitis

Morphological definition: Significant infiltrates of lymphocytes involve leptomeninges and perivas-cular spaces in the absence of demonstrable opportunistic pathogens.

Associated clinical syndrome: Aseptic/atypical meningtis (synonyms: atypical aseptic meningitis HIV-associated meningitis).

Diffuse poliodystrophy

Morphological definition: Diffuse reactive astro-gliosis and microglial activation involve the cerebral grey matter.

Possible associated clinical syndromes: HIV-1 associated cognitive/motor complex.

Cerebral Vasculitis including granulomatous angiitis

Morphological definition: Lymphocytic or granu-lomatous (lymphoplasmohistiocytic, with multi-nucleated giant cells) infiltration involves the walls of cerebral vessels, with or without accom-panying necrosis.

Possible associated clinical symptoms: Focal neurological deficit(s).

REFERENCE

Budka H, Wiley C A, Kleihues P, et al. HIV-associated disease of the nervous system: review of nomenclature and proposal for neuropathology-based terminology. Brain Pathol 1991; 1: 143–152

APPENDIX 4

CRITERIA FOR CLINICAL DIAGNOSIS OF CENTRAL NERVOUS SYSTEM DYSFUNCTION IN CHILDREN

HIV-1 associated progressive encephalopathy of childhood

Probable (must have each of the following):

1. Evidence for systemic HIV-1 infection:
   (a) Infants and children < 15 months
       (i)   virus in blood or tissues, or
       (ii) presence of HIV-1 antibody and evidence of cellular and humoral immune deficiency or other conditions meeting CDC case definition for AIDS.
   (b) Children > 15 months
       (i)   antibody or virus in blood or tissues.
2. At least one the folowing progresssive findings present at least 2 months:
   (a) Failure to attain or loss of development milestones or loss of intellectual ability, verified by standard developmental scale or neuropsychological tests

(b) Impaired brain growth (acquired mirocephaly or brain atrophy demonstrated on serial CT or MRI)

(c) Acquired symmetrical motor deficits manifested by two or more of the following: paresis, abnormal tone, pathologic reflexes, ataxia, or gait disturbance.

3. Evidence of another aetiology, including active CNS opportunistic infection or malignancy, must be sought from history, physical examination and appropriate laboratory and radiological investigation (e.g. lumbar puncture, neuroimaging). If another potential aetiology is present, it is not thought to be the cause of the above cognitive/motor/behavioural/developmental symptoms and signs.

Possible (must have one of the following):

1. Other potential aetiology present (must have each of the following):
   (a) As above (see Probable) # 1 and 2
   (b) Other potential aetiology is present but the cause of # 2 is uncertain.

2. Incomplete clinical evaluation (must have each of the following):
   (a) As above (see Probable) # 1 and 2
   (b) Aetiology cannot be determined (appropriate laboratory or radiological investigations not performed).

APPENDIX 5

CRITERIA FOR CLINICAL DIAGNOSIS OF HIV-1-ASSOCIATED PERIPHERAL NERVOUS SYSTEM DISORDERS

All of the following diagnoses require laboratory evidence of systemic HIV-1 infection (ELISA test confirmed by Western blot, polymerase chain reaction or culture).

I. HIV-1-associated acute inflammatory demyelinating polyradiculoneuropathy (HIV-1-associated Guillain-Barré syndrome)

Probable (must have):

1. Guillain-Barré syndrome by previously published criteria (Ann Neurol 1978; 565–567) except

(a) CSF mononuclear leukocyte count can be as high as 50 cells/mm^3.

Possible (must have one of the following):

1. Other potential aetiology present (must have each of the following):
   (a) As above (see Probable) # 1
   (b) Other potential aetiology is present and the cause of (see Probable) # 1 is uncertain.

2. Incomplete clinical evaluation (must have each of the following):
   (a) As above (see Probable) # 1
   (b) Aetiology cannot be determined (appropriate laboratory investigations not performed).

II. HIV-1-associated predominantly sensory polyneuropathy

Probable (must have each of the following):

1. Distal limb sensory symptoms (feet < hands) of a peripheral nerve nature (e.g. numbness, burning or pain).

2. Neurological examination confirming a distal relatively symmetrical polyneuropathy in which sensory abnormalities predominate.

3. Electrodiagnostic studies indicative of a polyneuropathy with features of both axonal loss and demyelination.

4. Normal CSF cell count and only minimal, if any, elevation of protein, with negative VDRL.

5. No other aetiology (including toxic exposure to ddI or ddC). Nerve biopsy may be indicated to rule out certain aetiologies such as amyloid, but is not a requirement.

Possible (must have one of the following):

1. Other potential aetiology present (must have each of the following):
   (a) As above (see Probable) # 1, 2 and 3
   (b) Other potential aetiology is present and the cause is uncertain.

2. Incomplete clinical evaluation (must have each of the following):
   (a) As above (see Probable) # 1 and 2
   (b) Aetiology cannot be determined (appropriate laboratory investigations not performed).

III. HIV-1-associated myopathy

Probable (must have each of the following):

1. Symptoms of proximal lower and/or upper extremity weakness, documented by physical examination.
2. No other aetiology (including toxic exposure to zidovudine). EMG and muscle biopsy may be necessary to rule out certain other aetiologies.

Possible (must have one of the following):

1. Other potential aetiology present (must have each of the following):
   (a) As above (see Probable) # 1
   (b) Other potential aetiology is present and the cause is uncertain.
2. Incomplete clinical evaluation (must have each of the following):
   (a) As above (see Probable) # 1

(b) Aetiology cannot be determined (appropriate laboratory investigations not performed).

APPENDIX 6

THERAPEUTIC PROTOCOLS

1. Antiretroviral agents – recommendations for usage
2. Use of cytokines in HIV infection
3. Treatment of specific infections common in immunodeficiency states
4. Useful antidepressant drugs in HIV infection
5. Drugs that cause psychiatric symptoms in HIV infection
6. Indications and costs of drugs commonly used in neurological patients with HIV infection
7. Disinfectants effective against HIV and HBV.

1. Antiretroviral agents – recommendations for usage

Clinical stage	Immune status	Previous antiretroviral therapy	Recommendations	Comments, trials
Asymptomatic or symptomatic	CD4 falling to < 300	On zidovudine (ZDV)	(a) Switch to ddI 200 mg b.i.d. or (b) continue ZDV or (c) Add ddI to ZDV or (d) add ddC to ZDV	ACTG 116A, 116B/117, 155 Note: No clear consensus of 'best' switch. May be based on ZDV tolerance and other adverse effects of ddI/ddC
Symptomatic: 'therapeutic failure'	CD4 50–500 falling or clinical progression or ZDV intolerance	Zidovudine	(a) ddI 400 mg/day or (b) combination therapy with ZDV + ddI or ZDV + ddC	
Symptomatic: 'therapeutic failure'	CD4 < 50 and falling or clinical progression or ZDV intolerance	Zidovudine	(a) Use ddI 500 mg/day or (b) ddC 0.75 mg t.i.d. or (c) discontinue	Heightened incidence of toxicities in advanced HIV infection and lack of benefit
Asymptomatic: zidovudine toxicity	CD4 > 500	Zidovudine with toxicity	Discontinue and observe	
Asymptomatic: zidovudine toxicity	CD4 50–500 stable	Zidovudine with toxicity	ddI 400 mg/day	ACTG 118, CPCRA 002, based on toxicity profile

ACTG, AIDS Collaborative Trial Group.
(Courtesy of John Phair; presented at ACTG meeting July 1993, see Sande et al 1993.)

2. The use of cytokines in HIV infection

Cytokine	Target cells	Clinical application	Starting dose	Time to response	Side-effects
G-CSF (filgrastim)	Committed neutrophils, multipotential haematopoietic cells	Neutropenia of HIV infection, chemotherapy or drug-induced neutropenia	0.5–0.1 μg/kg/day	ANCs increase within 1–2 days	Increased alkaline phosphatase, uric acid, LDH. Hypokalaemia, hypophosphataemia
GM-CSF	Committed neutrophils and macrophages	As with G-CSF	0.5–2.0 μg/kg/day	As with G-CSF	As with G-CSF, myalgias, fever, eosinophilia
Erythropoietin	Committed erythroid precursors	HIV-associated anaemia, chemotherapy or drug-induced anaemia	100–300 units/kg t.i.w. (better response if serum erythropoietin level is low)	1–2 weeks for reticulocytes, 5–6 weeks for increased haemoglobin	Burning and pain at injection sites
Interleukin-2	Progenitor cells of granulocytes, erythroid colonies and megakaryocytes	Not yet approved, may boost T lymphocyte numbers	NA	NA	Rash, delirium, encephalopathy

(Reproduced from Gabrilove & Jakubowski 1990)

3. Treatment of specific infections common in immunodeficiency states

Type	Diagnosis	Treatment	Prophylaxis
Bacterial			
Early syphilis (primary, secondary or latent syphilis < 1 year duration)	Serology	Benzathine penicillin G 2.4 million units i.m. (see algorithm)	None
Late, latent or syphilis of unknown duration	Serology	Benzathine penicillin G 2.4 million units i.m. for 3 weeks (see algorithm)	
Neurosyphilis (symptomatic and asymptomatic)	Serology CSF VDRL or WBC > 20/mm^3, protein > 50 mg/dl	Aqueous crystalline penicillin G 12–24 million units daily for 10–14 days or aqueous procaine penicillin G 2.4 million units i.m. daily + probenecid 500 mg p.o. q.i.d., both for 10 days	
Typical Gram-positive Gram-negative bacilli	Cultures and gram stains	Indicated antibiotics	None
Listeria monocytogenes	Gram stains, culture	Ampicillin 2–3 g every 4 hours Gentamicin × 4 weeks if blood culture positive	None
Viral			
CMV	Presumptive CMV encephalitis or radiculitis Blood or CSF cultures; immunostaining of tissues; or for retinitis: ophthalmoscopy	Ganciclovir 5 mg/kg every 12 hours × 14 days Alternative: foscarnet 60 mg/kg every 8 hours × 14 days (adjust for renal function)	Ganciclovir 5 mg/kg i.v. every 24 hours or foscarnet 90–120 mg/kg/day i.v. (adjust for renal failure)
Herpes simplex/zoster encephalitis	Viral cultures; immunostaining	Acyclovir 30 mg/kg/day i.v. in three divided doses for 14 days (adjust for renal failure)	None
Herpes zoster radiculitis (severe, multidermatomal)	Viral cultures, immunostaining	Acyclovir 30 mg/kg/day i.v. in three divided doses for 10–14 days (adjust for renal failure)	None
Herpes zoster dermatomal (non-complicated)	Viral cultures, immunostaining	Acyclovir 800 mg p.o. five times daily × 10 days	None
Papovavirus	Immunostaining histology	Cytosine arabinoside (anecdotal responses) 2–4 mg/kg i.v. × 5 days followed by 15-day 'rest' or intrathecal 50 mg via Ommaya reservoir	None

3.   *(contd)*

Type	Diagnosis	Treatment	Prophylaxis
Fungal			
Aspergillus	Cultures; histology	Amphotericin B 0.6 mg/kg/day × 4 weeks	None
Cryptococcus	Latex agglutination for antigen; cultures; India ink	Amphotericin B 0.6–1.0 mg/kg/day i.v. plus 5-fluorocytosine 100 mg/kg/day p.o. in four divided doses. Or, in mild cases, fluconazole 400 mg/day i.v./p.o.	Maintenance Fluconazole 200 mg/day p.o. or amphotericin 1mg/kg/week i.v.
Candida	Cultures; histology	Amphotericin B 0.6 mg/kg/day i.v.	None
Nocardia	Cultures; AFB stains; histology	Sulphamethoxazole 1 g t.i.d. or sulphisoxazole 1–2 g q.i.d. (for brain abscess achieve serum levels 150–200 µg/ml)	None
Coccidioidosis	Cultures; histology	Amphotericin B 0.6 mg/kg/day i.v. and intrathecal amphotericin B 0.25–1.0 mg three times weekly until CSF normalizes	
Mycobacteria			
M. avium intracellulare	Cultures; AFB stains	Choose 3–5 of: Clarithromycin 1 g p.o. b.i.d. Clofazimine 200 mg/day p.o. Ethambutol 15–25 mg/kg/day Ciprofloxacin 750 mg p.o. b.i.d. Amikacin 7.5 mg/kg i.v. every 12 hours Rifampin 600 mg/day p.o.	Rifabutin 150 mg p.o. b.i.d. or clarithromycin 500 mg p.o. b.i.d.
M. tuberculosis	Cultures; AFB stains	Isoniazid 300 mg/day + Rifampin 600 mg/day + ethambutol 15 mg/kg/day + pyrazinamide 15–30 mg/kg/day; two active drugs for > 9–12 months	Isoniazid 300 mg/day
Parasitic			
Toxoplasma gondii	Indirect immunofluorescence antibody; histology; empirical treatment of mass lesion	Pyrimethamine 50–75 mg/day plus sulphadiazine 6 g/day plus folinic acid 10 mg/day (clindamycin: alternative to sulphadiazine in sulpha-allergic)	Maintenance with pyrimethamine 50 mg/day plus clindamycin 300 mg b.i.d. or pyrimethamine 50 mg/day plus dapsone Folinic acid 5 mg/day

(After Pennington 1987)

4.   Useful antidepressant drugs in HIV infection

Drug	Starting dose HIV +	Usual daily dose	Therapeutic plasma level	Advantages	Most common side-effects
Nortriptyline	25 mg q.h.s. (increase dose every 3 days and check levels every 5 days)	75–100 mg q.h.s Titrate to level	50–125 ng/dl	Promotes sleep	Anticholinergic alpha blocking
Desipramine	25 mg q.h.s. (increase dose every 3 days and check levels every 5 days)	100–200 mg q.h.s. Titrate to level	125–200 ng/dl	May promote sleep	Anticholinergic alpha blocking
Fluoxetine	10 mg	20 mg q.d.	Unclear	Little sedation, few side-effects	Insomnia, agitation, nausea, anorexia
Trazodone	50–100 mg	150 mg for sleep 200–400 mg for depression	Unclear	Helps with fluoxetine induced insomnia	Sedation

(After Treisman, personal communication)

5. **Drugs that cause psychiatric symptoms in HIV infection**

Drug	Reactions	Comments
Acyclovir	Hallucinations, delirium, insomnia, depression	At high doses, particularly with renal impairment
Amphetamine-like drugs	Bizarre behaviour, hallucinations, paranoia, agitation, manic symptoms	Usually with overdose or abuse; depression can occur on withdrawal
Amphotericin B	Delirium	With intravenous or intrathecal use
Anabolic steroids	Aggression, mania, depression, psychosis	
Anticonvulsants	Agitation, confusion, delirium, depression	Usually with high doses or high plasma concentrations
Antidepressants, tricyclic	Delirium, confusion, hallucinations, mania	Mania or hypomania in about 10% of patients, also after withdrawal
Benzodiazepines	Rage, hostility, paranoia, hallucinations, delirium, depression, anterograde amnesia	During treatment or on withdrawal
Corticosteroids	Mania, depression, confusion, paranoia, hallucinations, catatonia	Especially with high doses; can occur on withdrawal
Dapsone	Insomnia, agitation, hallucinations, mania, depression	Several reports; may occur even with low doses
Dronabinol	Anxiety, disorientation, psychosis	More common in elderly
Fluoxetine	Mania, hypomania, depersonalization	Tremor and myoclonus can occur
Ganciclovir	Hallucinations, delirium, confusion, agitation	With renal dysfunction
Histamine H_2-receptor antagonists	Hallucinations, bizarre behaviour, delirium, depression	Usually with high doses; more common in elderly or with renal impairment
Interferon α	Delirium, depression, suicidal thoughts, anxiety	Occurs in up to 20%; depression treatable with fluoxetine
Iohexol/iopamidol	Confusion, disorientation	Infrequent
Isoniazid	Depression, agitation, hallucinations	Several reports
Ketoconazole	Hallucinations	Single case report
Loperamide	Delirium	Single case report
Methylphenidate	Hallucinations, paranoia	Several reports
Metoclopramide	Mania, depression, delirium	Several reports
Metronidazole	Depression, agitation, uncontrollable crying, disorientation, hallucinations	Several case reports, particularly with intravenous use
Narcotics	Nightmares, anxiety, agitation, euphoria, dysphoria, depression, paranoia, hallucinations	Usually with high doses
Non-steroidal anti-inflammatory drugs (NSAIDs)	Paranoia, depression, anxiety, disorientation, hallucinations	Uncommon; frequency varies among the NSAIDs
Procaine derivatives	Confusion, 'doom' anxiety, psychosis, agitation, bizarre behaviour	Many reports, especially with procaine penicillin G
Pseudoephedrine	Hallucinations, paranoia	Reported with overuse in adults
Salicylates	Agitation, confusion, hallucinations, paranoia	Chronic intoxication
Sulphonamides	Confusion, disorientation, euphoria	Several reports
Trimethoprim-sulphamethoxazole	Psychosis, depression, disorientation, hallucinations, delusions	Several reports
Zidovudine	Mania, paranoia, hallucinations	Infrequent, reported in two patients

(After *Medical Letter* 1993)

6.   Indications and cost of drugs commonly used in neurological patients with HIV infection
Average US wholesale prices from Medispan, May 1992

Drug	Indications	Typical regimen	Cost/week
Acyclovir	Herpes simplex, zoster	400 mg p.o. b.i.d.	$22.96
		800 mg p.o. × 5/day	$116.20
		2 g i.v./day	$1188.54
Amikacin	MAI	500 mg b.i.d.	$835.92
Amphotericin B	Fungal infections	50 mg/day × 3/week	$115.80
Ampicillin	Bacterial infections	500 mg p.o. q.i.d.	$3.64
Azithromycin	MAI (toxoplasmosis)	750 mg p.o. q.d.	$170.52
Buspirone	Anxiety (low abuse potential)	5 mg p.o. t.i.d.	$10.71
Clarithromycin	MAI	500 mg–1 g p.o. b.i.d.	$70.00
Clindamycin	Toxoplasmosis	300 mg q.i.d.	$59.92
		600 mg i.v. t.i.d.	$295.68
Clofazimine	MAI	100 mg p.o. b.i.d.	$2.80
Clotrimazole	Oropharyngeal candidiasis	10 mg p.o. × 5/day	$23.80
Dapsone	Toxoplasmosis prophylaxis	100 mg p.o. q.d.	$1.26
		50 mg p.o. q.d.	
ddI	Antiretroviral	200 mg p.o. b.i.d.	$40.04
		300 mg p.o. b.i.d.	
ddC	Antiretroviral	0.75 mg p.o. t.i.d.	$44.73
Ethambutol	MAI, MTB	400 mg p.o. t.i.d.	$24.78
Erythropoietin	Anaemia	6000 units × 3/week	$216.00
Fentanyl transdermal	Pain control	25 mg q.o.d.	
		75 mg q.o.d.	
		100 mg q.o.d.	
Fluconazole	Cryptococcosis	50 mg p.o. q.d.	$30.59
		10 mg p.o. b.i.d.	$96.18
		200 mg i.v. b.i.d.	$1661.38
Foscarnet	CMV retinitis, encephalitis, radiculitis	6 g i.v. q.d.	$513.31
Gamma globulin	Immune modulation	60 g i.v.	$3570/dose
Ganciclovir	CMV retinitis, encephalitis, radiculitis	350 mg i.v. q.d.	$170.52
G-CSF	Neutropenia	70 µg i.v. or s.c. q.d.	$135.00
GM-CSF	Neutropenia	70 µg i.v. or s.c. q.d.	$111.00
Haloperidol	Neuroleptic	2 mg b.i.d.	$1.75
Isoniazid	MTB	300 mg p.o. q.d.	$0.14
Interferon α	Possible treatment for PML	12 mU i.v. or s.c. q.d.	$755.00
Ketoconazole	Oropharyngeal candidiasis	200 mg p.o. q.d.	$16.24
Leucovorin (folinic acid)	Toxoplasmosis	10 mg p.o. q.d.	$37.94
Lorazepam	Anxiety	1 mg p.o. b.i.d.	$8.68
Methadone	Pain control		
Morphine sulphate	Pain control	30–60 mg b.i.d.	$32.62
Nortriptyline	Antidepressant	75 mg p.o. h.s.	$15.75
Prednisone	Myopathy	50 mg p.o. q.d.	$1.68
Fluoxetine	Antidepressant	20 mg p.o. q.d.	$13.51
Pyrimethamine	Toxoplasmosis	50 mg p.o. q.d.	$4.62
Zidovudine	Antiretroviral	100 mg p.o. × 5/day	$50.40
		200 mg i.v. t.i.d.	$327.60
Rifampin	MTB	600 mg p.o. q.d.	$27.58
Ritalin	Psychostimulant	10 mg p.o. t.i.d.	$7.98
Trimethoprim-sulphamethoxazole		1 DS p.o. q.d.	$0.47
		2 DS p.o. q.i.d.	$3.92
		250 mg (TMP) i.v. q.i.d.	$253.00

MAI, *Mycobacterium avium intracellulare*; MTB, *Mycobacterium tuberculosis*; PML, progressive multifocal leucoencephalopathy.
(After Bartlett 1992.)

7. Disinfectants effective against HIV and hepatitis B virus

Disinfectant	Concentration	Contact time (min)
Isopropyl alcohol	70%	5–30
Household bleach (sodium hypochlorite 5.25%)	1:10	10–30
Glutaraldehyde	2%	10–30
Heat	98°C	2

REFERENCES

Bartlett J G. A guide to HIV care from the AIDS Care Program of the Johns Hopkins Medical Institutions, Critical Care America 1992
Gabrilove J L, Jakubowski A. Hematopoietic growth factors: biology and clinical applications. J Natl Cancer Inst 1990; 10: 73–77
Medical Letter. Drugs that cause psychiatric symptoms. Med Lett Drugs Ther 1993; 35: 65–70
Pennington J E. Organ transplantation and associated infection. In: Bayless T M, Brain M C, Cherniack R M, editors. Current therapy in internal medicine – 2. Philadelphia: B. C. Decker, 1987: 189–193
Sande M A, Carpenter C J, Coggs G, et al. Antiretroviral therapy for adult HIV-infected patients. JAMA 1993; 270: 2583–2589

APPENDIX 7

GUIDELINES FOR INVASIVE PROCEDURES AND INFECTION CONTROL

Universal precautions

The Centers for Disease Control (CDC) (1988) has recommended that precautions for blood and body fluids be followed in the care of all individuals, whether known to be HIV seropositive or not. These guidelines, termed 'universal precautions', describe procedures that physicians and other health care workers should follow during clinical care and are intended to prevent the transmission of HIV and hepatitis B (Fig. 16.1). The CDC estimates that the risk of HIV infection following a single needle stick exposure to infected blood is less than 1% for HIV transmission, while it is 6–30% for hepatitis B. Universal precautions are intended to prevent percutaneous, mucous membrane and non-intact skin exposure of workers to HIV and hepatitis B. Precautions apply to blood, semen, vaginal secretions, cerebrospinal fluid and all tissues. They do not apply to urine, faeces, nasal secretions, sputum, saliva (except for dental workers), tears, sweat and vomitus.

1. Handwashing should be performed before and after all aspects of direct physical contact.
2. Gloves should be worn for handling blood, anything soiled by other body fluids, or for touching open lesions. Gloves should be worn for drawing blood, performing lumbar puncture, and collecting and handling specimens. Gloves should also be worn by any healthcare worker with cuts, skin breaks or open lesions on the hands.
3. Masks, goggles or face shields should be worn during procedures likely to generate droplets or aerosols of blood.
4. Gowns or aprons should be worn during procedures likely to generate splashes of blood and soiling of clothes.
5. Cardiopulmonary resuscitation. Resuscitation masks are advised when cardiopulmonary resuscitation is required.
6. Handling and disposal of needles and other sharps. To prevent needle stick injuries, needles should not be recapped , cut, bent or otherwise manipulated. Needles and other sharps should be disposed of in puncture resistant, leak-proof containers and disposed of by incineration.
7. Spills of blood/body fluids. Disposable gloves should be worn and disposable cleaning cloths used to clean up spills. Surface debris should be removed first and an appropriate disinfectant or a 1:10 solution of household bleach used to disinfect the area.

REFERENCE

Centers for Disease Control. Update: Universal precautions for prevention of transmission of human immunodeficiency virus, hepatitis B virus, and other blood-borne pathogens in health care settings. MMWR 1988; 37: 377–382

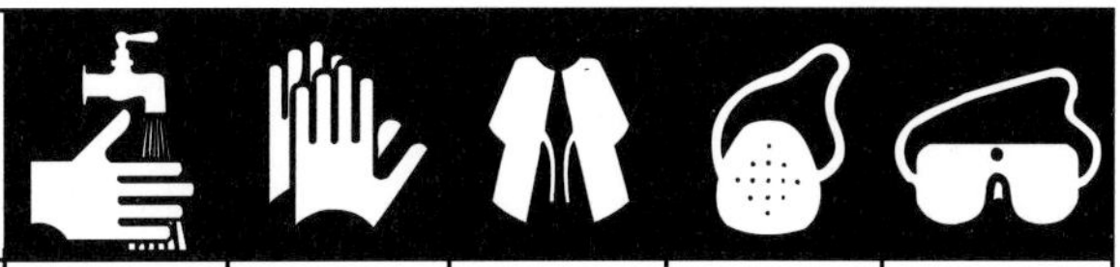

Procedure					
Talking to patient					
Adjusting IV fluid rate or non-invasive equipment					
Examining patient *without* touching blood or potentially infectious body fluids,* mucous membranes	✖				
Examining patient *including* contact with blood or potentially infectious body fluids,* mucous membranes	✖	✖			
Drawing blood	✖	✖			
Inserting venous access	✖	✖			
Suctioning	✖	✖	*Use gown, mask, eyewear if spattering by blood or potentially infectious body fluids* is likely*		
Inserting catheters	✖	✖	*Use gown, mask, eyewear if spattering by blood or potentially infectious body fluids* is likely*		
Handling soiled waste, linen, other materials	✖	✖	*Use gown, mask, eyewear only if waste or linen are extensively contaminated and spattering is likely*		
Intubation	✖	✖	✖	✖	✖
Inserting arterial access	✖	✖	✖	✖	✖
Endoscopy	✖	✖	✖	✖	✖
Operative and other procedures which produce extensive spattering of blood or potentially infectious body fluids*	✖	✖	✖	✖	✖

Fig. 16.1 Guidelines for universal precautions. Symbols refer to handwashing, gloves, gowns, masks and goggles. (From Johns Hopkins Hospital.)

APPENDIX 8

GUIDELINES FOR PREVENTION OF TRANSMISSION OF HIV-1 IN NEUROLOGIC PRACTICE

1. *Needles*
   Needles for venepuncture, lumbar puncture, or to instill local anaesthetic before lumbar puncture should not be recapped and after use should be placed in puncture-resistant containers for disposal.
2. *Sharp instruments*
   The use of sharp instruments, e.g. pins or sensory testing devices that might penetrate the skin or mucosa, should be limited and used with caution. Do not use pinwheels or lapel pins; a fresh pin should be used for sensory testing of each patient.
3. *Surface electrodes*
   Surface electrodes should be cleaned with a 1:10 dilution of household bleach or 70% isopropyl alcohol solution between patients. Electrodes contaminated with blood or body fluids should be thoroughly cleaned or discarded.
4. *Needle electrodes*
   Disposable needle electrodes should be used whenever possible. If reusable electrodes are indicated, electrodes should be manually cleaned of blood and particulate matter with disposable products and then placed in 70% isopropyl alcohol. After 90 minutes in isopropyl alcohol, electrodes should be sterilized in the routine manner. Insert needle electrodes with a technique that minimizes potential for accidental stick of the examiner. Needle electrodes should not be recapped after use but should be placed in puncture-resistant containers and sent for sterilization or incineration.
5. *Invasive Procedures* (e.g. nerve and muscle biopsy, myelography, arteriography)
   Use of gloves, goggles and other devices should be used as recommended by the US Public Health Service.
6. *Implementation of recommended precautions*
   In neurological practice, employers should ensure that all healthcare workers be oriented and educated as to the appropriate methods for handling potentially HIV-1-contaminated instruments as well as to routine use of universal blood and body fluid precautions for all patients. Equipment and supplies should be available to minimize the risk of transmission. Monitoring adherence to recommendations is advised.

Index

Acanthamoeba sp, 180
N-acetyl aspartate (NAA), 49
   choline ratios
      in AIDS dementia, 45, 46
      in white matter, 27
   creatine ratios, in AIDS dementia,
      45, 46
Acquired immunodeficiency syndrome
      (AIDS) *see* AIDS
Acyclovir
   in herpes simplex encephalitis, 136
Adenomas, pituitary, 193
Adenosine arabinoside (area-A), in
      PML, 147, 148
S-adenosylmethionine (SAM)
   CSF levels, 83
   SAH ratio, HIV infection, 83
S-adenylhomocysteine (SAH), SAM
      ratio, HIV infection, 83
Adrenal insufficiency, 215
Age
   and brainstem auditory evoked
      responses (AERs), 221
   and visual evoked responses (VERs),
      221
AIDP *see* Guillain-Barré syndrome
AIDS, 1
   defining criteria, CDC, 11
   dementia *see* Dementia complex,
      HIV-associated worldwide
      distribution, 1–2
   see also HIV: Paediatric AIDS
Akathisia, 214
Alprazolam, 59
Alzheimer's disease
   cognitive evoked potentials, 25
   prolonged P3 latencies, 223
Amantadine, in PML, 148
American Academy of Neurology,
      AIDS dementia criteria, 31, 32
Amitriptyline, 94, 95
Amoebiasis, cerebral, 180
Amphotericin B
   in coccidioidal meningitis, 129
   in cryptococcal meningitis, 125,
      126–127
   5-flucytosine combination, 125,
      126–127
   liposomal, 126

Amsler grid, vision self-testing, 210,
      217
Anaemia, pre-AIDS, and dementia
      development, 33–34
Analgesics, narcotic
   in neuropathic pain, 95, 96
   therapy guidelines, 96
   withdrawal signs/symptoms, 96
Angiitis, granulomatous, 245
Anticardiolipin antibody, 199, 205
Anticonvulsants (antiepileptic drugs),
      214
Antidepressants, in HIV infection,
      94–95, 96, 249
Antifungals, in cryptococcal meningitis,
      125–128
Antimicrobials, toxic neuropathy
      induction, 97
Antinuclear antibody (ANA), 199
Antiphospholipid antibodies, 199
Antiretroviral agents, use
      recommendations, 247
Antisaccadic eye movements, AIDS
      dementia, 37
Anxiety, generalized, 208
Apoptosis, and CD4 cell depletion, 8
Apraxia, 144
Arachidonic acid metabolites, CSF
      levels, 234, 235–236
Arachnoid cysts, 193
Arterial dissection, and strokes, 204
Arteritis
   necrotizing, mononeuritis multiplex,
      102
   septic, 203–204
   see also Angiitis
Aspergillus spp
   cerebral microabscesses, 131
   CNS blood vessels, 201
   meningitis, 130–131
Astrocytes
   in PML, 142, 144
   proliferation, AIDS dementia, 45,
      48, 49
Asymptomatic phase, 21–28
   and CDC stages II/III, 21
   cognitive impairment, 22–27
      studies over time, 24–25
   EEG studies, 26

MRI studies, 26–27, 224
nerve conduction tests, 230
neurological conditions, 21–22
peripheral nervous system
      abnormalities, 27–28
sensory neuropathy, 27–28
Ataxia, progressive, 106
Atheroma
   risk factors, 198
   and stroke in AIDS, 198–199
Atovaquone, in cerebral toxoplasmosis,
      179
Atrophy, cerebral, in dementia, 44,
      46
Auditory evoked potentials, 25–26,
      220–223
   AIDS dementia, 43
Autonomic neuropathies, 106

β_2-microglobulin, 7
   CSF, 42, 71, 233, 234–235
Baclofen, 95
Bacterial infections, 151–170
   recurrent, paediatric AIDS, 68
Bailey Scales of Infant Development,
      69–70
Basal ganglia
   calcification, paediatric AIDS, 73
   Toxoplasma abscesses, 171, 172,
      173–174
BCG vaccination, risks in AIDS, 162
Bell's palsy, 21, 105
Bicaudate ratio (BCR), 40
Biopsies
   brain, 191–192, 236–237
   muscle, 110–112, 116, 238
   nerve, 98, 101, 237
BK virus, 142
Blastomycosis, 130
Borrelia sp, 161
Botulism, 161
Brainstem auditory evoked potentials,
      220–221
   and age, 221
Breast feeding, HIV transmission, 66
Brown-Roberts-Wells stereotactic
      biopsy frame, 191, 237
Burkitt-like lymphoma, 185

255

BW-256U87, acyclovir pro-drug, 140

Calcium channel antagonists, 53, 59
Candidiasis, cerebral microabscesses, 130
Capsaicin, in sensory neuropathy, 94
Capsid proteins, HIV-1, 4, 5
Carbamazepine, 95
Cardiac embolism, 197–198, 203
Cardiac muscle, zidovudine effects, 112
Cardiomyopathy, 116
    HIV-associated, 215
Caudate atrophy, AIDS dementia, 40
CD4 count
    brainstem auditory evoked
        potentials, 221
    CIDP, 98
    CMV radiculitis, 105, 139
    CMV retinitis, 139
    coccidioidal meningitis, 128
    decline, 2, 7, 8
    disease staging, 11–13
    histoplasmosis, 129
    and HIV load, in dementia, 50, 51
    infection stage, 9–10
    Mycobacterium avium intracellulare
        infection, 166
    non-Hodgkin lymphoma, 186
    paediatric HIV infection, 66
    PML, 142
    sensory neuropathy, 92
    toxoplasmosis prophylaxis, 179–180
CD4 lymphocytes, immunological
    function, 8
CD4 receptors, HIV binding, 2, 4, 6
CD8 lymphocytes
    in CSF, 234
    HIV polymyositis, 111
Ceftriaxone, 160
Cellular immunity, and HIV, 7–9, 123
Central nervous system see CNS
Cerebral haemorrhage, 205
    drug abuse-associated, 203
Cerebral infarction
    meningovascular syphilis, 201, 202
    and zoster ophthalmicus, 200–201
Cerebral ventricles, expansion, AIDS
    dementia, 46
Cerebrospinal fluid (CSF) see CSF
Cerebrovascular disease, in AIDS,
    197–206
    aetiology, 197–204
    children, 73
    diagnosis, 204–205
    management plan, 205
Chemotherapy
    combination regimens, in non-
        Hodgkin lymphoma, 186–187
    radiotherapy combination, primary
        CNS lymphoma, 192–193
Children, HIV infection, 65–75
    CDC classification, 67
    cerebrovascular disease, 73
    clinical features, 66–72

CNS dysfunction, clinical diagnostic
        criteria, 245–246
    geographical spread, 65
    incubation period, 66–67
    neurological manifestations, 67–72,
        245–246
    opportunistic infections, 67, 68
    perinatal, 2
    progressive encephalopathy, 67–72,
        245–246
    strokes, 204
    systemic manifestations, 68
    transmission modes, 65–66
    vertical transmission, 66
    see also Paediatric AIDS
Chorioretinitis, Toxoplasma, 176
CIDP
    CD4 count, 98
    differences from Guillain-Barré
        syndrome, 98–99
Clindamycin, 177–178, 179
Clonazepam, 95
Clostridium botulinum, 161
Clostridium tetani, 161
CMV, 1
    and sensory neuropathy, 92
CMV antibodies
    encephalitis, CSF polymerase chain
        reaction, 42
    intrathecal, 138
CMV DNA, reverse transcriptase PCR,
    137
CMV encephalitis, 136–138
    clinical picture, 136–137
    imaging, 137
    neuropathological findings, 137–138
    paediatric AIDS, 73
CMV infection
    neuroimaging, 224
    treatment, 139–141
CMV myelitis, 78, 79
CMV radiculitis (radiculopathy) 89,
    103–105, 139–140
    differential diagnosis, 139–140
    neuropathology, 104–105
CMV retinitis, 138–139
CNS
    cytopathic effects of HIV, 52–53
    disorders, clinical diagnostic criteria,
        242–244
    gummatous disease, 156
    neurotoxic effects of HIV, 52–53
Cocaine, 45
    and cerebrovascular disorders,
        202–203
Coccidioidal meningitis, 128–129
Cognitive evoked potentials, 25–26
Cognitive impairment
    asymptomatic phase, 22–27
    definition variations, 24
    studies over time, 24–25
    tests, 23–27
Cognitive/motor disorder, minor, HIV-
    associated, 31, 32, 39, 55–56,
    243–244

Common peroneal nerve compression,
    105
Computed tomography see CT scans
Connective tissue disorders, 113
Cranial nerve palsies, 20, 21
Cranial neuropathies, 105
Creatine kinase (CK)
    in myopathy, 109–110
    in zidovudine myotoxicity, 111
Creatine phosphokinase (CPK)
    in myopathy, 109
    zidovudine myotoxicity, 112, 113
Crossed zoster syndrome, 199
Cryptococcal antigen
    CSF, 123, 128
    serum, 123–124
Cryptococcal meningitis, 3, 14
    antifungals, 125–126
    cerebrospinal fluid, 121, 122–123
    clinical features, 119–122
    CSF/serum cryptococcal antigen,
        123–124, 128
    epidemiology, 119
    fulminant, 120, 121, 128
    imaging, 122, 123, 124–125
    maintenance therapy, 128
    treatment, 126–128
Cryptococcomas, granulomatous, 119,
    122, 123, 128
Cryptococcosis, neuroimaging, 122,
    123, 124–125, 226
Cryptococcus neoformans, 119
CSF
    abnormalities, in HIV infection,
        230–232
    in AIDS dementia differential
        diagnosis, 42
    arachidonic acid metabolites, 234,
        235–236
    β_2 microglobulin, 233, 234–235
        p24 antigen correlation, 233
    in cerebral toxoplasmosis, 174–175
    in CMV radiculitis, 103
    in CNS aspergillosis, 201
    examination, 230–236
    glucose levels, 232
    HIV identification in, 232–233
    HIV IgG, 13
    HIV load in dementia, 50–51
    in IDP, 98
    intracranial volume, ratio,
        seropositive/seronegative cases,
        27
    lymphokines/monokines, 234–236
    p24 antigen levels, 233
    pleocytosis, 21–22, 230–232
        coccidioidal meningitis, 128
    in progressive encephalopathy,
        paediatric AIDS, 70–71
    serum/albumin ratio, 232
    in syphilis, 158–159
    in T. pallidum/HIV, 159
    in zoster ophthalmicus, 200, 204
CT scans
    in AIDS dementia, 43

CT scans (contd)
  cryptococcal meningitis, 122, 123,
    124–125
  see also Neuroimaging
Cubital tunnel syndrome, 105
Cyclobut, 140
Cytokines
  in CSF, 234–236
  and headache, 211
  and HIV replication, 8–9
  and HIV-infected macrophages,
    53–54
  myelosuppression, 34
  sensory neuropathy, 91, 92–93
  use in HIV infection, 248
Cytomegalovirus (CMV) see CMV
Cytopathicity, of HIV, CNS, 52–53
Cytoplasmic bodies, zidovudine
    myotoxicity, 112
Cytosine arabinoside (ara-C), in PML,
    147, 148
Cytotect, CMV-specific hyperimmune
    globulin, 140

Danazol, 115
Deafness, cryptococcal meningitis, 120
Dementia complex, HIV-associated,
    31–59
  AIDS defining event, 33
  associated disorders, management,
    58
  clinical diagnostic criteria, 242–243
  clinical features, 35–39
  coding/impairment level, 244
  CSF markers, 234–236
  diagnostic features, 38, 242–243
  differential diagnosis, 36, 38, 42–45
  early symptoms, 35–36
  EEG, 219
  epidemiology, 32–35
  established dementia treatment,
    56–58
  genetic factors, 51
  HIV load, 50–51
  host factors, 51
  immune activation, 49
  incidence, 33–35
  late features, 36–37
  long latency evoked potentials, 223
  and MHC, 51
  microscopic changes, 46–47
  multinucleated giant cell correlation,
    48
  neuroimaging, 226
  neuronal damage/dysfunction
    mechanisms, 52–55
  neuropsychological testing, 36,
    39–41
  p24 in CSF, 233
  pathogenesis, 50–55
  pathology, 45–49
  post-AIDS development, 33–34
  potential novel treatment, 58–59
  prevalence, 32–33

  prevention, 56
  prognosis, 39
  scales, 37–39
  SPECT, 227
  sub-cortical involvement, 35–36
  terminology/definitions, 31–32
  therapy, 55–59
  treatment monitoring, 228
Dementia, subclinical, 24
Demyelination
  and AIDS dementia, 44
  perivenular, and seroconversion, 22
  in PML, 142, 144
Depression, 208
  pseudodementia, 219
Desciclovir, 140
Desipramine, 94, 95
Developmental delay, paediatric HIV
    infection, 68–70
Dexamethasone, 58, 59
  in cryptococcal meningitis, 128
Dideoxycytidine (ddC), 6
  in AIDS dementia, 57
  toxic neuropathy, 89, 97
Dideoxyglyceropentofuranosyl
    thymidine (d4T), 6, 57, 97
Dideoxyinosine (ddI), 6
  in AIDS dementia, 57
  in progressive encephalopathy, 72
  toxic neuropathy, 89, 97
Dihydrofolate reductase inhibitors, 177
Dihydropteroate synthetase inhibitors,
    177
Disinfectants, for HIV/HBV, 252
Dizziness/faintness, 215
  drug-induced, 215
Doxepin, 95
Drug abuse, HIV and cerebrovascular
    disorders, 202–203
Drugs, indications/US costs (1992), 251
Dystonia, 214

EEG, 219–220
  in AIDS dementia, 42–43, 219–220
  in herpes simplex encephalitis, 133,
    134
  in progressive multifocal
    leucoencephalopathy, 145
  subclinical change, asymptomatic
    phase, 26
Electromyography (EMG), neurogenic
    weakness/myopathic weakness
    differentiation, 229–230
EMLA cream, in sensory neuropathy,
    94
Encephalitis
  CMV, 136–138
  giant cell, 48
  herpes simplex, 225
  HIV
    neuropathological diagnostic
      criteria, 244–245
    pathology, 47–48
  paediatric AIDS, 73

Encephalopathy, 207–208
  HIV, 31
  progressive
    laboratory studies, 70–71
    p24 in CSF, 233
    paediatric HIV infection, 67–72,
      245–246
    patterns, 68–70
    therapy, 71–72
  static, 68
Endocarditis, infective, 197, 198, 203
Endonuclease, HIV, 6
Entrapment neuropathies, 105
Envelope proteins
  antibodies, 9
  HIV-1, 4, 5
Erythropoietin, in zidovudine-
    associated anaemia, 57
Ethambutol, 166
Evoked potentials, 25–26, 220–223

Feet, pain, in HIV sensory neuropathy,
    88
Fentanyl, transdermal, in neuropathic
    pain, 95
FIAC/FIAU, 140
Fluconazole
  in coccidioidal meningitis, 129
  in cryptococcal meningitis, 125–126,
    127, 128
  dilantin (phenytoin) interaction, 126
5-Flucytosine
  amphotericin B combination, 125,
    126–127
  in cryptococcal meningitis, 125,
    126–127
Fluorescent treponemal antibody
    absorption (FTA-ABS) test,
    157–158, 159
Folic acid deficiency, 82, 84
Folinic acid, 177
Follicular hyperplasia, benign, 21
Foscarnet, 104, 138
  in CMV radiculopathy, 140
  in CMV retinitis, 139
  viral DNA polymerase inhibition,
    141
FTA-ABS test, CSF, 157–158, 159
  false positives, 159
Fungal infections, 119–132

Gait disturbances, causes, 214–215
Galactosyl ceramide, 4
Galactosyl sulphatide, 4
Ganciclovir
  in CMV encephalitis, 137–138
  CMV mutant resistance, 141
  in CMV radiculitis, 104, 140
  in CMV retinitis, 139
  foscarnet combination, CMV
    encephalitis, 138
  phosphorylation, 140
Ganglioneuritis, 106

Gay-related immunosuppressed disease (GRID), 31
General paresis, in syphilis, 156
Genomic structure, HIV, 5, 6
Gerstmann syndrome, 144
Gliomas, cerebral, 193
Gliosis, AIDS dementia, 49
gp120
  CD4 receptor binding, 7
    cell lysis, 8
  and cytokine production, 8
  neuronal toxicity, 53, 54
  vasoactive peptide inhibition, 54
Gracely and McGill Pain Questionnaire, 93
Graft-versus-host disease (GVHD), 10
Granulocyte colony-stimulating factor (G-CSF), 187
  in zidovudine-associated neutropenia, 57
Granulocyte macrophage-stimulating factor (GM-CSF), 187
Granulomatosis, lymphomatoid, 187–188
Guillain-Barré syndrome, 14, 20, 21, 98, 229
  differences from CIDP, 98–99

Haematological disorders, 199
Haematopoiesis, inhibition, and AIDS dementia, 34
Haemophilia, neuropathological features, in AIDS, 14
Headache
  causes, 211
  immunocompetent HIV-seropositivity, 211–212
  immunodeficient HIV-seropositivity, 212
  management protocol, 213
Hemiballismus, 214
Hemichorea, 214
Hepatitis B
  disinfectants against, 252
  immune complexes, mononeuritis multiplex, 102
Herpes group radiculitis, 103–105
Herpes simplex, 1
  myelitis, 78
Herpes simplex encephalitis (HSE), 133–136
  in AIDS, 134–136
  parenchymatous/periventricular changes, 135
  imaging, 133, 135, 225
Herpes zoster
  myelitis, 77–78
  radiculitis, 141
  and HIV, 103
  and stroke, 199–201
Histoplasma capsulatum, 129
Histoplasma polysaccharide antigen (HPA), serum/urine, 129–130

Histoplasmosis, 129–130
  clinical findings, 129
HIV, 1
  disease classification, 11, 12–13, 241–242
  identification in CSF, 232–233
  structure/life cycle, 3, 4–7
    and antiviral drug targets, 6, 7
  transmission, prevention guidelines, 252–254
HIV dementia see Dementia complex, HIV-associated
HIV DNA, 7
  CSF, 232, 233
HIV encephalitis, 31
HIV encephalopathy see Dementia complex, HIV-associated
HIV infection
  course, viral co-infection effects, 10
  and latency, 7
  staging/definitions, 11–13
HIV RNA, 7
  CSF, 232
  DNA ratio, and HIV disease state, 50
  in spinal cord macrophages, 82
HLA-DR5, and Kaposi's sarcoma, 153
HLA-DR/HLA-DQ, homology, 8
Hodgkin's disease, 193
Holotranscobalamin II, 55
Homocysteine, 55
Host response, to HIV infection, 9–10
HPMPA, 140
HPMPC, 140
HPMPG, in CMV infection, 140
HTLV-1
  paraplegia, and HIV myelitis, 78–79
  polymyositis, 110
Human immunodeficiency virus (HIV) see HIV
Humoral immunity, and HIV, 13–14
Huntington's chorea, 40
Hydrocephalus, 40
Hyperglobulinaemia, polyclonal, and IgG, 10
Hyponatraemia, cryptococcal meningitis, 123, 126
Hypotension, orthostatic, dizziness/faintness, 215

IDP see Polyneuropathies, inflammatory demyelinating
IgA antibodies, paediatric HIV infection, 66
IgG
  CSF, 232
  polyclonal hyperglobulinaemia, 10
IgG antibodies, toxoplasmosis in AIDS, 172, 175
IgG HIV antibodies, seroconversion illness, 19
IgM HIV antibodies, seroconversion illness, 19
Imaging see Neuroimaging

Imipramine, 95
Immunoglobulin, human, in IDP, 100, 101
Infant development, Bailey Scales, paediatric HIV infection, 69–70
Infection control, guidelines, 247, 252, 253
Infection risk, Western countries, group variations, 2
Inflammatory demyelinating neuropathies, sural nerve biopsies, 98, 99, 100
See also Polyneuropathies
Interferon-alpha
  in Kaposi's sarcoma, 184
  in PML, 147
Interferon-beta, in CMV encephalitis, 138
Interferon-gamma, production, and progression to AIDS, 10
Interferons, CSF levels, 235
Interleukin-1 (IL-1), 53–54
Interleukins, 8
  in AIDS dementia, 49, 51, 53–54
  CSF levels, 235
  production, and progression to AIDS, 10
Intervertebral disc, prolapse, 79
Intracranial pressure, raised, cryptococcal meningitis, 120–122, 128
Intravenous drug users (IVDUs)
  cerebral infarction, 203
  infective endocarditis, 197, 198
  long latency evoked potentials, 223
  mycotic aneurysms, 197, 198
  seropositive/seronegative, neurological symptoms, 25–26
  spinal epidural abscesses, 79–80
Invasive procedures, precautions guidelines, 247, 252, 253, 254
Investigations, 219–240
  see also various procedures
Involuntary movements, 214
Iron accumulation, HIV polymyositis, 111
Isoniazid, 166
  tuberculosis prophylaxis, 162
Itraconazole
  in coccidioidal meningitis, 129
  in cryptococcal meningitis, 126

JC virus
  detection in CSF, 147
  infection, screening, 28
  and progressive multifocal leucoencephalopathy, 142–148
Johns Hopkins HIV Dementia Scale, 37, 38

Kaposi's sarcoma (KS), 1, 89, 183–184
  cerebral, 205
  clinical features, 183–184

Kaposi's sarcoma (KS) (*contd*)
CNS involvement, 184
diagnosis/treatment, 184
incidence, 183
paediatric AIDS, 67
Ketoconazole
in cryptococcal meningitis, 126
dilantin (phenytoin) interaction, 126

Latex agglutination test, CSF, in
cryptococcal meningitis, 123
Lentiviruses, 3
Leskell stereotactic biopsy frame, 191,
237
Leucoencephalopathy, HIV
pathology, 47, 48–49
progressive multifocal *see* PML
Leucoencephalopathy, vacuolar, 245
Leukotrienes
CSF levels, 235
neuronal injury, 53, 58
Lidocaine cream
prilocaine combination (EMLA), 94
in sensory neuropathy, 94
Listeria monocytogenes, 167
Listeriosis, 167
Long terminal repeats (LTRs)
and neurotropism, 52–53
and neurovirulence, 52
Lower limb, SSEPs, 222
Lupus anticoagulant, 199
Lyme disease, 161
Lymphadenopathy, persistent
generalized, 21
Lymphocytic meningitis,
neuropathological diagnostic
criteria, 245
Lymphoid organs, HIV accumulation,
21
Lymphokines, in CSF, 234–236
Lymphoma
primary CNS (PCNSL), 187–193
cause of death, 192, 193
clinical features, 188–192
CNS, paediatric AIDS, 73
diagnosis, monoclonal antibodies,
191
differential diagnosis, 188–191
distinction from cerebral
toxoplasmosis, 173, 174
epidemiology, 187–188
incidence, in AIDS, 187
neuroimaging, 188–190, 226
periventricular spread, 190, 191
stereotactic brain biopsy, 191, 192,
237
supratentorial, 188
survival data, 192
treatment, 192–193
systemic
in AIDS, 184–187
incidence, 184–185
spinal cord compression, 79
see also various types

Macrophage colony-stimulating factor
(MCSF), 51
Macrophage-tropic HIV strains, 51–52
non-syncytium inducing (NSI), 11
Macrophages
HIV infiltration
cell activation, 234
neurotoxin production, 53
sensory neuropathy, 90–91
intravacuolar, 81–82, 245
lipid-laden, vacuolar myelopathy, 81
Magnetic resonance imaging *see* MRI
Mania, short-term, 36
Marinol, 59
Memantine, 59
Memorial Sloan Kettering Dementia
Scale, 38–39
Memory, short-term, AIDS dementia,
35–36
Meningiomas, 193
Meningitis, 21, 22
amoebic, 180
Aspergillus spp, 130–131
coccidioidal, 128–129
cryptococcal, 105, 119–128
fungal, management plan, 131
HIV-1, 13
lymphocytic, 245
lymphomatous, 105
syphilitic, 153–154
tuberculous, 163–164, 202
Meningoencephalitis
amoebic, 180
and seroconversion, 20
Meningomyelitis, syphilitic, 154
Meningovascular syphilis, 201–202
MENS (microcurrent electrical nerve
stimulation), 94
Mental status changes, 207–208
Methadone, in neuropathic pain, 95,
96
Methoxy mandelic acid (MMA), 55
5-methyltetrahydrofolate (MTHF),
CSF levels, 83
Mexiletine, in neuropathic pain, 95
MHC class II antigens, sensory
neuropathy, 91
Microglia, proliferation, AIDS
dementia, 45, 48, 49
Microglobulin-β$_2$, 7, 42, 71, 233,
234–235
Microhaemagglutination assay (MHA-
TP), 157, 158
Middle cerebral artery, in herpes
zoster, 199–201
Migraine, 198–199, 211–212
Mitochondria, abnormal, zidovudine
myotoxicity, 112, 113
Monoclonal antibodies, in primary
CNS lymphoma diagnosis, 191
Monokines, in CSF, 234–236
Mononeuritis multiplex, 101–103
nerve conduction tests, 229
Morphine, in neuropathic pain, 95, 96
Motor disorders, short-term, 36, 37

Movements, involuntary, 214
MR spectroscopy (MRS), 226
in AIDS dementia, 44, 45, 46, 49
MRI
in AIDS dementia, 43–44, 45
in CMV radiculitis, 103, 104
in cryptococcal meningitis, 122, 123,
124–125
in HIV infection asymptomatic
phase, 26–27
in lymphoma, 188–190, 226
in PML, 145–146, 224
interpretation protocol, 225
in toxoplasmosis, 173–176, 225–226
in vacuolar myelopathy, 83, 84
white matter/CSF volumes, 224
Multinucleate giant cells
AIDS dementia, 46, 48
HIV encephalitis, 47–48
Multiple sclerosis, 14
and HIV infection, 22
Muscle
biopsies, 238
infections, 115
wasting, 114, 115
Muscle disorders, 109–117
biopsy findings, 109
management plan, 116
see also Myopathy
Muscle evoked potentials (MEPs),
220–223
flexor policis longus, latency, 223
magnetic stimulation, 222
Muscle fibre atrophy, 110
Myalgia, polymyositis, 110
Myasthenia gravis, 14
Mycobacterium avium intracellulare
(MAI) infection, 68, 166–167,
187
clinical features, 166–167
treatment, 167
Mycobacterium tuberculosis, 161, 202
Mycotic aneurysms, 197, 198
Myelin basic protein, loss, and AIDS
dementia, 44
Myelin pallor, AIDS dementia, 44, 46,
48–49
Myelitis
herpes virus group, 77–78, 79
HIV-associated, 77
inflammatory necrotic, 79
Toxoplasma, 176
Myelography, CMV radiculitis, 103
Myelopathy
HIV-associated, clinical diagnostic
criteria, 243
HLTV-1-related, 14
paediatric HIV infection, 72, 73
and paraparesis, 20
see also Vacuolar myelopathy
Myelopathy, in AIDS, 77–85
definition, 80
differential diagnosis, 77
types, 77
Myoclonus, 214

Myoglobinuria, 110
Myopathy, 109–117
    paediatric HIV infection, 72
    toxic, zidovudine-related, 109,
        111–115

Naegleria spp, 180
National Institute of Mental Health
        (USA)
    neuropsychological battery, 40
    neuropsychological test
        recommendations, 228
nef protein, 53
Neoplasms in AIDS, neurological
        aspects, 183
Neopterin, 7, 42, 71
    CSF, 234, 235
Nerve biopsies, 237–238
Nerve conduction studies, 229–230
    asymptomatic phase, 27–28
Nerve growth factor (NGF), 93
Neurocognitive disorder, mild, 32
    see also Cognitive/motor disorder, minor
Neuroimaging, 223–227
    in AIDS dementia differential
        diagnosis, 42, 43–45
    CMV infection, 224
    cryptococcosis, 226
    herpes simplex encephalitis, 225
    HIV-associated dementia complex,
        226
    intracranial lesions, 15
    lymphoma, 226
    PML, 224–225
    spinal cord, 226
    toxoplasmosis, 225–226
    white matter/CSF volumes, 224
Neuroinvasiveness, 13, 51
Neuronal loss, AIDS dementia, 45, 49,
        50
Neuropathological diagnostic criteria,
        244–245
Neuropathy, HIV-associated
    in children, 72
    diagnosis, 101
    new terminology, 47
Neuropsychological impairment,
        asymptomatic phase, 22–27
Neuropsychological testing, 227–228
    AIDS dementia, 36, 39–41
    battery criteria, 227
    cognitive impairment severity, 40
    HIV CDC stages II/III, 23–27
    test types/uses, 228
Neurosyphilis, in HIV infection
    asymptomatic, 153
    clinical features, 152–157
    CSF changes, 158–159
    disease spectrum, 157
    epidemiology, 151–152
    laboratory diagnosis, 157–159
    meningovascular, 201–202
    ocular manifestations, 153, 154–155,
        156

treatment
    adequacy, 159–160
    guidelines, 160–161, 162
    response measurement, 160
Neurotoxicity, of HIV, CNS, 52–53
Neurotropism, 13, 51–52
    and long terminal repeats (LTRs),
        52–53
Neurovirulence, 13, 51
    and long terminal repeats (LTRs),
        52
Nimodipine, 59
Nitric oxide, gp120 neurotoxicity
        mediation, 54
NMDA antagonists, 53, 59
Nocardia asteroides, 130
Nocardiosis, 167
Non-Hodgkin lymphoma (NHL),
        184–187, 188
    aetiopathogenesis, 186
    clinical features, 185–186
    differential diagnosis, 186
    epidemiology, 184–185
    Epstein-Barr virus, 185, 186
    incidence, 184–185
    neuroimaging, 185, 186
    opportunistic infection prophylaxis,
        187
    sites, 185
    treatment, 186–187
Nordihydroguaiaretic acid, 59
Nortriptyline, 94, 95
NSAIDs, in neuropathic pain, 94
Nutrition, and sensory neuropathy, 92
Nutritional/vitamin deficiencies, AIDS
        dementia, 54–55

Occupational exposure, 2
Oculomotor palsies, 210
Oligodendrocytes, inclusion bodies, in
        PML, 142, 143, 144
Opportunistic infections, 13–14
    bacterial, 151–170
    CNS, paediatric AIDS, 73–74
    fungal, 119–132
    and headache, 212
    mental status changes, 207–208
    paediatric HIV infection, 67, 68
    parasitic, 171–181
    prophylaxis, and NHL, 187
    treatment protocols, 248–249
    and vasculitis, 199
    viral, 133–150
Optic neuritis, syphilitic meningitis,
        153, 154
Oxetanocin, 140

p24 antigen
    CSF
        in AIDS dementia, 51
        detection, 233
        in progressive encephalopathy, 70
    and HIV load assessment, 50

and HIV seroconversion, 19, 20
Pachymeningitis, syphilitic, 154
Paediatric AIDS
    case definition, 67
    indicator diseases, 67
    neurocognitive abnormalities, 70
    neuropathology, 73
    primary CNS lymphoma, 192
Paediatric strokes, 204
Papilloedema, cryptococcal meningitis,
        120, 121
Paraplegia, and myelitis, 78
Parasitic infections, 171–181
Parkinsonism, 214
Parkinson's disease, 40
Pentoxifylline, 58
Peripheral neuropathy, 87–96
    in asymptomatic phase, 27–28
    paediatric HIV infection, 72
    syndromes, 87
    and vacuolar myelopathy, 82
    see also Sensory neuropathy; Toxic
        neuropathy
Personality changes, short-term, 36
Phenytoin (dilantin), 95
    antifungal interaction, 126
Plasmacytoma, spinal cord
        compression, 79
Plasmapheresis, in IDP, 100, 101
Platelet activating factor (PAF)
    antagonists, 59
    CSF levels, 236
    neuronal injury, 53, 58
PML, 141–148
    associated disorders, 141–142
    cerebrospinal fluid PCR, 147
    differential diagnosis, 146
    focal neurological deficits, 144
    management plan, 148
    neuroimaging, 145–146, 147,
        224–225
    neuropathological diagnostic criteria,
        245
    posterior fossa lesions, 146
    presenting symptoms, 144
    treatment, 147–148
Pneumocystis carinii pneumonia (PCP),
        1, 187
    in children, 67, 68
Pneumonia
    lymphocytic interstitial (LIP), in
        children, 67, 68
    see also Pneumocystis carinii
        pneumonia
Poliodystrophy, diffuse, 49, 245
Polymyositis, HIV-associated, 14, 109,
        110–111
    steroid therapy, 111
    zidovudine myotoxicity comparisons,
        113–115
Polyneuropathies, inflammatory
        demyelinating (IDP), 97–101
    pathogenesis, 100
    sensory neuropathy comparisons,
        101

Polyneuropathies, inflammatory demyelinating (IDP) (contd)
 treatment, 100–101, 101
 see also CIDP; Guillain-Barré syndrome
Polypharmacy, mental status changes, 207–208
Polyradiculopathy, syphilitic, 156
Positron emission tomography (PET), 226
 in AIDS dementia, 44
Prednisone, in zidovudine myotoxicity, 114, 115
Prilocaine cream, lidocaine combination (EMLA), 94
Primary CNS lymphoma, 187–193
 see also Lymphoma
Progressive multifocal leucoencephalopathy see PML
Proposagnosia, 144
Prostaglandin E$_2$, 42
 CSF, 234, 235–236
Protease
 HIV, 6
 inhibitors, 6
Proviruses, 4
Psychiatric/psychological symptoms, 208–209
 drug-induced, 209, 250
 treatment, 209, 249
Pyrazinamide, 166
Pyridoxine (vitamin B$_6$), toxic neuropathy, 97
Pyrimethamine, in cerebral toxoplasmosis, 176–178, 179

Quantitative sensory testing (QST), nerve function, 88, 89–90, 91
Quinolinic acid, 42
 CSF levels, 234, 236
 AIDS dementia, 54

Radiculitis
 CMV, 139–140
 herpes group, 103–105
Radiculomyelitis, progressive, CMV-associated, 92
Radiculopathy, and sciatica, 20
Radiotherapy, in primary CNS lymphoma, 192–193
Ragged red-type fibres, in zidovudine myotoxicity, 111–112
Rapid-plasma-reagin (RPR) test, 157, 158
 false positives, 158
Replication, HIV
 point mutations, 10–11
 regulating genes, 5–6
Retina, cotton wool spots, in AIDS, 139
Retinitis, CMV, 138–139
Retroviruses, 3
 replication, 3

Reverse transcriptase, 4
 inhibitors, 6
 PCR, HIV load in CSF, 233
Rhabdomyolysis, 110
Rhombencephalitis, listerial, 167
Rifabutin, 166
Rifampicin, zidovudine interaction, 166
Risk factors, and CNS infections, epidemiological features, 14

Sciatica, radiculopathy and, 20
Seizures, 212–214
 anticonvulsants, 214
 causes, 213
 investigations, 213–214
Sensory neuropathy, HIV-associated, 87–96
 in asymptomatic phase, 27–28
 course, 88–89
 diagnostic criteria, 88, 246–247
 differential diagnosis, 89, 101
 dying-back axonal neuropathy, 90, 91–92
 evaluation, 89–93
 IDP comparisons, 101
 neurodiagnostic testing, 88–90, 91
 pain quantification, 93
 pathogenesis, 92–93
 pathology, 90–92
 and polymyositis, 114
 signs and symptoms, 88
 treatment, 93–96
 unmyelinated fibre loss, 91–92
Seroconversion, 19–21
 dermatological manifestations, 19
 mononucleosis-like illness, 19
 neurological manifestations, 19, 20
 window, 9, 19
Serological markers, 9
Seropositivity
 early CNS impairment, testing, 25
 infants, mental/psychomotor development, 70
 neuropsychological tests, 23–24
Serotonin deficiency, 236
Sexually transmitted diseases (STDs), as HIV transmission co-factors, 151
Single-photon emission computed tomography (SPECT), 226–227
 in AIDS dementia, 44–45
Sinusitis, and headache, 211, 212
SIV, 3, 13
 infection, CSF pleocytosis, 231
Slow viruses, 3
Somatosensory evoked potentials (SSEPs), 25–26, 220–223
 Erb's point stimulation, 221
 and peripheral nerve potential, 221
 posterior tibial, latency, 222
Spastic paraplegia, tropical, and HTLV-1 myelopathy, 82, 83
Spatial disorientation, 144

Spinal cord
 and AIDS, 77–85
 compression, 79, 154
 infarction, 79
 syphilis, 153–154
Spinal epidural abscesses, 79–80
 causative agents, 79, 80
Staging, 11–13
Status epilepticus, 214
Stavudine (d4T), 6
 in AIDS dementia, 57
 toxic neuropathy, 97
Stereotactic brain biopsies, PCNSL, 191–192, 237
Strokes
 antiphospholipid antibodies, 199
 arterial dissection, 204
 cocaine-related, 202–203
 and HIV seropositivity, 197–205
 paediatric, 204
Sulphadiazine, in cerebral toxoplasmosis, 177, 178
Sural nerve biopsies, inflammatory demyelinating neuropathies, 98, 99, 100
Syncytia
 and cell lysis, 8
 and HIV course, 11
Syntex Laboratories, vision self-testing advice, 216–217
Syphilis
 as AIDS risk factor, 151–152
 general paresis, 156
 incidence, 151
 meningovascular, 155–156, 201–202
 myelitis, 78
 post-treatment
  CSF abnormalities, 159
  treponemal seroreactivity, 158, 160
 spinal cord, 153–154
 stages, 152
 see also Neurosyphilis
Syphilitic meningitis, 153–154

T cell tropic, syncytium inducing (SI), HIV isolates, 11
T helper lymphocytes, CD4 receptors, HIV binding, 2, 4
Tabes dorsalis, 156
Tarsal tunnel syndrome, 105
tat protein, 53
TENS (transdermal electrical nerve stimulation), 94
Tetanus, 161
Thalidomide, 58
Thallium scans, 227
 primary CNS lymphoma, 190, 191
Therapeutic protocols, 247, 248–251
Thromboxane B$_2$, CSF levels, 236
Todd's paresis, 202
Toxic epidermal necrolysis, 74
Toxic neuropathy, 93, 97, 98
Toxoplasma chorioretinitis, 176

Toxoplasma gondii, 171
  seroprevalence in AIDS, 172
Toxoplasma myelitis, 176
Toxoplasmosis, 164, 165
  cerebral, 171–180
    abscesses, 3, 13, 171, 172,
      173–174
    biopsies, 176
    clinical features, 172–173
    cysts, 171–172
    diagnosis, PCR, 175–176
    differentiation from primary CNS
      lymphoma, 188–189, 190
    imaging, 173–176
    induction therapy, 176–178
    and lymphoma, 173–174
    maintenance therapy, 178
    management plan, 180
    neuroimaging, 225–226
    prognosis, 178
    prophylaxis, 179–180
    reactivation in AIDS, 172
    signs/symptoms, 172–173
    treatment, 176–179
  intramedullary, spinal cord, 79
  skeletal muscle, 115
Transient ischaemic attacks (TIAs),
    antiphospholipid antibodies,
    199
Tremor, 214
Treponema pallidum, 152
Triazoles, in cryptococcal meningitis,
    125
Tricyclic antidepressants, in
    neuropathic pain, 94–95, 96
Tropism, HIV and dementia, 51–52
Tuberculomas
  spinal epidural abscesses, 79, 80
  in TB meningitis, 164, 165
Tuberculosis, and AIDS, 161–166
  abscesses, 164
  CSF studies, 163
  diagnosis, 164–166
  ethnic aspects, 161
  meningeal, 202
  multi-drug resistance, 162, 166

neuroimaging, 163–164, 165
neurological complications, 163–166
prevalence 161, 162
treatment, 165, 166
Tumour necrosis factor (TNF-α),
    53–54, 167, 211
  AIDS dementia and, 49, 51, 53–54
  CSF levels, 234, 235
  and HIV replication, 8–9
  and muscle wasting, 115
  progressive encephalopathy, 71
Tyrosine, phosphorylation, gp120-
    regulated, 53

US, AIDS prevalence, regional
    differences, 2
Uveitis, syphilitic, 154

Vacuolar leucoencephalopathy,
    neuropathological diagnostic
    criteria, 245
Vacuolar myelopathy, 80–84
  clinical features, 81
  histological diagnostic criteria, 81,
    245
  investigations, 83–84
  non-AIDS, 82
Varicella zoster, 141
Vasculitis
  cerebral, 245
  HIV mononeuritis multiplex, 102
  in HIV and opportunistic infections,
    199
VCAM-1, 51
VDRL test, 157
  CSF
    sensitivity/specificity, 157–158
    and treponemal load, 158
Vincristine
  in Kaposi's sarcoma, 184
  neurotoxicity, 89
Viraemia, and infection stage, 9–10
Viral infections, opportunistic,
    133–150

Virchow-Robin spaces, cysts, 119, 122
Virion, HIV-1, 4–5
Vision, self-testing, 210, 216–217
Visual acuity, changes, 210–211
Visual analogue scale (VAS), pain
    assessment, sensory neuropathy,
    94
Visual changes, 209–211
  causes, 209
Visual evoked potentials, 25–26,
    220–223
Visual field deficits, 209–210
Visual impairment, neurosyphilis, 154
Vitamin B$_{12}$, deficiency, and AIDS
    dementia, 54–55
Vitamin B deficiency, 82, 83, 84

Wallerian degeneration, sural nerves, in
    AIDS, 91
Wasting, in AIDS, 114, 115
White matter
  atrophy, MRI, 224
  in dementia, 43–44, 49
  in PML, 142–143, 146

Zidovudine, 6
  AIDS dementia delay, 56
  and AIDS dementia incidence, 35
  drug holiday, and myotoxicity, 111,
    114–115
  in established dementia, 56–58
  headache induction, 212
  optimal dosage, in AIDS dementia,
    56–57
  in paediatric progressive
    encephalopathy, 71–72
  resistance, 57–58
  toxic myopathy, 72, 109, 111–115
    HIV polymyositis comparisons,
      113–115
    post-exercise delayed recovery,
      112–113
Zoster ophthalmicus, 199–201
  angiography, 202, 204